Mineralized Collagen Bone Graft Substitutes

Woodhead Publishing Series in Biomaterials

Mineralized Collagen Bone Graft Substitutes

Edited by

Xiu-Mei Wang

Zhi-Ye Qiu

Helen Cui

ELSEVIER

WP
WOODHEAD
PUBLISHING
An imprint of Elsevier

Woodhead Publishing is an imprint of Elsevier
The Officers' Mess Business Centre, Royston Road, Duxford, CB22 4QH, United Kingdom
50 Hampshire Street, 5th Floor, Cambridge, MA 02139, United States
The Boulevard, Langford Lane, Kidlington, OX5 1GB, United Kingdom

British Library Cataloguing-in-Publication Data
A catalogue record for this book is available from the British Library

Library of Congress Cataloging-in-Publication Data
A catalog record for this book is available from the Library of Congress

ISBN: 978-0-08-102717-2 (print)

ISBN: 978-0-08-102739-4 (online)

For Information on all Woodhead Publishing publications
visit our website at https://www.elsevier.com/books-and-journals

Publisher: Matthew Deans
Acquisition Editor: Sabrina Webber
Editorial Project Manager: Naomi Robertson
Production Project Manager: Sojan P. Pazhayattil
Cover Designer: Mark Rogers

Typeset by MPS Limited, Chennai, India

Contents

List of Contributors

Wei Ai Beijing Allgens Medical Science and Technology Co., Ltd., Beijing, P.R. China

Helen Cui Beijing Allgens Medical Science and Technology Co., Ltd., Beijing, P.R. China

Yun Cui Beijing Allgens Medical Science and Technology Co., Ltd., Beijing, P.R. China

Qi Ding Beijing Allgens Medical Science and Technology Co., Ltd., Beijing, P.R. China

Zhi-Min He Beijing Allgens Medical Science and Technology Co., Ltd., Beijing, P.R. China

Yan-Li Hu Beijing Allgens Medical Science and Technology Co., Ltd., Beijing, P.R. China

Zhi-Ye Qiu Beijing Allgens Medical Science and Technology Co., Ltd., Beijing, P.R. China

Tian-Xi Song Beijing Allgens Medical Science and Technology Co., Ltd., Beijing, P.R. China

Xiu-Mei Wang School of Materials Science and Engineering, Tsinghua University, Beijing, P.R. China

Zi-Rui Wang Beijing Allgens Medical Science and Technology Co., Ltd., Beijing, P.R. China

Preface

Mineralized collagen is a biomimetic composite material that simulates the chemical composition and microstructure of natural bone matrix. Based on the understanding of natural mineralized collagen and its formation process, many studies have been performed to prepare biomimetic materials mimicking natural mineralized collagen. Until now, there have been a number of bone substitute materials developed via different methods based on mineralized collagen. Some of these materials have been commercialized and approved by governmental administrations as medical device products. As a biomimetic artificial bone repair material that is most similar to human natural bone in terms of composition and microstructure, mineralized collagen demonstrates good bone regeneration effects in repairing bone defects at different parts of the body. And it is increasingly recognized by clinicians, medical researchers, and medical regulatory authorities.

This book introduces the structure, principles, properties, biomimetic preparation methods, characterization, and clinical applications of mineralized collagen as a model for bone repair materials. Compared with similar books, the advantages of mineralized collagen as a new bone tissue repair material are introduced systematically. Compared with traditional bone grafts made of metals or ceramics, mineralized collagen possesses many advantages, such as biomimetic composition, biodegradation, better biocompatibility, and better biomechanics. It provides a safer and more reliable material for bone tissue repair, and it lays a theoretical and practical foundation for researchers in this field.

Chapter 1

Natural Bone Tissue and Its Biomimetic

Zhi-Ye Qiu[1], Yun Cui[1] and Xiu-Mei Wang[2]
[1]Beijing Allgens Medical Science and Technology Co., Ltd., Beijing, P.R. China, [2]School of Materials Science and Engineering, Tsinghua University, Beijing, P.R. China

1.1 NATURAL BONE COMPOSITION AND HIERARCHICAL STRUCTURE

1.1.1 Bone Composition

Bone is mainly composed of cancellous bone and dense bone. Fig. 1.1 is a schematic diagram of the structure of long bones. The epiphysis at both ends is composed of cancellous bone; the middle is called the backbone, and is composed of compact bone. Structural units of dense bone constitute the Haversian system, as shown in Fig. 1.1 in cross-section. The longitudinal section of the bone is the orientation of mineralized collagen fibers. The structure of cancellous bone is a three-dimensional trabecular frame. Bone is one of the most complex biomineralization systems. Its inorganic components are mainly hydroxyapatite and carbonated apatite, accounting for about 65% of the total mass; the organic component is mainly type I collagen, and a small amount of noncollagen protein, polysaccharides, lipids, etc. account for about 34% of the total weight; the rest is water [1].

1.1.1.1 Inorganic Minerals

Bone has the most complex inorganic system, that is, a calcium phosphate system. Its complexity is mainly reflected as follows:

1. Bone inorganic type with polymorphism. The most important inorganic phase in bone is hydroxyapatite (HA, molecular formula $Ca_{10}(PO_4)_6(OH)_2$), but it contains impurity ions such as CO_3^{2-}, Cl^-, F^-, Na^+, Mg^{2+}. CO_3^{2-} can replace OH^- or PO_4^{3-} to form alpha or beta carbonated apatite (CHA). In addition, various mineral phases such as amorphous calcium phosphate (ACP), octa-calcium phosphate (OCP), and

Mineralized Collagen Bone Graft Substitutes. DOI: https://doi.org/10.1016/B978-0-08-102717-2.00001-1

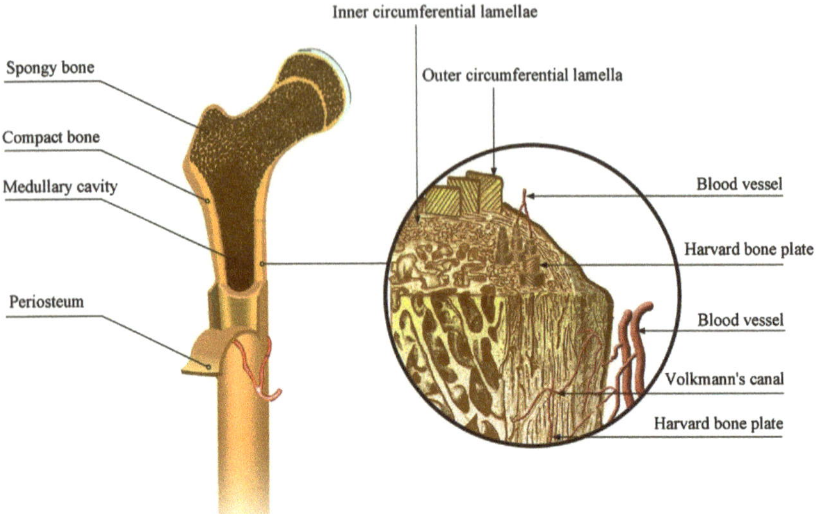

FIGURE 1.1 Long bones hierarchical structure diagram.

di-calcium phosphate dibasic (DCPD) are present in the bones, which are believed to exist as precursors to apatite. The relevant evolution mechanism is as follows [2–4]: first ACP forms, and then it transforms into OCP, and finally it forms into −HA. Next DCPD is formed, which is badly crystallized, but then gradually matures and transforms into HA.

2. Calcium phosphate system between each phase has very close crystal diffraction peaks, which makes the identification of the phase difficult. The main crystal forms of calcium phosphate are hydroxyapatite (HA): $Ca_{10}(PO_4)_6(OH)_2$, hexagonal structure; OCP: $Ca_8H_2(PO_4)_6H_2O$, triclinic structure; di-calcium phosphate dibasic (DCPD): $CaHPO_4 \cdot H_2O$, monoclinic structure; tricalcium phosphate (TCP), $Ca_3\ (PO_4)_2$, monoclinic structure.

1.1.1.2 Organic Substances [5]

The most important organic component of bone is type I collagen, which usually accounts for 85%−90% of the total protein. Other proteins are called noncollagens. Bone noncollagen protein content is small, but there are many types. More than 200 species of noncollagens have been reported, among which 12 species constitute the majority. Collagen is the main bone matrix protein, a class of glycoproteins secreted by connective tissue cells. Table 1.1 lists the main proteins in bone organic components.

1.1.1.3 Osteocytes

The main cells involved in the growth and development of bone include osteogenitor cells, osteoblasts, osteocytes, and osteoclasts. Fig. 1.2 is a schematic illustration of cells in the bone. These cells exert their own function

TABLE 1.1 Composition of Bone Matrix Organic Phase

Extracellular Matrix Components	Properties and Functions
Collagen I	Provides a scaffold for bone structure and matrix mineralization
Osteonectin	Glycoprotein: bind Ca++ and type I collagen; promotes the formation of hydroxyapatite nucleus
Osteocalcin	Skeletal Gla protein: a marker phenotype of the late osteogenic phase that is associated with remodeling of the bone and possibly through which the mineralization process has been controlled
Fibronectin	Osteoblast adhesion matrix
Osteopontin	Sialoprotein: binding line composition, involved in bone remodeling
Bone sialoprotein	Sialoprotein: binding line composition

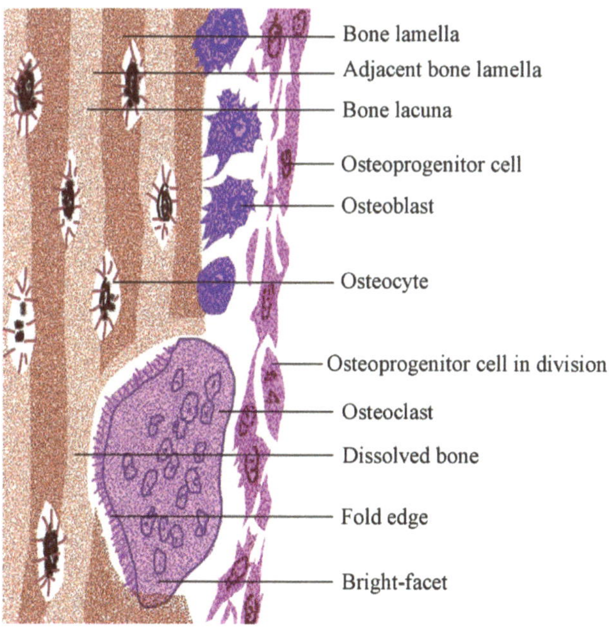

FIGURE 1.2 Bone cell and distribution.

TABLE 1.2 Bone Cell Types and Their Functions

Cell Type	Morphology	Location	Function
Osteogenitor cells	Fusiform, smaller	Periosteum, cortical bone, periosteum, and bone surface	They are the stem cells in bone tissue; proliferate and differentiate into osteoblasts
Osteoblast	Cubic or short columnar, with protrusions	Generally arranged in a single layer covering the surface of new bone	Secrete osteoid, release matrix vesicles, promote osteoid calcification
Osteocytes	Small cells, flat oval, multiple protrusions	Scattered in the bone plate or between the plates	Have a certain osteolytic and osteogenic role and participate in regulating calcium and phosphorus balance
Osteoclasts	Large, polarized cells, with multinuclear	Bone tissue edge	Release a variety of hydrolases and organic acids, dissolve bone; phagocytosis of the decomposition of bone matrix

and play an important role in the balance of healthy bone tissue. As shown in Table 1.2, the growth, maintenance, and absorption of bone are due to the synergistic effect of these four kinds of cells.

Osteoprogenitors

Osteoprogenitor cells (osteoprogenitor cells), also known as osteoblastic cells, are mainly in the periosteum, the periosteal surface of these bones. The thickness of cell layer varies with the age and the location of the bone surface. Osteoprogenitor cells in the periosteum originate from the poly differentiation potency mesenchymal cells in the periosteum. Previous studies showed that pericytes in the perivascular blood vessels also have the same capability to differentiate into osteoblasts. There are a large number of osteoprogenitors in bone marrow stromal cells. The bone marrow progenitor cells differentiate from stromal stem cells that have a multidirectional potency in bone marrow. Periosteum and bone marrow-derived osteoprogenitors differentiate into osteogenic bone directly without the presence of other inducers. Osteoprogenitor cells with this property are called determined osteoprogenitor cells (DOPC). In contrast, there is a class of osteoprogenitors in the body present in pathological situations, such as heterotopic ossification and fracture repair, which come from undifferentiated mesenchymal cells throughout the body. These osteoprogenitors after osteoinductive factors such as bone morphogenetic proteins BMP, can differentiate into osteoblasts, and their osteogenic pattern is also different from derterminedosteoprogenitor cell DOPC, but through ossification of cartilage osteogenesis, so we call such osteoprogenitors inducible osteoprogenitor cells. Osteogenic progenitor cells have the ability to split propagation and further differentiate into specialized functional cells, and further differentiate into osteoblasts. The observation of light microscopy showed that the morphological changes of osteoprogenitor cells were similar to those of fibroblasts and endothelial cells. Both of them showed long cells with oval or elongated nuclei and light staining of nucleus and cytoplasm. Under electron microscopy, osteoprogenitor cells have some endoplasmic reticulum and undeveloped Golgi, more mitochondria, and free ribosomes. In addition, there are also findings that osteoprogenitors may also be transformed into osteoclasts.

Osteoblasts

Osteoblasts are cells that form bone tissue. Osteoblasts can synthesize and secrete bone matrix and participate in the mineralization of bone to regulate the balance of calcium and phosphate ions in developing bone. Osteoblasts are derived from osteoprogenitor cells. Many factors affect the conversion of osteoprogenitors, such as various hormones and local released bioactive substances after fracture. In the presence of these factors, osteoprogenitors can multiply in large numbers and begin to differentiate into osteoblasts that perform osteogenic functions. Osteoblasts belong to functional cells and therefore rarely undergo division and proliferation.

Osteoblasts are morphologically diverse, usually cubic, round or flat, cylindrical, with a diameter of $20 \sim 50\ \mu m$. Osteoblasts in full-fledged phase were full-fledged with alkaline cytoplasm, which may be related to the presence of a large number of nucleosomes and rough endoplasmic reticulum in the cytoplasm of osteoblasts. Cytoplasm has a round or oval, bulky, but lighter-staining nuclei, the nucleus usually has 1–3 nucleoli. The nuclei of osteoblasts are usually located on the side far from the new bone.

Osteoblasts are usually found on the surface of new bone, arranged in a monolayer. There are a lot of hairy short protrusions on the surface of osteoblasts that are connected to adjacent cells and penetrate the surrounding bone-like tissue, forming a network structure. When the bone-like tissue completely buries osteoblasts, it gradually transforms into osteocytes, the cytoplasm located in the tubules. The study of the cell microstructure shows that the organelles in the cytoplasm of osteoblasts are abundant, the cytoplasm is filled with well-developed rough endoplasmic reticulum, and a large number of nucleosomes and free ribosomes are attached to the rough endoplasmic reticulum. The osteoblast Golgi enlarges and forms vacuoles, located in the middle of the cell. Osteoblasts have round mitochondria, in addition to lysosomes, vacuoles, and glycogen granules. These structural features of osteoblasts indicate that osteoblasts are robust.

1.1.2 Bone Structure

The bones of any structure are superior to that of saturated fibers with minerals, because of the complex hierarchical structure of the bones. The mechanical properties of bones derive from their structure, and hydroxyapatite (usually a carbonaceous apatite) forms on collagen fibers, proteoglycans, and many other protein substrates. The initial position of mineralization is in the gap between collagen molecules. The crystallographic orientation of this flaky crystal is related to the orientation of organic matter. Recent observations show that the crystals are often arranged in parallel along the collagen fibers, which are consistent with the adjacent collagen fibers, resulting in long-range order, which gives the skeleton unusual breaking properties. The structure of mammalian bone significantly affects the mechanical properties of the bone. The density of the mineralized fibers and the direction and size of the arrangement control the strain, as well as the mode of propagation of the strain in the bone. Neutron diffraction studies of human scapula show that the hydroxyapatite *c*-axis preferentially lies in the direction of stretching along the muscles that are attached to it. In some areas, the two muscles act in different directions and it was found that the orientation of the crystal in the bone was divided into two groups, corresponding to the stretching directions of the two muscles, respectively.

The composition and structure of the material determines the properties of the material. Bone tissue as a natural biomineralized material is no exception. The main function of the bone is to provide structural support for the body. It is generally believed that the mechanical characteristics of the macrostructure of the bone depend on its shape and size, as well as the nature of the material and the way in which the material is arranged in space. Bone has a multilevel hierarchical structure, and each level of the structure is built on a microstructure of the next level, as shown in Fig. 1.3.

1. The structural unit of the bone on the microscale is the Haversian unit. The typical bone unit has a diameter of about 150–250 μm. A bone unit is a 3–7-μm-thick layer, composed of 4–20 layer plates concentrically

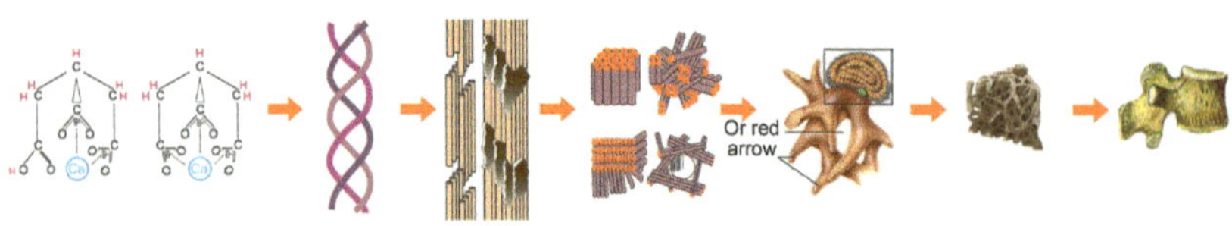

FIGURE 1.3 Hierarchical structure of human cadaver bone.

arranged around the Haversian tube. The bones in this level are staggered through the lacunae, the tubules, and the Volksmann tubes, which are connected directly to the bone marrow to transport the metabolites in the bones.

2. The layered bone plate is further composed of collagen fibers. The collagen fibers in each bone plate are arranged in parallel to each other, and the collagen fibers in the adjacent bone plates are oriented at an angle to each other. Weiner believes, for the cortical Haversian system, that the plate also has a finer structure, which consists of two layers with different thickness. The collagen fibers in the thick layer are oriented at an angle to the long axis of the bone. The orientations of the thick collagen fibers in the adjacent plates are at an angle. The *c*-axis of collagen fibers and mineral crystals in all the thin layers is perpendicular to the length of the bone axis direction [6–8].
3. Collagen fibers include collagen microfibers and hydroxyapatite. In the bone, the collagen fibers are regularly arranged to form a gap, overlapping periodic structure regions with a period of about 67 nm, in which the overlapping regions alternate with each other. This kind of structure provides a template for mineral deposition, with preferentially nucleates in the interstitial region. The bone mineral crystal is flaky with 2–5 nm in thickness, 20 nm in width and 40–60 nm in length usually. The length of the apatite crystals can reach 170 nm due to the growth from the gap zone to the overlapping region [9]. The apatite crystals of bone mineral have a preferred orientation with crystallographic *c*-axes parallel to the axial direction of collagen fibers [10]. All those features together form the basic bone structure: mineralized collagen fibers.
4. A procollagen molecule in three-strand helical structure, arranged in parallel to form collagen microfibrils. The bone's Haversian system is derived from the process of bone remodeling and reconstruction [11], and the formed bone unit is also called the second bone unit. In a typical bone formation process, bone formation begins with the extracellular assembly of collagen molecules secreted by the cells and collagen templates, followed by the deposition of minerals on collagen templates. Unlike other mineral tissues, there is a secondary remodeling process in the bone, which involves the formation of a vascular tube in the established bone and mineralization again to form a Haversian structure. In addition, the bone is continuously resorbed through the osteoblasts and osteogenesis to adapt to changes in the external stress. Therefore, the mineralization of bone is a continuous process. The final mature bone is formed by the bones of various stages. They have different composition, mineral density, and mechanical properties. This feature adds difficulties to the study of bone mineralization.

The three-stranded helical structure of procollagen molecules (level 1) and hydroxyapatite crystals self-assemble into collagen fibers (level 2), which in turn are organized into lamellar structures (level 3) instead of being arranged in another staggered structure. The bone cell assembly layers on adjacent layers are stacked together in parallel arrays (layered bones) or concentrically arranged cylindrical structures, the bone units (level 4). Each layer of bone has fibers arranged in the alternating direction. At a relatively long scale, bone units are grouped into Haversian systems as the basic building blocks for a variety of bone microstructures (level 5). These structures include a porous framework (cancellous bone) and a relatively tight structure (cortical bone). Each structure has similar constituent motifs but different spatial organization, depending on the specific structure/function relationship throughout the bone. Finally, at the macrolevel, each bone has a specific topography and structure (level 6) to function as a whole [12].

The macroscopic appearance of different types of bones is dictated by the cell differentiation during embryogenesis. For example, the shape of the long bones on the legs prior to mineralization is a soft, degradable, nonmineralized cartilage matrix with a large amount of water. Cells first deposit on the cartilage matrix, then assemble around it and differentiate into osteoblasts, which secrete collagen. Bone mineralization occurs in collagen, forming a mineralized ring around the cartilage. Interestingly, the bone ring does not provide nutrients to the cells in the cartilage matrix and, as a result, degenerates into a bone marrow-containing cavity. The newly formed bone is then remodeled into different structures [13]. Bone has a multilevel hierarchical structure from the molecular scale to the macroscopic scale. Cell and mineralized collagen sheets are the basic constitutive elements of various microstructures. The entire macroscopic appearance has been determined by the biodegradable cartilage model during the embryonic period.

1.2 NATURAL BONE FORMATION PATTERNS AND BONE REPAIR

1.2.1 Bone Generation Model

There are three main types of bone generation: membrane osteogenesis, intraochondrogenic, and additional osteogenesis [14].

1.2.1.1 Membrane Osteogenesis

Intramembranous ossification occurs in the skull and part of the skull base, facial bone, clavicle, and some parts of the mandible where there is bone formation without cartilage. Intramembranous ossification produces the intercellular matrix and rapidly ossifies into original trabecular bone. These cells are transformed into osteocytes in the mineralized osteoid and most of the remaining cells remain in the periphery as osteoblasts. The original trabeculae radiate parallel to a specific skull surface. These primitive trabeculae increase in length by free end growth. Eventually producing bone tissue with a primary ossification center. The ossification center, on the one hand further forms or augments the peripheral trabeculae, and on the other hand rapidly expands upon fusion with the bone island appearing in the primordial fibroblasts. Oppositely expanded, peripheral trabeculae become more and more regular and connected to each other, the centrifugal expansion speed slows down. At this time skull vault, covered with a special layer of membrane, begins a new osteogenic process. The membrane structure from the outside to inside is as follows: a thin layer of surface fiber, mitotic cell layer, fibrovascular layer, and more mature osteoblast layer. This is the main osteogenic process of intramembranous ossification.

During membrane osteogenesis, the mesenchymal cells in the membrane differentiate into osteoblasts as early as possible. The osteoblasts secrete the interstitial cells of the bone, embedding themselves therein, and the cells project long protrusions in contact with each other. Fine fibers and matrix fill in between cells. The matrix is eosinophilic. At this point is the formation of the naive matrix, known as the osteoid, and the osteoid surface is attached with alkaline phosphatase osteoblasts. With the thickening and mineralization of osteoid, osteoblasts form more osteoids, and a large number of osteoblasts are embedded in the newly formed bone and converted into osteocytes. These osteocytes remain in contact with each other through their cell protrusions and connect with the surface osteoblasts, forming a complete nest-tubule system. The new bone formed at this time is acicular trabecular bone, woven into each other, forming the original cancellous bone. Some of the original cancellous bone is transformed into dense bone. Osteoblasts continue to make new bone on the surface of the existing trabecular bone, to form the bone deposition, resulting in trabecular gap filling. Under the compression of adjacent trabecular bone, the outside of the original braided bone is converted into trabecular at the surface, forming irregular concentric layers of bone, which constitute the original Haversian system. The original Haversian system is different from the mature Haversian, with irregular shape, uneven distribution of bone cells, and collagen fibers randomly distributed. While some of the original cancellous bone continued to exist as cancellous bone, in these primitive cancellous bone, the thickness of trabecular bone is no longer increased. The connective tissue between trabecular bone is differentiated into bone marrow hematopoietic tissue, while the osteoblasts and mesenchymal cells near the bone surface are converted into bone intima, and the connective tissue outside the bone forms the bone outer membrane. After the adventitia is formed, the inner cells of the adventitia may continue to differentiate into osteoblasts. The external surface area of the bone is continuously thickened and expanded to form dense bone on the outside of the flat bones. The dense bones on the inside are also formed in the same way.

1.2.1.2 Cartilage Osteogenesis

Endochondral ossification is the initial development of trunk and limb bones. In the normal repair of the bone fracture, callus formation and maturation take place as well as the in endochondral ossification process. Endochondral ossification takes place in the site of bone formation, first by mesenchymal tissue differentiation into hyaline cartilage, which is later gradually replaced by bone. This process occurs slowly, starting from the fetus, and is complete at adulthood.

The development of long bones in the embryo is typical of endochondral ossification [15], which is a process in which cartilaginous primordia are replaced by bone to form osteochondral complex. First, undifferentiated mesenchymal cells aggregate, secrete cartilage matrix, and are differentiated into chondrocytes. Then the hyaline cartilage and perichondrium are formed, constituting the contour of the bone base. The cartilage model will be replaced by bone later. Ossification begins at the middle of cartilaginous membrane. The central chondrocytes begin to hypertrophy, followed by cartilage matrix calcification, perichondrium into periosteum, and the formation of the original bone collar. The original bone collar is invaded by the fibrocystic vascular tissue; new bone replaces the calcified cartilage and forms the original bone center. The center is constantly evolving and expanding at both ends. Various precursor cells enter the center through vascular tissues and differentiate. Osteoblasts secrete bone matrix on the mineralized cartilage matrix. Osteoclasts absorb calcified cartilage and immature bone tissue, and the central portion of cartilage membrane is absorbed to form the bone marrow cavity.

Endochondral ossification occurs in short bones, flat bones, and irregular bones, such as scapula, carpal bones, phalanges, and vertebrae. In the process of endochondral ossification, the earliest ossification site, called the primary ossification center, can develop a new ossification center in other corresponding sites as the ossification progresses, which is called the secondary ossification center.

1.2.1.3 Additional Osteogenesis

Additional osteogenesis occurs in the process of bone membranous enlargement and remodeling. It is an osteoblast that is arranged and secreted by the osteoblasts on the surface of the existing bone, followed by calcification into lamellar bone. In the development and growth of bone, the osteogenic primordium is formed by endochondral ossification or intramembranous osteogenesis. The surface is covered with periosteum. Subperiosteal osteoblasts directly increase new bone by excreting osteoid on the surface of bone. It is the same model in the bone remodeling, caused by osteoblast and osteoclasts bone resorption and the secretion of new bone.

1.2.2 Fracture Healing and Bone Remodeling

Bone has a self-healing function: bone fracture began to self-healing. Fracture healing refers to the tissue repair between the fracture ends. This reaction manifests itself in the healing reaction, which ultimately restores the normal structure and function of the bone. Fracture healing is an extremely complex biological process, influenced by many factors. Fracture healing is based on the proliferation and differentiation of bone-forming cells in the periosteum. Fracture healing can be divided into the following several alternating evolution processes [16]:

1. Hematoma period: the periosteum, bone, and bone tissue are damaged after fracture, while there is damage to the small blood vessels around the skeleton. This causes rupture of blood vessels, hemorrhage, the formation of hematoma, then coagulation, followed by fibrin deposition. As a framework, this initially plays the role of temporary fixation.
2. Inflammation and debridement: hematoma contains a large number of red blood cells, white blood cells, polymorphonuclear neutrophils, macrophages, and so on. Macrophages phagocytose necrotic tissue, cell debris, residual organelles, etc., and are dissolved, digested, and absorbed in the cell body.
3. Fiber callus formation: there are newborn capillaries from the periosteum, fibroblasts, and bone formation invasive hematoma. Fibroblasts secrete a large number of collagen fibers, and after differentiation, the hematoma forms a fibrous callus. The fracture can be joined and surrounded by broken ends, forming fusiform spindle. Fiber callus, also known as temporary callus, is relatively soft, and is divided into epidural callus, bridge callus, connected callus, and closed callus according to the location.
4. The initial formation of bone callus: the process of fiber callus evolving into the bone callus includes the deposition of calcium salts around the fibroblasts, directly transforming them into the bone cells. The process is mainly through the differentiation of bone-forming cells into chondrocytes and osteoblasts, secreting matrix-like osteoid, and gradually replacing the fibrous callus. Collagen fibers were initially secreted cross-link, irregularly distributed trabecular. The mineralized trabecular is braided bone.
5. Secondary bone callus formation: there is a layer of osteoblasts in the newly formed braided bone surface, which continuously secrete bone-like tissue. The internal voids are gradually filled with nascent bone tissue, with the trabecular bone fusion. The Haversian system appears, and braided bone gradually evolves into the lamellar bone. Bone lamella is formed by the mature lamellar bone callus, also known as the final callus. At the same time, chondrocytes proliferate to form cartilage callus, then evolve into bone callus through the cartilage internal osteogenesis.
6. Bone rebuilt and remodeled: with the gradual increase in the range and density of bony callus, the medullary cavity is also filled with bony callus. Finally, the bony callus is connected with the cortex, and the fracture gap disappears to reach the fracture healing. In this newly formed bone

tissue, along with limb movement, edema, and periosteal muscle groups, the callus is rearranged to meet the biomechanics needs. Osteoclasts absorb excess callus, and make the marrow cavity recanalization. The insufficient callus is supplemented through the membrane osteogenesis. The final fracture site is restored to normal structure and function.

Bone remodeling changes the shape of the skeleton, while remodeling only adjusts the internal structure of the bony tissue. Bone is a highly active tissue that sustains its own microdamage through sustained remodeling and maintains the homeostasis of the structure, load, and calcium. About 10% of bone is remodeled every year [1]. The homeostasis balance of the skeletal system is achieved by bone remodeling. Bone remodeling varies between cancellous and cortical bone, but both rely on the activity of osteoblasts and osteoclasts, the balance and coordination between bone formation and bone resorption. In cancellous bone, remodeling is performed on the surface of the trabecular bone. The osteoclasts form the Howship's lacuna, and osteoblasts migrate and undergo additional osteogenesis. This phenomenon is called "crawling replacement." In the case of cortical bone, the osteoclasts absorb bone into the interior of the bone as though tunneling. The vascular tissues and osteoblasts, or their precursors, in turn penetrate. The osteoblasts secrete on the surface of the absorbed bone and deposit, forming new laminar bone. The new Haversian system forms when the multilayer concentric plates form around the blood vessels, also known as the second bone unit [17,18]. The ability of the bone to repair itself is limited. It is difficult to self-heal when there is a large defect in the bone, which involves the treatment of bone defects.

1.3 BONE DEFECT REPAIR MATERIALS

Bone defect, meaning the integrity of the phalanx structure is destroyed, is a common clinical symptom. The main causes of bone defects include trauma, bone tumors, degenerative diseases, infections, osteomyelitis, and a variety of congenital diseases. According to statistics, there are 20 million orthopedic surgeries per year in the world, 70% of which require to use of bone implant material for bone defect filling and repair. Smaller bone defects (usually less than 8 mm) are likely to heal themselves. However, it is difficult to heal completely by self-healing when bone defects are too large, or bone defects are in smaller bones. This requires surgical intervention. For different parts of the different bone types, there will be different needs in terms of bone substitutes. Clinically, the defects of long bones often require reconstructive surgery to restore their shape and function. Most clinical procedures include autologous graft or allograft as well as the use of synthetic materials.

Autologous bone graft takes healthy bone from other parts of the patient's body. The most common bone resources are ilium, tibia, and fibula to provide cancellous, cortical, or total bone, respectively. Autologous bone graft produces no rejection, has the maximum biological potential, with the strongest bone induction, and the effect is also the most satisfactory. Autologous has been used as the gold standard for the treatment of bone defects. Autologous bone graft is one of the best clinically effective treatments at present, but there are also some problems of limited sources and side effects caused by the bone [19]. Allograft, which is healthy bone from the donor's body, is used for the transplantation of bone defects. Although donors are more readily available, they are at risk of disease transmission and are therefore less commonly used clinically. Therefore, there is an urgent need in the clinic for a more reliable and richer bone substitute to replace or repair damaged bone. Metals and bioceramics have been used clinically as permanent substitutes, but each has its own drawbacks. An ideal bone substitute that can simultaneously meet both the needs of urgency and the patient's full recuperation needs to be studied. One possible solution to these problems is to use bone tissue engineering.

1.3.1 Bone Tissue Engineering

Tissue engineering was first introduced in the 1980s by Langer and Vacanti. It is a principle and technique that applies engineering and life sciences to the design and manufacture of a structure that rebuilds or repairs tissues and organs and maintains or enhances tissue functions. It is an interdisciplinary research field [20]. Three key elements of bone tissue engineering are signaling molecules (bone growth factors, osteoinductive factors), matrix materials, and target cells. The matrix material serves as a carrier for the signaling molecules, which are transported to the defect site, meanwhile provides a scaffold for the growth of new bone. The target cells of the induction factor are the perivascular walking, undifferentiated mesenchymal cells, which have the characteristics of multidirectional differentiation potential, that can differentiate into muscle tissue, fibrous tissue, adipose tissue, and bone tissue. But under the action of osteoinductive factors, mesenchymal stem cells will be irreversible differentiation towards the direction of cartilage cells, bone cells, thus supplemented into osseous cells to meet the needs of a wide range of defect. Bone growth factor can stimulate osteoblastic mitosis, resulting in a large amount of new bone. This osteogenesis approach becomes "osteogenesis-inducing." Therefore, the basic starting point of bone tissue engineering is to realize the repair and regeneration of bone in a way of "inducing osteogenesis" instead of simply "crawling replacement." Tissue engineering bone is expected to be the first tissue engineering product.

The classic work on osteogenesis was done by Urist and Reddi et al. As early as 1965, Urist [21] found that the formation of new bone was observed within 2 weeks after the inactivated demineralized bone matrix was implanted in the muscle of experimental animals. He called this *osteogenic.*

Reddi et al. [22]. showed a series of tissue-induced reactions that induce osteogenesis. When the decalcified bone matrix is implanted into the muscle or the skin, undifferentiated mesenchymal cells are activated and migrate to the site of implantation. Those cells adhere to the matrix and differentiate through mitosis proliferation and form cartilage. Then the cartilage mineralizes, with vascular invasion. The osteoblasts differentiate to form and secrete bone matrix, and finally bone matrix mineralizes and bone marrow is formed.

In 1981, Sampath and Reddi [23] completed a very important experiment. They found that signal molecules extracted from decalcified bone matrix that are osteoinductive but inactivated, must be recombined with appropriate carrier materials to restore bone induced activity. The carrier material they used was a collagen matrix, of which the main constituent is cross-linked type I collagen. In 1984, Urist et al. [24] used β-TCP as a carrier of inducer and implanted it into the muscle. He found that the new bone yield was 12 times higher than that of the new bone implanted with the inducer alone. These experiments revealed that the material plays a decisive role for the efficient use of signal molecules.

In recent years, the application research of bone tissue engineering has been booming in many fields such as orthopedics, oral surgery, and craniofacial surgery. The current international researches related to bone tissue engineering focus on four aspects: (1) the basic research of signaling molecules including BMP series and new kinds of growth factors, such as cell biology and molecular biology, especially with genetic engineering [25,26]; (2) the use of a variety of new biomimetic bone substitute material as a carrier and its applications; (3) the research and application of stromal stem cells; (4) clinical trials of new materials and BMP complex. Among them, the effective transport modes of signal molecules, and the application of these factors in the design and manufacture of new bone substitute materials are the key aspect at present.

Analysis shows that, under the guidance of the basic principles, the strategy of bone tissue engineering can be divided into two types. In the first one, the carrier material and the signaling molecule are implanted into the body, and the differentiation of osteoblasts is induced by the signaling molecule leading to the growth of new bone. The second involves the use of in vitro cell culture technology to obtain a sufficient number of osteoblasts, assembled in vitro with the carrier material and then implanted into bone defects site. A wide range of carrier materials are involved, including polylactide (PLLA, poly-L-lactide; PLGA, copolymers of glycolide and lactide), PEO/PBT copolymers, collagen, hyaluronic acid, bovine bone, hydroxyapatite, bioactive glass, complex of PLGA and HA, complex of HA and collagen, complex of HA and β-TCP, coral skeleton, and porous titanium implant with calcium phosphate salt membrane. In the form of the carrier, except for a few particles, microspheres, and films, most of them are made into a porous structure of block.

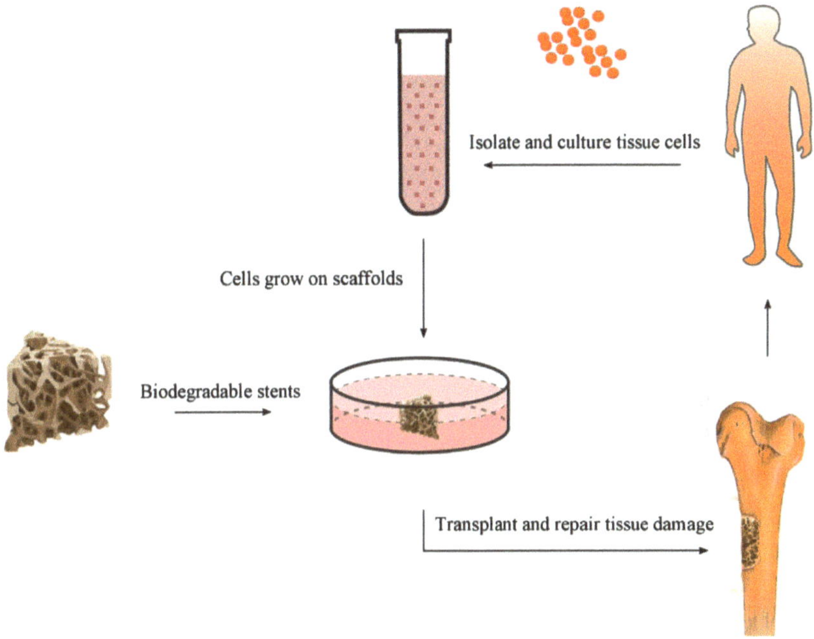

FIGURE 1.4 Bone tissue engineering diagram.

Fig. 1.4 Professor Cui Fuzhai was invited to contribute an annotation of bone tissue engineering biomedical engineering encyclopedia [27]. First of all, osteoblasts or growth factors were implanted on the surface of biodegradable scaffold material. Then as shown in the arrow, the scaffold material was implanted into the bone defect site. The scaffold material then gradually degrades with the formation of new bone and finally the scaffold material is completely degraded, and the bone defect site is gradually replaced by new bone tissue.

The emergence of bone tissue engineering brings new hope for bone tissue repair, but there are still many problems that need to be addressed [28]. First, the source of seed cells. This is because allogenic cells often cause immune rejection, resulting in graft failure. Therefore, the tissue engineering seed cells need to come from the patient, which will inevitably lead to secondary trauma to the patient. In addition, the somatic cells as seed cells exist in limited sources, are difficulty to obtain, and cannot yield unlimited proliferation. Adult stem cells are currently the focus of tissue engineering seed cells. These cells have stronger proliferation characteristics and can differentiate into different tissue cells under certain conditions. However, the regulatory mechanism of such cells is still not fully understood. Second, compound tissue engineering issues. Most parts of the body are a combination of many different tissues. The defects are often multiple tissue defects, or even at the same time, are the loss of the tissue of the embryonic germ layer. In the traditional tissue engineering method it is difficult to form complex composite tissue engineering products. Traditional tissue engineering technology needs to be expanded in cell culture, with differentiation induced by stem cells, composite culture of cell scaffold, and in vivo culture. The process is complicated, time-consuming, and requires high technical requirements, and is especially not suitable for the repair of acute injury.

Recently there are promising applications for collagen-based composites. One type is to mechanically mix collagen with calcium phosphate ceramics or the inject collagen into porous ceramics. This biomimetic material has seen more progress than ever before. Another type is partly bionic in composition and structure, and mineralize collagen fibers in vitro, to form close proximity to the natural bones of the body. Kikuchi [29] and Itoh [30], using cold pressure, and Chang [31], using glutaraldehyde crosslinking method, made a lumpy material used for various types of bone defect repair. The material obtained by cold pressing has low porosity, small pore size, and good strength, but it is unfavorable for cell growth as a framework material. The glutaraldehyde cross-linked material has poor formability, no compressive properties, and the residual glutaraldehyde has a negative impact on the biocompatibility of the material. The greatest advantage of the collagen-based material is that it is very good biocompatible material, and is a natural base for cell growth. Based on the research of mineralized collagen, professor Fuzhai Cui, the Department of Materials Science and Technology of Tsinghua University, prepared a nanohydroxyapatite-collagen composite by using collagen sponge as the mineralized base. This material has good flexibility but poor moldability and low compressive strength. To solve this problem, they further introduced the principle of biomimetic preparation, trying to prepare porous framework materials for bone tissue engineering. So that the complex material can maintain the excellent biocompatibility with certain strength and ease of forming properties, to meet the clinical application requirements.

1.3.2 Bone Defect Repair Materials

In view of the above shortcomings of traditional tissue engineering techniques, Shimizu first proposed the concept of in situ tissue engineering technique in 1998. The basic method of in situ tissue engineering is to use the basic principles of tissue engineering to induce the migration, proliferation, and differentiation of local cells (including somatic cells and adult stem cells) in defect tissue through various methods to form a new tissue repair defect. In situ tissue engineering consists of three basic elements: scaffolds materials, seed cells, and growth factors.

A variety of materials can be used as scaffolds for bone tissue engineering [32]. They can be divided into five categories, according to their sources: natural polymers, bioderived bone framework materials, bioactive ceramics, synthetic multipolymer materials, and composite bone substitute materials.

1.3.2.1 Natural Polymer

Naturally degradable polymers are naturally derived polymeric materials from animals or plants. This includes collagen, phospholipids, fibrin, chitosan, starch, hyaluronic acid, and polyhydroxybutyrate. The main advantages of these materials are their biocompatibility, potential bioactivity, their ability to interact with host tissues, and the availability of materials such as chitosan and starch, as well as their wide variety of sources and their low cost.

1.3.2.2 Biologically Derived Bone Framework Material

Natural bone materials include both autologous and allogenic bone tissue. Allogeneic bone tissue in turn includes allogeneic and xenogeneic bone tissue. Bioderived frame material is the natural bone material to remove cellular components, and primarily eliminate the antigenicity. But it still completely or partially preserves the original structure and part of the physiological activity of the tissue, so its application is very extensive.

1.3.2.3 Bioactive Ceramics

There are a variety of biological ceramics that have been developed and used in clinics in recent years. Bioactive ceramics can be divided into three categories according to their performance: (1) hydroxyapatite, representing the surface active ceramic; (2) TCP, representing the biodegradable ceramics; and (3) coral hydroxyapatite. They are similar to natural bone salts in composition and structure with good biocompatibility, osteoconductivity, and bone-binding capacity coupled with nontoxic side effects. Bioactive ceramics have been widely used as hard tissue repair materials and bone filling materials for physiological scaffolds. The disadvantage is that they are brittle and difficult to shape. At present, most researchers believe that calcium phosphate ceramic artificial bone is not easy to degrade or degrades slowly in the body. That might lead to barriers in the bone healing and reconstruction. Therefore, we should seek to faster absorb and degrade the framework materials.

1.3.2.4 Synthetic Polymeric Materials

Polymers are formed by polymerizing many low molecular weight monomer structures together, containing many repeating monomer structures. At present, the polymers that can be used as osteoblast implanting matrix are mainly polylactic acid (PLA), polyglycolic acid, polyphosphazenes, polyorthoester, polycaprolactone, polyesterurethane, poly anhydride-*co*-imides, polyhydroxybutyrate, and its polymers.

1.3.2.5 Bone Substitute Material

Hydroxyapatite has drawn much attention in bone tissue engineering due to its excellent biocompatibility and bioactivity. However, its mechanical properties and processability have limited its application. To improve the mechanical properties of materials and speed up the formation of new bone, HA is often complexed with other materials. It can be divided into three categories according to the different composition:

HA/Metal Bone Substitute Material

It must meet the four basic requirements for medical metal material: human body adaptability, corrosion resistance, appropriate mechanical strength, and surface biocompatibility. Medical metal materials, which have high mechanical strength and fatigue resistance, are widely used as implant materials in clinics. But they are poor in terms of corrosion resistance and biocompatibility. Currently medical metal is mainly used as bone plate, bone screws, crowns, etc. The use of metal implants has reached 2 million or more pieces in the United States each year. Spraying HA coating on the surface of the metal material is commonly practiced to overcome its poor biocompatibility. The most common spraying technique is to convert HA to smoke at temperatures above 1000°C and spray directly onto the metal surface to form a coating.

HA/Organic Synthetic Polymers

Organic synthetic polymers include bioinert polyethylene, polymethyl methacrylate and biodegradable absorbent PLA, polyhydroxy butyric acid, and other toughening materials. Bioinert material cannot be degraded in the body, reducing the binding force of HA and bone, so there is a tendency to be eliminated.

HA/Natural Biopolymer

Studies have shown that collagen-based bone growth scaffolds rarely cause toxic side effects. Collagen is the main organic component in bone tissue. After being complexed with hydroxyapatite, the composition and the hierarchical structure are very close to natural bone and therefore have excellent biocompatibility with human tissues. The research results of the HA/collagen complex show that collagen has a chemotactic and differentiation promoting effect on mesenchymal stem cells during osteogenesis. HA acts as a nucleus, a scaffold, and participates in matrix calcification, promoting new bone formation. In the past, we prepared nanohydroxyapatite/collagen/PLA biomimetic composite scaffolds, and simulated natural bone from both the structure and composition. We obtained good experimental results and got SFDA registration approval in 2011. According to the bionics ideas to prepare the structure and composition of biomimetic, biocompatible material is the future development direction of tissue engineering materials frameworks.

An appropriate three-dimensional framework is an essential part of tissue engineering and should have the following properties:

Safety

Tissue engineering materials belong to a class of biomedical materials, and as such need to be implanted in patients, which is different from the general industrial and agricultural products. The safety is directly related to the patient's health and life. Therefore, safety is the primary property of tissue engineering materials. Biological hazards caused by biomedical materials fall into two categories: one is the biological hazards caused by the material; another is biological damage caused by mechanical failure of biomedical materials. For the preparation of tissue engineered materials, the first type of hazard is to be avoided. The use of safe and reliable raw materials and preparation methods, in particular, is important to avoid cross-infection of animal infectious agents and cause immune rejection.

Biocompatibility

The framework materials should have good biocompatibility and be able to integrate into the host's tissue without causing any immune rejection. This is mainly reflected in two aspects: the surface properties and degradation products. The surface properties directly affect the short-term behavior of cells and tissues that have been implanted at the time of implantation. The degradation products affect the long-term effects of surrounding tissues on their response after the framework material is gradually degraded. The surface properties of materials, including chemical and topological structures, can affect the cell adhesion and proliferation. The surface chemical properties of the material affect the function of the protein adsorption and thus affect the cell activity, while its topological structure mainly affects the osteoconductivity [33].

Porous

Tissue engineered scaffolds must have open, interconnected pore structures to provide a large surface area for cells to grow into and distribute, which facilitates vascularization of the structure. Porousness and connectivity also play a crucial role in the replenishment of nutrients and oxygen and in the excretion of metabolic waste, an extremely important property in particular for bone tissue engineering. In the process of bone metabolism, even in the in vitro culture environment, a large amount of material transmission is constantly carried out. However, the porosity also affects other properties of the frame, such as mechanical properties. The pore size is generally determined in balance with the mechanical properties and the tissue to be replaced.

Pore Size

Pore size, like porosity, is also one of the important properties of the frame. Many researchers have discussed the relationship between the structure of the framework and histocompatibility. Human osteoblasts can pass through larger than 20 μm pore size; larger pore size will be more conducive to the passage of human osteoblasts. Pore sizes greater than 50 μm facilitate the growth of new bones into these holes [34]. The minimum pore size required for the framework is 80–100 μm for osteoconduction [35]. The mechanical properties often decline with the increase of porosity [34]. Therefore, the framework is usually prepared to jointly consider these two factors.

Mechanical Properties

The framework needs sufficient mechanical strength to resist fluid stress and to maintain the necessary space for cell growth and matrix production in vitro. There are two kinds of forces that the bone defect needs to bear in vivo. One is sustained supportive force, especially the stress that the lower extremity bone needs to bear; the other is the stress of the surrounding muscles and other tissues associated with the muscle. After bone defect, the surrounding soft tissue and muscle can easily press into the defect site and hinder the bone regeneration. The mechanical strength of the framework also affects the tension generated within the cytoskeleton, which plays an important role in controlling the shape and function of the cells. The tough surface of the frame is conducive to the arrangement of the tension fibers, the expansion, and differentiation of cells. The compliance of the framework affects the connection and aggregation of cells.

Degradation

Degradability is an important property of tissue engineering materials. The scaffold materials gradually degrade with the growth of new tissue. If the degradation is too fast, it will collapse before the new tissue grows into the body, then it will not be able to guide the regeneration of the tissue. If it degrades too slowly, it will hinder the growth of the new tissue and is not conducive to the repair of the defect. Generally, the material degradation rate and mechanical properties can be achieved by control of the molecular weight of polymer materials, components, and distribution of different polymer blends; or blends of natural polymer materials with synthetic polymer materials, polymer materials with ceramic materials, or use hybrid technology. Degradation products also have a significant impact on the tissue repair process. It affects the ability of the cells to regain their normal physiological status after prolonged proliferation. Good biodegradable scaffold materials produce nontoxic small molecules by hydrolysis or enzymatic degradation, which the pH value close to the body environment, through metabolism or secretion and excreted.

Biological Activity

According to the interaction between materials and tissues, biomaterials can be divided into four categories [36]: (1) the material is toxic and can cause necrosis of the surrounding tissues; (2) the material is nontoxic, but will be replaced by the surrounding tissue through dissolution; (3) the material is inert, nontoxic, and bioinert, and will form a certain thickness of the cyst at the interface of the material, separating the material and tissue; (4) bioactive material, that is, nontoxic material with biological activity. The material and the normal tissue can be well bonded through the interface. Obviously, the most beneficial for tissue repair should be biologically active material.

REFERENCES

[1] F.Z. Cui, X.M. Wang, H.D. Li, Assembly mechanism of mineralized collagen, Mater. china. 28 (4) (2009) 34–39.

[2] J.D. Termine, A.S. Posner, Infrared analysis of rat bone: age dependency of amorphous and crystalline mineral fractions, Science. 153 (3743) (1966) 1523–1525.

[3] T.G. Spiro, Calcium in Biology, Wiley, 1983.

[4] J.D. Termine, E.D. Eanes, Comparative chemistry of amorphous and apatitic calcium phosphate preparations, Calcified Tissue Res. 10 (1) (1972) 171–197.

[5] R.P. Gehron, The biochemistry of bone, Endocrinol. Metab. Clin. North Am. 18 (4) (1989) 858–902.

[6] S. Weiner, P. Zaslansky, Structure-Mechanical Function Relations in Bones and Teeth, Springer, Netherlands, 2004.

[7] S. Weiner, T. Arad, W. Traub, Crystal organization in rat bone lamellae, FEBS Lett. 285 (1) (1991) 49–54.

[8] L.B.S. Relations, Lamellar bone: structure - function relations, J. Struct. Biol. 126 (3) (1999) 241–255. Special Issue.

[9] W.J. Landis, M.J. Song, A. Leith, et al., Mineral and organic matrix interaction in normally calcifying tendon visualized in three dimensions by high-voltage electron microscopic tomography and graphic image reconstruction, J. Struct. Biol. 110 (1) (1993) 39–54.

[10] N. Matsushima, M. Akiyama, Y. Terayama, Quantitative analysis of the orientation of mineral in bone from small-angle X-ray scattering patterns, Jpn. J. Appl. Phys. 21 (1) (1982) 186–189.

[11] J.D. Currey, The Mechanical Adaptations of Bones, Princeton University Press, 2014.

[12] S.S. Liao, The Study on Mineralized Collagen Based Materials for Bone Tissue Engineering, Tsinghua University, 2003.

[13] J.G. Carter, Microstructure and Mineralization of Vertebrate Skeletal Tissues., American Geophysical Union, 2013.

[14] J.A. Buckwalter, M.J. Glimcher, R.R. Cooper, et al., Bone biology, J. Bone Joint Surg. -Am. Vol. (2009).

[15] D.G. Pechak, M.J. Kujawa, A.I. Caplan, Morphological and histochemical events during first bone formation in embryonic chick limbs, Bone 7 (6) (1986) 441–458.
[16] Z.J. Liu, Osteoarthropathy, People's Medical Publishing House(PMPH), 2000.
[17] J.A. Buckwalter, M.J. Glimcher, R.R. Cooper, et al., Bone biology. I: Structure, blood supply, cells, matrix, and mineralization, Instr. Course Lect. 45 (8) (1996) 371–386.
[18] J.A. Buckwalter, M.J. Glimcher, R.R. Cooper, et al., Bone biology. II: Formation, form, modeling, remodeling, and regulation of cell function, Instr. Course Lect. 45 (11 Suppl. 3) (1996) 387–399.
[19] F.R. Rose, R.O. Oreffo, Bone tissue engineering: hope vs hype, Biochem. Biophys. Res. Commun. 292 (1) (2002) 1–7.
[20] R. Langer, Tissue engineering, Science 260 (5110) (2000) 920–926.
[21] M.R. Urist, Bone: formation by autoinduction, Science 150 (3698) (1965) 893–899.
[22] A.H. Reddi, C. Huggins, Biochemical sequences in the transformation of normal fibroblasts in adolescent rats, Proc. Natl. Acad. Sci. USA 69 (6) (1972) 1601–1605.
[23] T.K. Sampath, A.H. Reddi, Dissociative extraction and reconstitution of extracellular matrix components involved in local bone differentiation, Proc. Natl. Acad. Sci. USA 78 (12) (1981) 7599.
[24] M.R. Urist, A. Lietze, E. Dawson, Beta-tricalcium phosphate delivery system for bone morphogenetic protein, Clin. Orthopaed. Relat. Res. (187) (1984) 277. &NA.
[25] V. Vicente, L. Meseguer, F. Martinez, et al., Ultrastructural study of the osteointegration of bioceramics (whitlockite and composite beta-TCP + collagen) in rabbit bone, Ultrastruct. Pathol. 20 (2) (1996) 179–188.
[26] D.Y. Suh, S.D. Boden, J. Louis-Ugbo, et al., Delivery of recombinant human bone morphogenetic protein-2 using a compression-resistant matrix in posterolateral spine fusion in the rabbit and in the non-human primate, Spine 27 (4) (2002) 353–360.
[27] F.Z. Cui, T.F. Jiang, Tissue-Engineered Bone, John Wiley & Sons, Inc, 2006.
[28] R.E. Horch, Future perspectives in tissue engineering, J. Cell. Mol. Med. 10 (1) (2010) 4–6.
[29] M. Kikuchi, S. Itoh, S. Ichinose, et al., Self-organization mechanism in a bone-like hydroxyapatite/collagen nanocomposite synthesized in vitro and its biological reaction in vivo ☆, Biomaterials 22 (13) (2001) 1705–1711.
[30] S. Itoh, M. Kikuchi, Y. Koyama, et al., Development of an artificial vertebral body using a novel biomaterial, hydroxyapatite/collagen composite, Biomaterials 23 (19) (2002) 3919–3926.
[31] M.C. Chang, T. Ikoma, M. Kikuchi, et al., Preparation of a porous hydroxyapatite/collagen nanocomposite using glutaraldehyde as a crosslinkage agent, J. Mater. Sci. Lett. 20 (13) (2001) 1199–1201.
[32] W.R. Dong, Y.Q. Xiao, Y.J. Piao, et al., In vivo tissue engineering: a new concept, Acad. J. First Med. Coll. PLA 24 (9) (2004) 969.
[33] J.E. Davies, Mechanisms of endosseous integration, Int. J. Prosthodont. 11 (5) (1998) 391.
[34] J.X. Lu, B. Flautre, K. Anselme, et al., Role of interconnections in porous bioceramics on bone recolonization in vitro and in vivo, J. Mater. Sci. Mater. Med. 10 (2) (1999) 111–120.
[35] O. Gauthier, J.M. Bouler, E. Aguado, et al., Macroporous biphasic calcium phosphate ceramics: influence of macropore diameter and macroporosity percentage on bone ingrowth, Biomaterials 19 (1-3) (1998) 133.
[36] L.L. Hench, J. Wilson, Surface-active biomaterials, Science 226 (4675) (1984) 630–636.

Chapter 2

Preparation and Characterization of Biomimetic Mineralized Collagen

Yun Cui[1], Helen Cui[1] and Xiu-Mei Wang[2]

[1]*Beijing Allgens Medical Science and Technology Co., Ltd., Beijing, P.R. China,* [2]*School of Materials Science and Engineering, Tsinghua University, Beijing, P.R. China*

2.1 THE BASIC PRINCIPLES OF BIOMINERALIZATION

Biomineralization is widespread in the biological world, from organisms in bacteria to oysters, corals, ivories, bones and teeth—that is, from nanoscale to the macrocosm. It includes a new chemical mechanism that combines hard and soft materials, inorganic and organic materials together. Recently, Ehrlic has reviewed the number and variety of biomineralized products, and has now identified about 128,000 molluscs; about 800 corals; over 5000 sponges (including 525 glass sponges); more than 700 calcium-containing green algae, red algae, brown algae; more than 300 kinds of deep-sea foraminifera; and more than 200,000 kinds of diatoms. This process of building inorganic-based structures in life is called biomineralization.

Biomineralization material refers to the natural biological ceramics and biopolymer composites such as bones, teeth, pearls, shells, and antlers, which are synthesized by living systems. Although the major inorganic components that make up biomineralized materials are widely found in nature, some minerals, such as calcite and hydroxyapatite, are the same in composition and crystallization as the corresponding minerals in the lithosphere, but once controlled by this particular life process, they have the unparalleled benefits of conventional ceramics, such as high strength, high fracture toughness, excellent damping properties, good surface finish, and many other special features. These unusual properties come from the ingenious assembly of materials and the fine microstructure that they have under certain biological conditions.

Biominerals provide not only structural support and mechanical strength, but also an organ. Biology is a natural architect, and the biominerals that are built contain many important biological functions such as protection,

Mineralized Collagen Bone Graft Substitutes. DOI: https://doi.org/10.1016/B978-0-08-102717-2.00002-3

exercise, biting and grating, buoyancy, optics, magnetism, gravity sensing, storage, and more. Numerous facts have shown that this advanced feature stems from the evolution of special organizations and that such structures must function fully within the body as part of the entire body.

The peculiarity of biomineralization is that it is a naturally occurring and highly controlled process modulated by the mechanisms within the body of the organism. Biomineralization can achieve crystal shape, size, structure, orientation and alignment from the molecular to the mesoscopic level, and precise control and assembly, resulting in a complex hierarchical structure, which has special optical, magnetic, and mechanical properties.

Many biomineralized tissues, including bones, are bioceramic composites synthesized through a cell-controlled process that involves fine-tuning the nucleation and growth of mineral crystals at the molecular level, as well as the organic and microassembly of inorganic members. Life system biomineralization materials assembled in an aqueous environment using materials widely found in nature such as calcium carbonate, calcium phosphate, silicon oxide, iron oxide, etc., have unique structures and incomparable properties with conventional materials. Understanding the basic laws of biomineralization process and applying and implementing the biomimetic synthesis strategy of materials can enable people to design and synthesize advanced materials with specific structures and functions at molecular level, including biomaterials, advanced ceramics, semiconductors, and optical materials with excellent light, electricity, magnetic properties of nanomaterials, and therefore subject to material science, physics, chemistry, biology, medicine, and even the electronics industry and many other areas of concern. Although much detail remains to be seen, several basic principles of biomineralization have been recognized:

1. Biomineralization occurs in specific subunit compartments or microenvironments where crystals can only nucleate and grow at specific functional sites. Compartment dimensions are dictated by the spatial distribution of organic matrices secreted by the cells, and usually these organic matrices self-assemble into a matrix of preferred orientation fibers or serves as a template for mineralization growth that contains functional domain structures that control the formation of crystals. Mineralization occurs outside of the mineralized active compartment by a series of molecular processes. Supersaturation in the compartment is governed by several example transport mechanisms or ion pumps, including mechanistic vesicles, polyelectrolytes, phosphoproteins or other Ca^{2+} binding proteins, phospholipids, and enzymes. The increased density of these biomineralized materials is achieved through the clear organic template and then the space created by the mineralization filling.
2. The specific biominerals have a definite grain size and crystallographic orientation, which is determined by the organic matter's prestructure and its chemical properties. Most crystals grow inside the matrix structure; some matrix molecules can then be integrated into the crystal lattice of the mineral. In some cases, minerals can be absorbed and remodeled through the processes of cell regulation.

3. Macroscopic growth is achieved by the assembly stacking of a large number of growth cells, thereby forming a composite material and providing the conditions required for further growth and repair of the biological tissue.

The basic feature of biomineralization process is the growth of crystals under the modulation of organic matrix. The regular prestructuring of organic macromolecule matrix not only provides the structural framework for mineralization and sedimentation, but also provides various functional groups and suitable interaction between inorganic ions at the environment and interface, which directly controls the nucleation and growth of minerals. The interaction at the organic–inorganic interface is called "molecular recognition," mainly in the matching of lattice geometry, electrostatic potential interaction, polarity, stereochemistry, space symmetry, and surface topography. From the study of abalone shells, there are two main types of control roles in the biomineralization process. One is the matrix protein, polysaccharide matrix, which first by its own self-assembly or cross-linking process forms a complex ordered structure, and then guides the crystal orientation assembly. The other is a soluble functional protein, especially its polyanionic group, which has a wide range of regulation to inhibit or promote nucleation, crystal phase orientation, crystal orientation, morphology, and crystal growth.

2.1.1 Biological Mineralization Interface Control

An important advance in biomineralization research over the past two decades has been to recognize the modulating effect of organic templates on inorganic crystals, where molecular recognition at the organic–inorganic interface plays a key role in the orderly assembly of crystals, growth, and microstructures. The most representative is Mann's organic–inorganic interface molecular recognition theory.

Based on the phenomenon of directional nucleation guided by organic templates in biomineralization, Mann [1,2] employed a molecular ordered assemblage of Langmuir monolayers as a growth substrate to simulate the $CaCO_3$ mineralization system and to explore the proposed solution environment composition, pH value and functional groups of solution, the structure and morphology of the ordered body, the charge state of the polar head on the membrane surface, and the chemical potential difference between the inner and outer surfaces of the lipid bilayer on the formation and growth of the crystal to study the Mineralization molecular recognition process and control. The study suggests that the choice of organic macromolecule templates for the nucleation of inorganic ions involves the molecular reaction on the surface and the protein adsorption process at the interface, which is an interfacial process. Molecular recognition between organic and inorganic interfaces is thought to be due to size, charge, and molecular shape matching resulting from structural, stereochemical, and kinetic relationships, and is a result of weak intermolecular forces, spatial geometry, and stereochemical matching synergies. The rules of molecular recognition in organic–inorganic interface are described as follows:

1. Lattice geometry matching: The atomic arrangement of organic nuclei on the organic macromolecule is required to be matched with the formed solid phase lattice.
2. Electrostatic potential interaction: Polyanion nucleation is assisted by providing the electrostatic interaction between the negatively charged surface and the positive ions. The distribution of polycations on the template also provides a stereochemical template that absorbs the anionic layer, thus controlling the nucleation, phase sites, and phases.
3. Stereochemistry: The spatial structure size of organic macromolecules and inorganic crystals at the interface.
4. Matrix morphology and polarity, spatial symmetry: The organic matrix morphology through the impact of space charge distribution in the mineralization process, the polarity of the organic surface, and the spatial symmetry all affect the mineralization process.

Subsequently, the Nancollas team at New York University's Department of Chemistry also conducted a series of templates to investigate the heterogeneous nucleation of calcium phosphate mineralization systems [3,4]. It is demonstrated that heterogeneous nucleation of hydroxyapatite on the surface depends not only on the relative concentration of the precipitated phase but also on the surface properties of the substrate. The key contributor to the nucleation event is not the contact angle of the embryos on the wetted solid surface but the surface work.

Recognition of the organic–inorganic interface molecular recognition has been used to prepare complex three-dimensional structures, especially semiconductors and electronic devices [5–7].

Due to the limitations of experimental methods, all observed nucleation facts of the present day are based on relatively large crystal sizes. There is a lack of an ideal description of the molecular forces operating at the organic–inorganic interface, as well as knowledge of the critical structures (periodic, amorphous), size, and composition of initial reactions and large-scale nucleation events involving ionic bonds.

2.1.2 Natural Bone Formation and Mineralization

Natural bone is composed of mineralized collagen (MC) by a series of self-assembly and molecular rearrangement and subsequent processing and modification of the formation. The natural bone formation and biological mineralization are closely related. Biomineralization is the basis of bone formation, and the self-assembled MC fibers formed by biomineralization are the basic raw materials that form the skeleton network [8–12]. The self-assembly of collagen is also the basis of the basic microstructure of bone. Biomineralization can be regarded as the initial stage of the process of bone formation, and has been accompanied by the entire process of bone formation. The process of bone formation is a continuous process of biological mineralization and related regulation [13–19]. The MC and MC bundles produced by the process are connected with each other through self-assembly, rearrangement, and recombination to form different hierarchical structures of the bone. Different hierarchical structures form the bone tissue through complicated combination and modification [20]. In summary, biomineralization is the theoretical basis for bone formation.

The basic form of bone formation is also the main process of bone formation. Liu et al. [21] found that the special mechanical and physiological properties of natural bone tissue are largely dependent on the nanosize and molecular level of collagen fibers and corresponding apatite crystals' multilevel self-assembly structure and rearrangement of composite structure. Apatite crystals in the early mineralization of collagen molecules have been generated with the interface identification and binding effects. They have a decisive impact on the structure and properties of subsequent biomineralization and tissue formation products. Studies have shown that the regulation of biomineralization and bone formation has already begun and has a profound impact in the early stages of biomineralization. In addition, the experimental results also show that nanoscale MC molecules' self-assembly will have its periodic spacing structure. This is the basis for the self-assembly of collagen molecules to form a matrix structure of highly ordered MC and is also the key to determining the mechanical properties and bioactivity of the final mineralized product. These provide the theoretical basis for the future research of bone repair and bone regeneration materials. Uskoković [22] in the observation of apatite crystal nucleation and growth process found, in the presence of matrix protein, apatite and collagen fibers will have a unique combination of structural and orientation of the growth. This shows that the framework of the bone tissue structure is constructed from the self-assembly of collagen molecules and the combination of biomineralized crystal products. This also confirmed that the diversity of bone tissue was born in the mineralization process of different crystalline phases and different forms of mineralized crystal products. The experimental results also pointed out that biomineralization is not only the basis of bone formation, but also the basic mechanism of bone tissue to maintain a stable biological mechanism, and also to promote bone formation and stability of bone roots. Bone tissue in vivo is in a stable homeostasis. The aged bone tissue is removed, the newly formed bone tissue is added in place of the lost part daily, and the nascent bone component comes from the mineralization of the mineralization.

Enamel is formed by a typical grading process. This process is accomplished under the strict control of ameloblasts and their secreted extracellular matrix. First, at the nanoscale, gene regulation expresses some proteins (mainly amelogenin) that self-assemble into nanospheres. The nanospheres formed by the protein then interact with the specific crystal facets of the hydroxyapatite crystallites, thereby regulating the crystal growth. Crystals are grown and fused into microfibers. Ameloblasts control the orientation of hydroxyapatite crystals and thus form the typical structure of enamel: enamel. The hydroxyapatite crystals are arranged parallel to each other in the middle part of the glaze along the long axis of the glaze. As it moves away from the center of the glaze, the orientation of the hydroxyapatite crystals begins to turn toward the edge of the glaze, and the ordering of the alignment begins to decrease. The part between the glazes is called the enamel sheath, in which the orientation of the hydroxyapatite crystals becomes messy and the content of the organic matrix is significantly increased. Glaze columns are long columns that usually resemble "keyhole" shapes when viewed cross-sectionally. Under macroscopic dimensions, the glaze columns are closely arranged in different ways in different areas of the enamel. The formation of these arrangements are related to some special protein and cell activity of enamel development.

Hierarchical structures exist widely in many natural or synthetic biological materials. Weiner's and other observations based on the results of Scanning electron microscopy (SEM) and transmission electron microscopy (TEM), proposed a seven-level hierarchical structure of human bone, and have been widely recognized by the scientific community. Similar hierarchies also exist in the zebrafish bone structure. Some materials mainly composed of mineralized calcium carbonate also exist in a strictly ordered hierarchical structure, the most typical example of which is rock. Not only that, some of the materials synthesized by self-assembly also have a hierarchical structure. To study biological self-assembly, Tsinghua University Biomaterials Research Group has formed MC nanofibers, and reported the characteristics of multilevel assembly of this fiber.

2.2 BIONIC MINERALIZATION RESEARCH

2.2.1 Hierarchical Structure

Based on the observations of Atomic Force Microscope (AFM), SEM, and high-resolution transmission electron microscopy (HRTEM), the Biomaterials Group of Tsinghua University [23,24] proposed a new view on enamel structure: there is a multilevel structure of enamel, and a schematic diagram of the hierarchical structure is given. As shown in Fig. 2.1, enamel consists of seven levels of grading structure: seventh grade: enamel; sixth grade: glaze array; fifth grade: enamel/enamel interstitial continuum; fourth

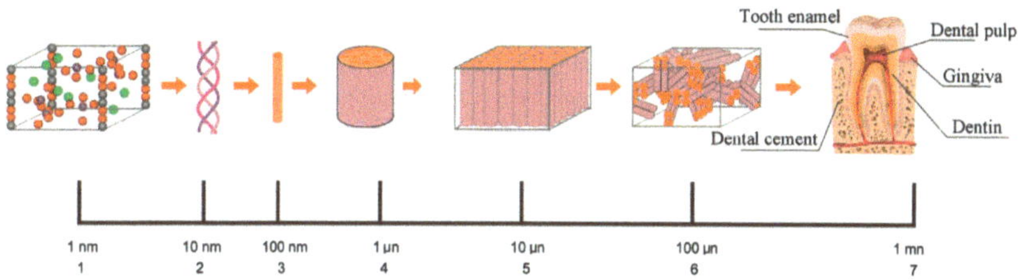

FIGURE 2.1 Enamel hierarchical structure diagram.

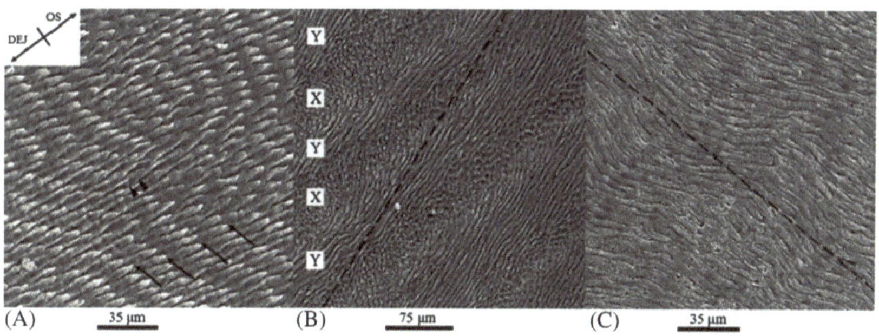

FIGURE 2.2 Enamel array. In Fig. 2.2A, it can be seen that the enamel of the 1/3 outer layer of the enamel is radially arranged [24]. Fig. 2.2B shows that the enamel has 2/3 of the inner layer and that the enamel is wavy. The structure of the enamel was observed along the dotted line as shown in Fig. 2.2C [24]; in the 2/3 region of the enamel inner layer, the enamel columns were oriented alternately [(XY) Ie HSB structure]. The enamel structure observed along the dotted line is shown in Fig. 2.2B [24].

grade: hydroxyapatite crude crystal crude fiber; third grade: hydroxyapatite crystal fibers; second grade: hydroxyapatite crystal nanofibers; first grade: the main component, nanohydroxyapatite crystals and a small amount of organic matrix. The results of the grading of enamel were as follows.

Seventh grade, dental enamel: enamel is the structure that covers the outermost layer of the tooth; its thickness can reach 2 mm.

Sixth grade, prism array (prism array): Enamel is composed of different structures of the glaze array. As shown in Fig. 2.2, enamel has a so-called radial structure in the 1/3 enamel surface, with the enamel orientation perpendicular to the occlusal surface. In addition, the typical Retzius line (shown by the black arrow) and the periodic structure of the glaze (black triangles) can be seen in the figure. In the inner 2/3 area of the enamel, enamel is wavy (Fig. 2.2B). If the enamel is cut longitudinally, a typical Hunter–Schreger band (HSB) can be seen, as shown in Fig. 2.2C.

Fifth grade, enamel prism/interprism continuum: Fig. 2.2 is a typical AFM topograph of unpolished enamel. Glaze column diameter is 6–8 μm. Glaze columns are the basic units of a glaze array that are closely aligned with one another and separated by an intermediate, organic enamel sheath.

Fourth grade, hydroxyapatite crude fiber (hydroxyapatite crystal fiber): Fig. 2.2 shows a typical SEM morphology of the structure of the glaze acid corrosion. The figure shows that the glaze column is made of hydroxyapatite composed of crude fibers (indicated by arrows). These fibrous structures are defined as the fourth grading of enamel and the first of the graded enamel columns. The diameter of the fiber is 600–1000 nm. Crude fiber structure is composed of a number of closely arranged fine fibers, and enamel third hierarchical structure.

Third grade, hydroxyapatite crystal fibrils: They are considered to be the basic constituent units of enamel. Hydroxyapatite microfibers are formed by the close arrangement. Such a fibrous structure is currently defined as the third hierarchical structure of enamel. The diameter of the fiber is 90–130 nm, and the cross-sectional shape of the fiber is irregular.

Second grade: hydroxyapatite crystal nanofibril, as well as first level, major component: the basic compositional structure of enamel is generally recognized as nanoscale microfibrils, that is, the second level of enamel hierarchy. The width of the microfiber crystal is 20–40 nm. Microfibers along the long axis of the glaze column are closely arranged to form a third hierarchical structure. The first hierarchical structure of enamel, hydroxyapatite crystals, make up these microfibrils. In enamel, hydroxyapatite is up to 96%.

In our laboratory, the microstructure of the zebrafish vertebrae has been carefully studied and similar grading characteristics have also been found in relatively simple fish vertebrae [25]. Therefore, zebrafish can be used as a model for studying the microstructure and bone diseases of human bones. As shown in Fig. 2.3, in zebrafish systems, the basic unit of bone material is MC fibers (level 2), which is a composite of hydroxyapatite crystals and collagen fibers (level 1). MC fibers are usually arranged in parallel along the long axis to form MC bundles (level 3). These MC bundles are usually assembled together in two ways: parallel arrangement and plywood-like arrangement (level 4). At a higher level of assembly, the initially deposited bone tissue undergoes internal remodeling to form a ring-shaped, multilayered structure surrounding the central notochord and the nerve and vessel arches extending to the back and abdomen (level 5). Levels 6 and 7 are the vertebrae and the entire vertebra, respectively. In the study of transgenic animals, we found that some gene changes will change the arrangement and assembly of collagen, thereby affecting the development of bone and the exercise of function. Studying the effect of collagen on mineralization in transgenic animals may provide the basis for future gene therapy and help us to understand the self-assembly codon for the assembly of MC in vivo. In the study of 1i1 mutant in zebrafish vertebra [26], after the gene mutation, the arrangement of collagen fibers was mainly arranged in parallel, the cross-linking effect between fibers was reduced, resulting in a large number of microcracks; the collagen fibers became coarse and the arrangement was

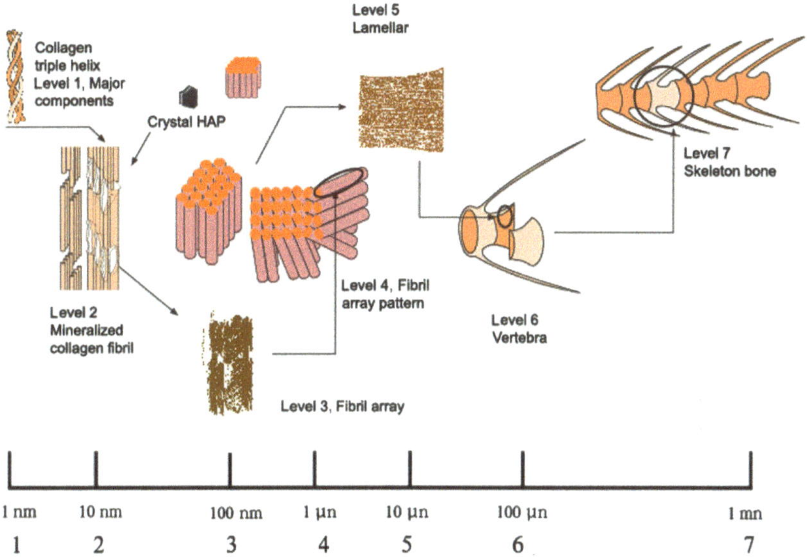

FIGURE 2.3 Zebrafish spine hierarchical structure diagram.

loose, and bending. These changes in collagen cause mineralization, crystal crystalline/maturity is reduced, and thus affect the mechanical properties of bone. Our study of Axin2-lacZ knockout mouse found that AxinII knockout resulted in high expression of β-Catenin in Wnt signaling pathway, which promoted cell proliferation and differentiation, especially increasing the osteoblast activity and inhibiting the activity of osteoclasts. In this knockout mouse femur, the amount of trabecular was significantly increased, collagen secretion was increased in trabecular bone and arranged more closely, and thus the degree of mineralization increased. Since the osteoblasts were stronger than osteoclasts, the mouse did not appear osteoporotic after resection of ovary; on the contrary, the bone mass increased and cortical bone mechanical properties significantly increased.

2.2.2 Prebuilt

The hierarchical structure of bone is based on the ability of organic matrices to regulate mineralization in the long evolutionary process of biological tissues. The macromolecular framework and the cells together participate in the construction of structures that trigger much greater complexity compared with the single cells. Another possibility is that the preformed mineral structure units are self-assembled in situ. In this way, vesicles and other associated minerals in biomineralization must be incorporated into cellular processes to increase the size and complexity of the structure. In addition, since vesicles associated with cellular features (scaffolds, microscopic, etc.)

can be used to create discrete, complex shapes such as curved needles and disks, the prefabricated mineralogical units form specific shapes and sizes.

In general, minerals deposited within vesicles can migrate to specific areas around the cell, or are released to extracellular sites through the cell membrane and then organized into highly ordered structures. Therefore, one of the basic concepts in vesicle-based biomineral construction involves the migration of prefabricated mineral structural units. In some cases, mineral-containing vesicles are used only as biological transporters to package and transport minerals to and from extracellular sites instead of assembling them directly into an ordered structure. For example, the formation of braided bones and the initial mineralization of turkey tendons are associated with acicular hydroxyapatite crystals encapsulated in bilayer phospholipid vesicles, the stromal vesicles. Vesicles are assembled at a distance from the mineralization site in the extracellular space and are quickly filled with hydroxyapatite as they approach the collagen matrix. At the mineralization front, they rupture and release internal inclusions to the collagen matrix. What will happen next is a highly controversial topic: Will the released crystals enter the pores of collagen fibers? Or do they dissolve, increase local supersaturation, and begin to nucleate crystals in the pores of collagen fibers? Researchers are still arguing about this issue [27].

However, in unicellular organisms, there is much more evidence that mineral-containing vesicles are used to construct prefabricated mineral building blocks that are more ordered structures. In this process, vesicles are not only involved in the appearance of discontinuous mineralized structures and their transport to distant locations, but also associated with the released units and the structure surrounding the entire extracellular space. For example, a foraminiferal construct is a mineralized shell with interconnected lumens, whereas in the calcitubapolymorpha shell it consists of calcite crystals formed within the vesicle. Needle-like crystals, 1–2 μm in length, are bundled in large vesicles and transported from the cytoplasm to compartments closed by the organic outer layer. The crystal is released as a complete building block to the mineralization front, so the thickness of the shell gradually increases. Although the crystals that first reach the organic shell are arranged in parallel along the surface, the subsequent crystals are randomly arranged in the wall [28].

In conclusion, vesicles containing preformed biological minerals can be migrated into cells or extracellularly to form larger structures.

2.2.3 Highly Ordered Self-assembly

In many unicellular organisms, vesicles transport not only minerals but also structural units that assemble into ordered structures. For example, *Stephanoeca diplocostata Ellis* is a unitary, carapace-shaped dinoflagellate that is commonly found in coastal waters of Europe and the Mediterranean.

This cell has a colorless protoplast, on the front is a flagellum surrounded by tentacles. This protoplast lies in an open-ended reticular basket that consists of 150–180 silicon bands. Although curved silicon ribbons were initially formed in intracellular vesicles, they ultimately formed an attractive extracellular basket structure outside the cell. High-resolution electron microscopy images of a single ribbon show an irregular amorphous lattice with no noticeable periodicity. There is no short-range order of more than about 1 nm (about 3 Si–O–Si units), a phenomenon that shows that silicon forms a continuous, disordered gel-like structure. Moreover, these images also show a random network structure composed of SiO_4 units connected by Si–O–Si bonds of different bond angles instead of the microcrystalline block structures randomly arranged by the microcrystal polyhedrons.

How is this basket structure formed? High-resolution optical microscopy can be used to observe protozoan activities. The results showed that mature cells cling to a fully formed pocket and swim around, trapping bacteria with small trawls. Although the pocket is intact, the cells continually generate extra small rods that enter the intracellular space and are held in the form of small aggregates at the open end of the basket, looking like mature bananas. Once enough sticks have accumulated, about 150 or so cells begin to divide, and the daughter cells and additional sticks squeeze together at the open end of the complete pocket and enter the environment. Within 3 minutes, a new pocket is built around the daughter cells through a series of phases, such as cell assembly and placement of the sticks. Although many details are not clear, the basket is made up of cells pushing outward. In the process, individual rods slide out of the bundle one by one along the sides and are locked in the frame. It is worth noting that these rods are bonded together in head-to-head or T-shape from unknown compounds of silica and some organic material. This method can keep the basket intact under pressure in the seawater environment. The connection between the two silicon ribbons is glued together during the bonding process and the electron density of the connecting material is usually lower than in the silicon ribbon.

High-resolution electron micrographs have shown that silicon and some organic substances make up this connection, indicating that the flow of organic polymers allows silicon to be added before the chain is hardened. Interestingly, the silicon-rich zone is metastable and can slowly dissolve into the liquid medium. The mineral decomposition depends on the physical growth conditions: at 20°C, mineral decomposition in the activated solution is completed within 10 days. Research on the decomposition of silicon mineralization is very important in explaining the local chemical environment of silicon in silicon ribbons. Assuming that these regions are composed of high-solubility silicon, the first step in mineral decomposition occurs at the center of the local area along the central axis of the belt. Alternatively, the surface silicon may be well protected by a thin layer of organic film. Over time, the reaction centers accelerate mineral decomposition until they extend along the central axis to connect together, forming a friable, filling band. As the mineral decomposition proceeds, the central control section continues to expand until the outer edge of the band shows signs of mineral decomposition until it becomes the final depression, and the interesting phenomenon of this preferential dissolution is that the band becomes hollow but its mechanical strength has not decreased significantly. So the silicon basket still maintains its function, although the silicon has experienced a serious mineral decomposition, but is still intact as before. Bending and breaking occur only when the pipe wall becomes very thin. The mechanical design of biosilica then becomes a structural feature associated with biological functions. Interestingly, the silica rod is metastable, dissolving slowly in seawater to form a complete hollow rod rather than a planar etch zone. The advantage of this preferential dissolution center over the stick's surface is that the ordered structure is stable over a certain time frame. This is because under certain boundary conditions, the decrease in mechanical strength between the solid rod and the hollow cylinder is very small. For similar reasons, tubular rods, rather than solid rods, were used as a scaffold for construction.

In addition to the mineral sticks and needles, intracellular microdomains and disks are also used as building blocks for highly ordered assemblies of multicellular organisms. For example, the curved microdots in the golden algae resemble roofing tiles on the cell walls. Similarly, the ball of stone is also assembled into the famous hollow shell structure, which we will discuss in detail in the next section.

In summary, the controlled release of vesicular-derived biogenic minerals from protozoa and algae organisms leads to the self-assembly of extracellularly highly ordered structures.

2.3 MULTILEVEL PROCESS

As a general principle, it can be considered that the construction of biomineralization with multilevel structure is a multistage process including multiscale construction stage. To illustrate the principle of this multistage process, we now discuss the different stages in the construction of calcite pellets by *Emiliania huxleyi*. With this model, we can propose a general framework for understanding the construction phase associated with biomineralization structures [29].

2.3.1 Ball

The calcite crystals produced by the single-cell algae *E. huxleyi* make up a spherulite disk, which is interconnected into a hollow spherical structure called a spherulite. A complete sphere has a diameter of about 6 μm, as shown in Fig. 2.4. We mention that the spherulites originate in intracellular vesicles, which migrate to the cell membrane and are released and fused into a pellet. Here we analyze the various phases of the construction of the spherulites, illustrating the complexity of the biomineral structure in unicellular organisms. We start with *E. huxleyi*'s ball of stone and dissect the structure to reveal its construction. Each disk is oval, with from 30 to 40 crystal structure units formed by the diameter of the tubular ring. Our next step is to analyze a single ball of stone. To do this, first sonicate in water for a few minutes, and thereby the individual structures within the disk are released. These micron sized crystals have unusual morphology (Fig. 2.5). It is important to note the fine fiber structure of the 3–4 μm pellet. As long as the structural elements are arranged around the oval ring, a bilateral ball stone plate is formed (Fig. 2.6).

A key question is: what is the crystallographic nature of this peculiar structure? Due to the very small size of individual cells, it is necessary to use electron diffraction analysis. The results show that each unit is a calcite single crystal, the crystallographic *c*-axis and *a*-axis, respectively, parallel and perpendicular to the ball and stone surface. After establishing the single-crystal unit cell crystallography of spherulites, we also need to know how these crystals grow and eventually form such highly oriented, highly ordered assemblies. Obviously, we need a lot of spherulites during growth, but this is not easy to do because the structure itself is not stable and is usually hidden inside the cells. Using the electron microscope, to take the "needle in the haystack" path of studying the ball, the initial stage of the construction process has been clearly stated. It turns out that the assembly of the rings takes place during the initial stages of ball formation, and geometrically circular

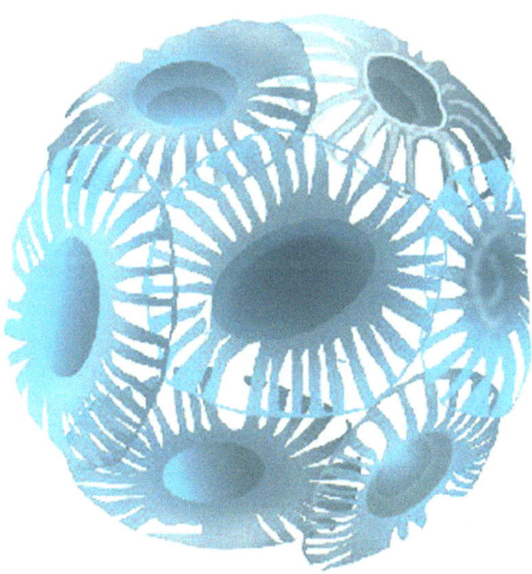

FIGURE 2.4 Hollow structure of *Emiliania huxleyi* spheres.

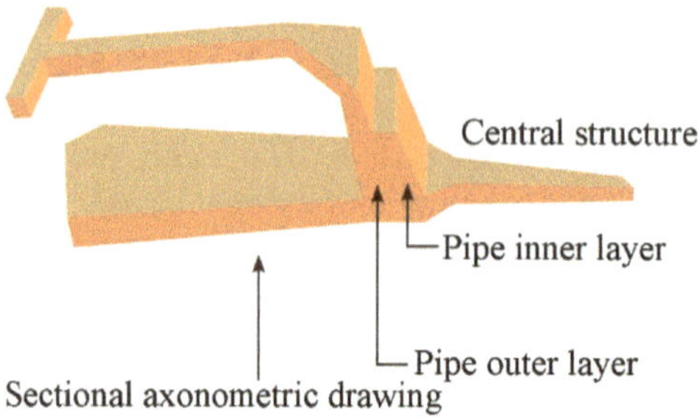

FIGURE 2.5 Single structural unit of a stone plate.

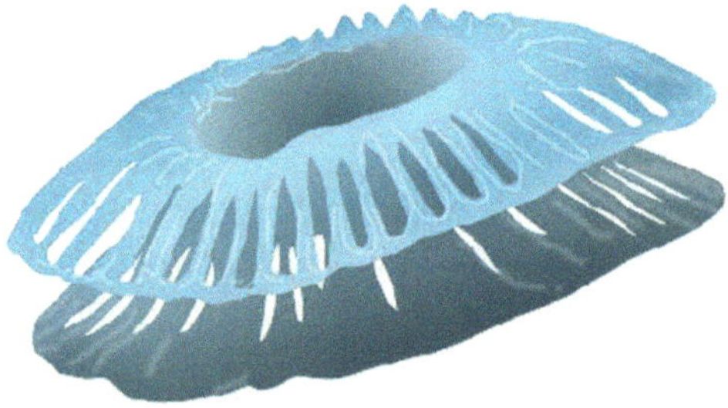

FIGURE 2.6 Spherical plate structure diagram.

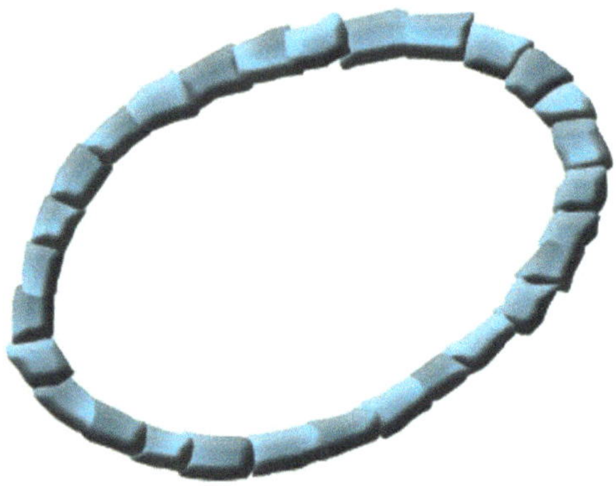

FIGURE 2.7 *Emiliania huxleyi*'s initial stage of spherulite formation.

necklace-shaped calcite crystals are formed before the structural units (Fig. 2.7). Initially, each crystal unit was a 40-nm-thick rhombohedron that grew to 100 nm in height and grew into a product that radially grew from the top and bottom along the *c*-axis to form a z-shaped ring of crystals, the crystal ring of the stone corresponds (Fig. 2.8A). The z units are interconnected and grow selectively so that adjacent crystals overlap each other and

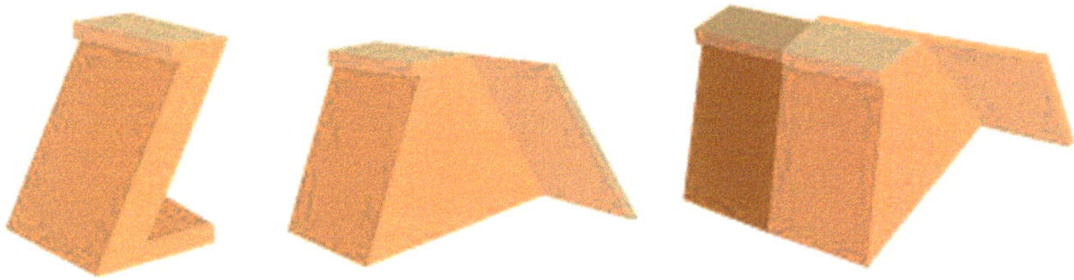

FIGURE 2.8 Structural unit in a spherical ring: (A) initial z-shaped crystal; (B) laterally extending; (C) overlapping and interlocking with each other.

interlock with each other (Fig. 2.8B and C). Because the lateral extension always looks in one direction and in the anticlockwise direction in the axial direction, the construction process develops into a morphological chirality.

However, we still have not elucidated what happened during the initial nucleation stage, which is still unknown. We do not know exactly how z-shaped crystals are arranged around the stones. We only know that each crystal is contained in a vesicle, which in turn is assembled around the organic disk. One possibility is that the edges of the organic disk contain functional groups that can induce the calcite crystal orientation nucleation through the interface molecular recognition process. To illustrate the crystallographic orientation observed, planes perpendicular to a must have preferentially nucleated on the organic disk so that the c-axis lying in the plane will emit emissive arrangements [30]. In addition, as a mature crystal is also perpendicular to the ball and stone ring, the original nucleation surface may be a zigzag facet as shown in Fig. 2.8. These observations suggest that the nucleation of spherulites is more complicated than initially thought.

2.3.2 Construction Phase

The entire assembly process of spheres is clearly a very complex multistage process involving several stages of construction spanning different length scales. Although not as special a case of biomineralization as bone, seaweed cells take such a complex build process that one can expect to find common principles in this example to help us explain a theoretical framework that can be used to solve the mysteries of other mineralization systems.

The first stage of ball formation involves the assembly of vesicles around the organic substrate before mineralization. We can equate this with supramolecular preorganization as shown in Table 2.1, which can be applied to different types of supramolecular assemblies, including the organization of collagen fibers. Once the vesicles have been established around the edge of the organic substrate, the second phase of the ball building begins. Including the directional nucleation of a single calcite crystal in each vesicle, we see

TABLE 2.1 Supramolecular Assembly in Biomineralization

Assembly	Ingredient	System
Nano aggregation	Glaze gene	Enamel
	Ice nucleated protein	Bacterial cell wall
Nanocapsules	Ferritin	Mammals, bacteria
Vesicle	Phospholipid	Magnetic bacteria
		Diatoms
2-D template	Surface protein	Bacterial cell wall
	β-sheet glycoprotein	Shell
3-D crystalline nets	Collagen	Bone
3-D macromolecular network	α/β-Chitin	Hat shell teeth
		Crab skin
	Cellulose	Plant surface
	Mucopolysaccharides	Bacterial cell wall

this as a general principle, in which the supramolecular preassembled tissue in interface molecule recognition is encoded by effective information that directs along some of the crystallographic direction of the nucleation. Some possible interface types may illustrate a great degree of molecular specificity at the surface of organic matrices. After nucleation, the third stage of construction begins, including in the sphere of stone, the crystal eye that grows in the predetermined direction to form a complex form of crystals. The principle here is the vector specification, including the morphological mechanism we discussed. Finally, the pebble plate migrates to the cell wall and forms a highly ordered assembly of the pebbles as a prefabricated structural unit. From a broader perspective, this is similar to the hierarchical structure of bone, where a series of related bone structure elements are embedded as the length scale increases [31].

As a general model for further development, we can consider the biomineralization structure to be a multilevel structure containing at least four stages of construction: supramolecular preorganization, interfacial molecular recognition, vectoring, and highly ordered assembly.

A popular analogy may help to understand: it is like building a house. First, make a building plan and find a location. This means cleaning up a space and setting the boundaries. This allows you to unify the perception of size, traits, and the connection between individual details (stage 1) before beginning the construction process. Also, this ensures safety when approaching the site, so that the material can be guaranteed in the subsequent stages of supply. Next, you need to base your ground on a plan or blueprint that contains information that builds the basic styles (stage 2). Once done, the house can be constructed as scheduled. The next step involves determining if a window, roof, etc. will be placed in the right position (stage 3). If a series of construction sites were set up in one place, the result would be more than just one individual house, but instead a street full of highly ordered houses (stage 4). In terms of further grading, houses are embedded in streets, with streets in towns or cities, and cities in countries. This analogy may provide a reference for our understanding of the biological mineral structure in living organisms.

2.4 MINERALIZED COLLAGEN NANOFIBERS MULTILEVEL SELF-ASSEMBLY AND ITS APPLICATION IN THE REGENERATION OF BONE ENGINEERING

Early collagen mineralization and the research of biomimetic surface nucleation sites for the preparation of hydroxyapatite (HA) mineralization of collagen fibers. Biomimetic preparation of hydroxyapatite MC fibers is a long-sought bone graft material in many laboratories because of its composition, structure, and properties. Natural bones are similar and have good bioactivity and biodegradability. There are many reports on the structure, properties, synthesis mechanism, and application of collagen/ hydroxyapatite [32–35]. However, the MC fiber structure of human bone has not been reported in vitro because its assembly mechanism is not yet clear. It is now known that there is not a simple mechanical mixing between collagen and hydroxyapatite, with the −COO...Ca coordination between collagen and hydroxyapatite [36]. Ca^{2+} and collagen molecules joined together cause the collagen molecules wider, shorter, when the Ca^2 concentration reached 1.0 mol/L, the neutral solution of collagen will not be able to assemble into fibers. This shows that during the formation of collagen/ hydroxyapatite, Ca^{2+} is the site of interaction between organic and inorganic phases. Our laboratory [37] showed that the carboxyl and carbonyl groups on collagen are two types of nucleation sites for hydroxyapatite biomineralization. Oxygen atoms on both groups coordinate with Ca^{2+} in solution to become the core of heterogeneous nucleation, and then nucleate and grow up. The formation of inorganic minerals, all or part of the nucleation sites wrapped CO and COO−, resulting in amides I, II, and III reducing the infrared absorption peak intensity, and the amide I band redshift. The laboratory [38] used the method of molecular simulation, combined with the traditional crystal growth theory and the basic theory of biomineralization, to establish a theoretical model for the collagen/calcium phosphate coprecipitated mineralization system, and studied the collagen fibers in the mineralization process of nucleation sites and crystal growth of organic template role. The results showed that in the early stage of collagen mineralization, collagen microfibers adsorbed calcium ions in solution to induce mineralization, resulting in the accumulation of calcium ions on the surface of collagen microfibrils. At the same time, these calcium ions have a large number of structural states similar to hydroxyapatite, the angle between the *c*-axis of the hydroxyapatite crystal, and the long axis of the collagen fiber is significantly aggregated in a large angle region (70–90 degrees). These results demonstrate the carbonyl site nucleation sites on collagen fibers and the modulation of collagen on hydroxyapatite crystal formation and preferential orientation. However, the details of the subsequent nucleation and growth process are unclear, such as the size of the nucleus from amorphous to crystalline, or the ability to directly grow apatite nanocrystals, are not yet clear.

In the research of biomineralization, attention has been paid to the modulation effect of organic molecules on nucleation and growth of inorganic crystals. In fact, biomineralization is the interaction between the two. However, few studies have found that the process of nucleation and growth of inorganic crystals can also cause the conformational changes of organic macromolecules. Recently, our laboratory used circular dichroism to obtain evidence that the pitch of collagen alpha helix in MC changed significantly [39]. However, the current data is still difficult to give a quantitative description.

2.4.1 Transmission Electron Microscopy

In 2003, our laboratory made a breakthrough in the research field of MC fibers in human bone in vitro. The conditions for the self-assembly of MC fibers in human bone were found, namely, providing suitable pH, temperature, and ion concentration environment for the solution to prepare human bone MC fibers by self-assembly of collagen calcium phosphate [39,40]. The laboratory designed and prepared the graded self-assembly of mineralized collagen nanofibers. Fig. 2.9 is a MC hierarchical assembly schematic. TEM observation at different magnifications confirmed that the composite contains multiple levels of hierarchical structure. As can be seen from the TEM photograph of Fig. 2.10, the composite consists of intertwined collagen fibers of more than 1 μm in length. Each collagen fiber is surrounded by a layer of hydroxyapatite nanocrystals. Hydroxyapatite nanocrystals are grown on the surface of collagen fibers. Electron diffraction analysis showed that in the observed MC fiber samples, the crystallographic *c*-axes of hydroxyapatite are preferentially aligned parallel to the long axis of the collagen fibers. To directly study the relationship between newly formed crystals and collagen fibers, our laboratory also performed HRTEM analysis at lattice level. HRTEM analysis of paralleled MC fibers showed that crystalline lattices were found not only in the region of both sides of the collagen but also in

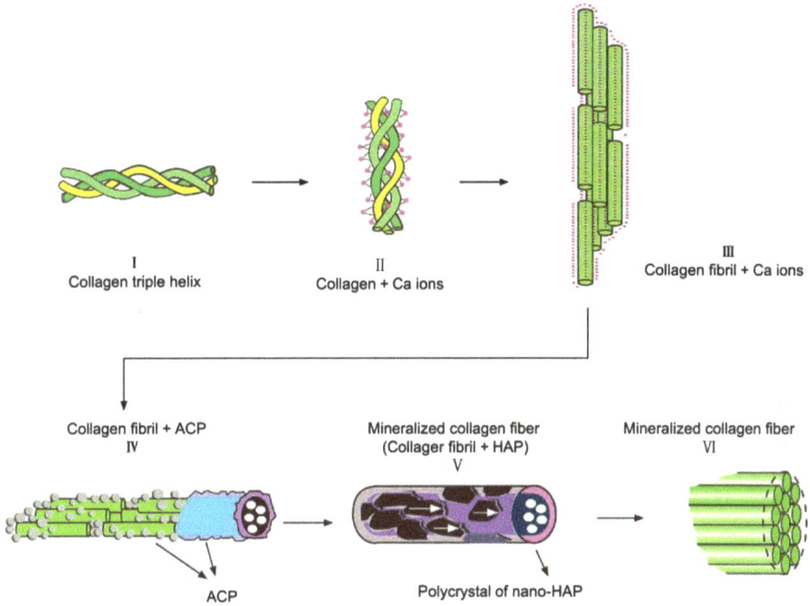

FIGURE 2.9 Mineralized collagen fibrillar grading assembly schematic (arrow in the V shows nanocrystalline hydroxyapatite c-axis).

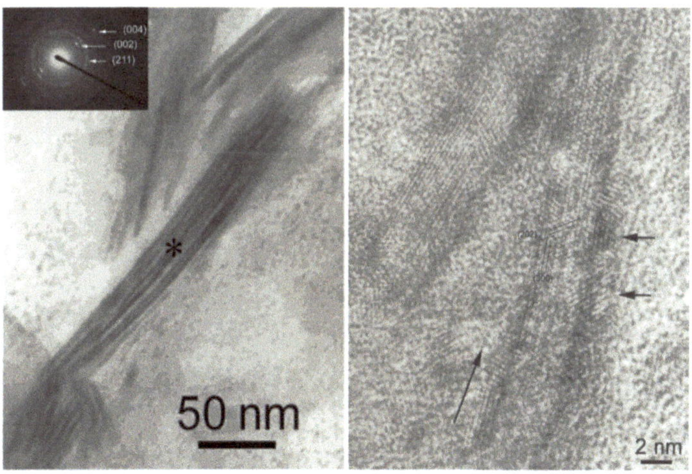

FIGURE 2.10 The photo on the left shows the transmission electron microscopy image of the mineralized collagen (MC) fibers. The asterisk in the figure is the center of the selection area. The diameter of the diffraction area is about 200 nm. The inserted image is the selected area electron diffraction of MC fibers. The photo to the right shows a high-resolution transmission electron micrograph of MC fibers, with the long arrow pointing out the long axis direction of collagen fibers. Two short arrows point to two hydroxyapatite nanocrystals.

the middle region of the collagen fibers and the electron density on the surface of the collagen fibers was higher than in the middle region. These results show that hydroxyapatite crystals grow on the surface of the collagen, surrounding the fibers. Hydroxyapatite grains have a size of 2–4 nm. Measurement and calculation of the crystal lattice of the hydroxyapatite crystals distributed on the collagen surface in the HRTEM photograph showed that the interplanar spacing was 0.27 nm corresponding to the (300) crystal plane of apatite and the interplanar spacing was 0.26 nm on the (202) crystal plane, the angle between them was measured as 49.8 degrees, whereas in the synthesized hydroxyapatite crystal, the calculated angle was 51.8 degrees. Hydroxyapatite crystals attributed to [010] with axis. Therefore, hydroxyapatite *c*-axis was preferentially arranged parallel to the collagen fibers. These results are consistent with the results of electron diffraction. SEM results show the adjacent MC fibers with their long axis parallel to each other form a MC fiber bundle.

2.4.2 Scanning Electron Microscopy

MC fibers in the three-dimensional network structure of calcium phosphate crystals covered the surface of collagen fibers. Fig. 2.11 shows a scanning electron microscopy of MC fibers. MC fibers are arranged parallel to each other along their long axis. MC fibers range in diameter from 77 to 192 nm. The experimental phenomena observed for the aggregation of calcium phosphate nanocrystals on the surface of collagen fibers are consistent with the results of TEM.

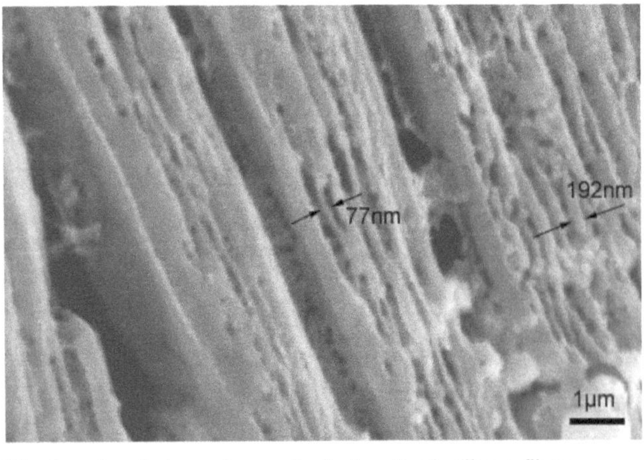

FIGURE 2.11 Scanning electron micrograph of mineralized collagen fibers.

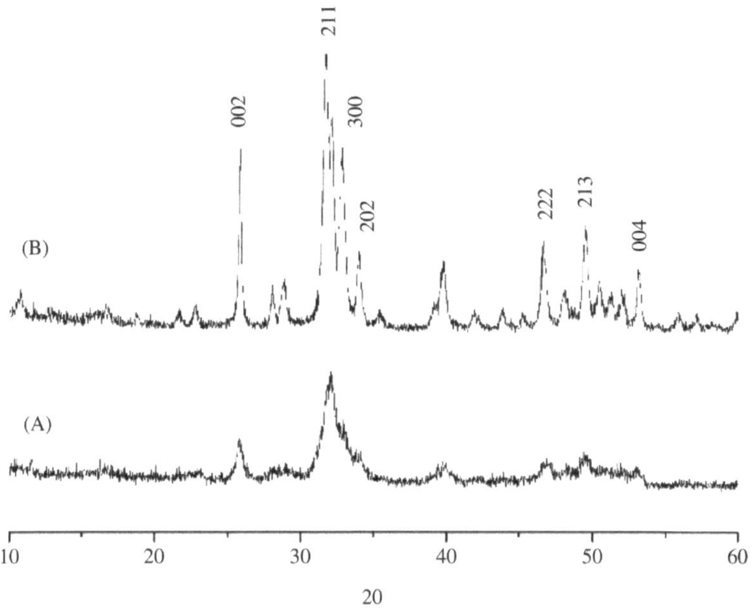

FIGURE 2.12 X-ray diffraction comparison of mineralized collagen fibers (A) with commercially available hydroxyapatite (B).

2.4.3 Crystal Structure

Crystal structure of calcium phosphate was done by infrared spectroscopy and X-ray diffraction studies. Fig. 2.12 shows the X-ray diffraction pattern of the MC X-ray diffraction pattern and the commercially available hydroxyapatite powder with good crystallinity. The inorganic phase of the MC fibers can be judged as apatite from the graph and no diffraction peak of other calcium phosphate crystals is observed. The result of X-ray diffraction is consistent with the result of electron diffraction mentioned earlier. The intensity of each diffraction peak is proportional to the diffraction peak intensity of pure hydroxyapatite. This shows that the mineral in the MC powder sample used in the X-ray diffraction experiment is randomly oriented and has no texture.

Fig. 2.13 shows the infrared spectra of MC fibers, calcium phosphate crystals deposited in the absence of collagen under the same experimental conditions as collagen mineralization, and three samples of reconstituted collagen fibers. Infrared spectroscopy of MC fibers appears to be a combination of collagen fibers and deposited calcium phosphate infrared spectroscopy. Both MC fibers and deposited calcium phosphate have typical phosphate vibration peaks in hydroxyapatite crystals. The location of the phosphate vibration peak is reported in Table 2.2. As can be seen from the table, the phosphate peak in the mineralized fiber is located almost identically to the

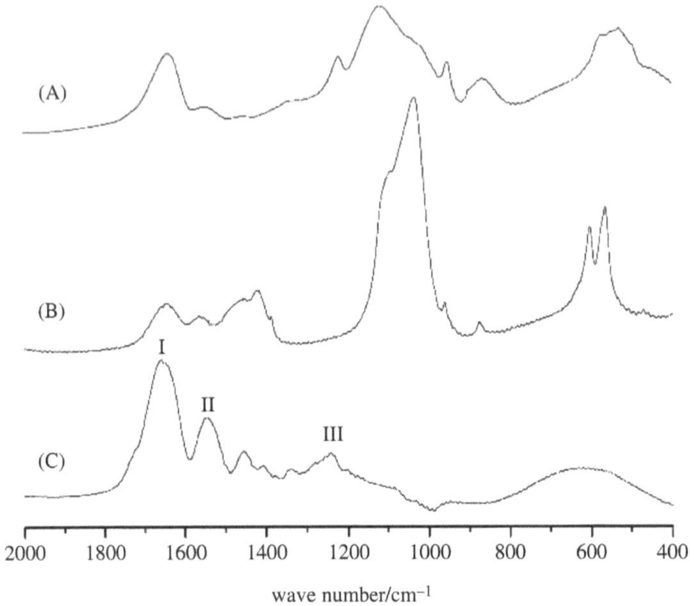

FIGURE 2.13 Mineralized collagen (A), hydroxyapatite precipitate (B) versus reconstituted collagen (C) Infrared.

TABLE 2.2 Calcium Phosphate Precipitation, Mineralization of Collagen Fibers in the Infrared Spectrum Peak Position Compared With the Literature Hydroxyapatite and Octacalcium Phosphate Comparison

Calcium Phosphate	Mineralized Fibrils	Hydroxyapatite [42]	Assignment
562	568	571	ν4
601		602	ν4
		632	OH librational mode
961	950	962	ν1
1031	1029	1050	ν3
1089	1113	1089	ν3

The wave number in cm^{-1} is given.

deposited calcium phosphate, but with some differences from pure hydroxyapatite. Weak peaks of carbonate at 1417 and 870 cm^{-1} were found on the infrared spectra of the deposited calcium phosphate and MC fibers. The inclusion of carbonate in the MC fibers is reasonable [41] because of the potential for carbon dioxide in the air to be incorporated into the solution during mineral deposition.

In the reconstituted collagen fibers, the amide I band observed at 1657 cm^{-1} is mainly attributable to the stretching vibration of C=O. On MC fibers, the amide I band moved to 1651 cm^{-1}. The red shift of the amide I band indicates that the intensity of the C=O bond in the peptide chain is weakened because of the formation of a new coordination bond between the C=O bond by the calcium ion. This result shows that the carbonyl group on the surface of collagen molecules is the nucleation site of calcium phosphate. In MC fibers, the intensity of the amide I, II, and III bands sharply diminished and the peaks of amide II and III bands almost disappeared. Calcium phosphate crystals grow on the surface of collagen fibers, completely or in part, covering these nucleation sites, resulting in a decrease in the amide I, II, and III band intensities.

2.5 HIGH-STRENGTH MINERALIZED COLLAGEN ARTIFICIAL BONE

Existing porous mineralized collagen (MC)-based artificial bone grafts have only limited strength similar to human cancellous bone that could only serve as filler for bone defects at nonloadbearing sites or in concert with additional fixation, rather than be used to provide mechanical support at human load-bearing sites by itself. In this study, a MC-based artificial bone with a high strength comparable to human cortical bone was developed.

The artificial bone was fabricated according to an in vitro biomimetic mineralization technique and a cold compression molding process under a certain pressure, so as to obtain a dense biomimetic MC composite similar to the natural cortical bone in terms of both composition and microstructure. Mechanical properties of this dense MC were tested and biocompatibility was evaluated by cell culturing and animal experiments.

2.5.1 General Observation and Density Measurements

The appearance of the dense MC artificial bone (MC-1000) is shown in Fig. 2.14. It is seen that the material is white (left, Fig. 2.14A) or presents as ivory white under the sunlight (right, Fig. 2.14B). The surface of the dense MC is smooth and glossy without any impurity or defect. Higher pressure of 400–1000 MPa effectively densified MC material, and the density of products reached 1.6–1.7 g/cm^3, which was in accordance with that of the natural cortical bone tissue in terms of either theoretical analysis or actual measurement.

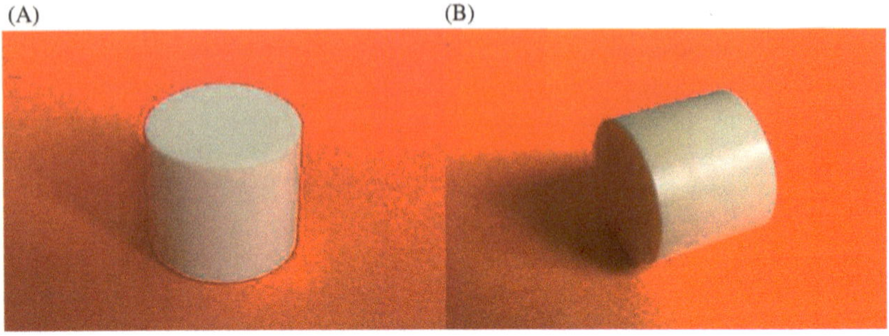

FIGURE 2.14 Appearance of the dense mineralized collagen.

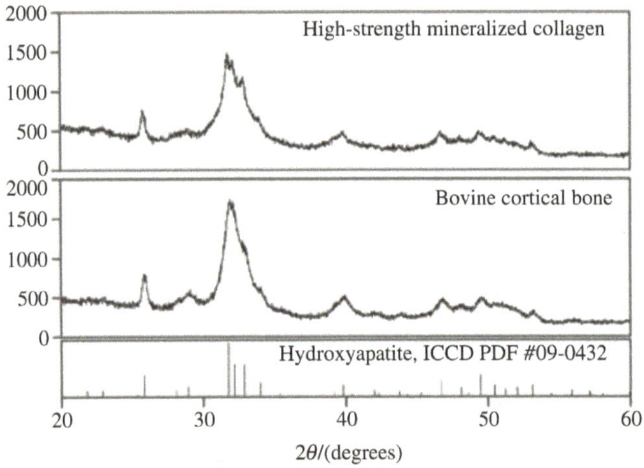

FIGURE 2.15 X-ray diffraction pattern comparison between the dense mineralized collagen and the bovine cortical bone.

2.5.2 High-Strength Mineralized Collagen of Phase

The X-ray diffraction patterns shown in Fig. 2.15 indicate that the phase and composition of dense MC artificial bone was similar to the natural cortical bone. The diffraction peaks corresponded to characteristic peaks of hydroxyapatite (ICDD PDF #09-0432), and no other peaks were observed. Therefore, the main phase of the dense MC was composed of hydroxyapatite, which was in conformity with the major inorganic component of the animal's bone tissue.

2.5.3 High-Strength Mineralized Collagen Molecular Structure

Fig. 2.16 shows the Fourier transform infrared (FTIR) spectrum of high-strength MC, MC, collagen, and hydroxyapatite, and the position of the

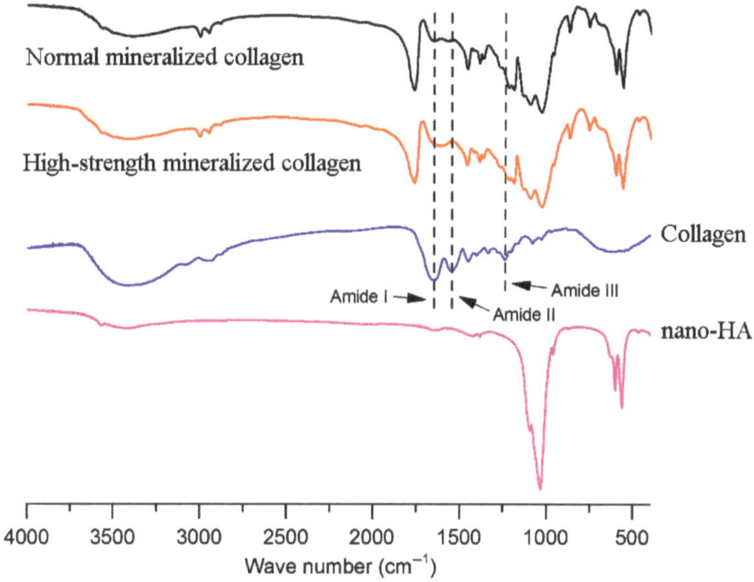

FIGURE 2.16 Fourier transform infrared spectrum contrast.

amide I absorption peak in the FTIR spectral line (red) of high intensity MC (red) with respect to the FTIR spectrum of the normal MC moves in the direction of the low wave number and overlaps with the amide II. This obvious redshift may be caused by the increase of hydrogen bonds in the collagene-folding, indicating that, under the pressure of the press, MC intermolecular and intramolecular forces are enhanced, which is beneficial to the formation of high mechanical strength of MC materials. In contrast, the absorption peak position and strength of amide III were not significantly different in the FTIR spectrum of common MC and high-strength MC materials, indicating that the process of forming materials had no effect on the c-n and n-h on the MC amide bonds.

2.5.4 The Microstructure of High-Strength Mineralized Collagen

The surface and internal SEM observations of high strength MC materials are shown in Fig. 2.17. Fig. 2.17A is the surface morphology of the material. It can be seen that the material surface is smooth and the roughness is low (depending on the surface roughness of the mold), and the material is evenly distributed without obvious defects. The material section shown in Fig. 2.17B shows that a large number of micron-sized and submicron-sized MC fibers are connected to each other to form a network structure, which has a certain contribution to the strength formation of the densified MC material.

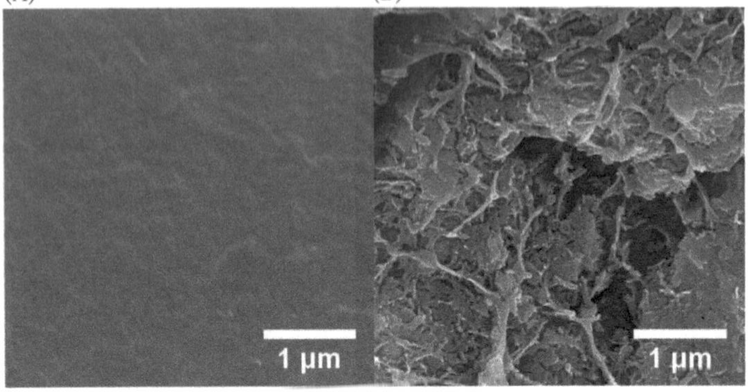

FIGURE 2.17 Scanning electron miscroscpy.

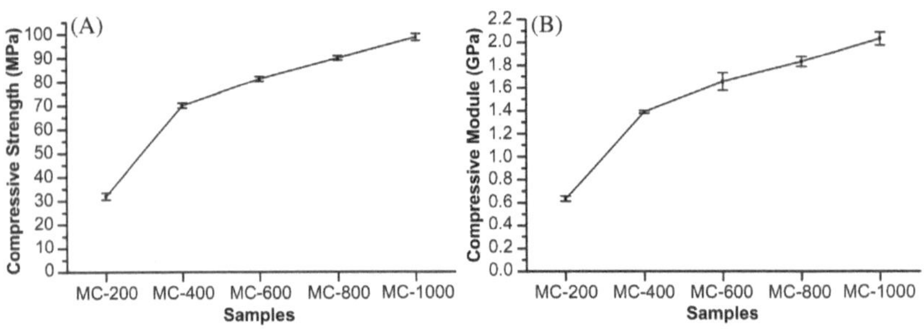

FIGURE 2.18 (A) Compressive strength and (B) compressive modulus of the dense mineralized collagen samples prepared with different compression molding pressures.

2.5.5 Mechanical Properties

Compressive strength and compressive modulus of the dense MC are shown in Fig. 2.18. Both of them increased with the pressure within the compression molding process. The compressive strength from MC-400 to MC-1000 presented a good linear relationship with the modeling pressure, while MC-200 had a rather lower compressive strength (Fig. 2.18A). MC-1000 reached a compressive strength of approximately 100 MPa, which was comparable to human cortical bone of 100–150 MPa. Similar to the compressive strength, the compressive modulus also showed a fine linear increasing trend for the samples of MC-400 to MC-1000 (Fig. 2.18B). It is noticeable that the compressive modulus values were much lower than that of human cortical bone and were close to human cancellous bone, indicating that there would be no stress shielding effect by using such dense MC materials in biomedical applications.

2.5.6 In Vitro Biocompatibility

As a biomimetic material, MC should possess good biocompatibility. The MC sample with the highest mechanical strength (MC-1000) was used for

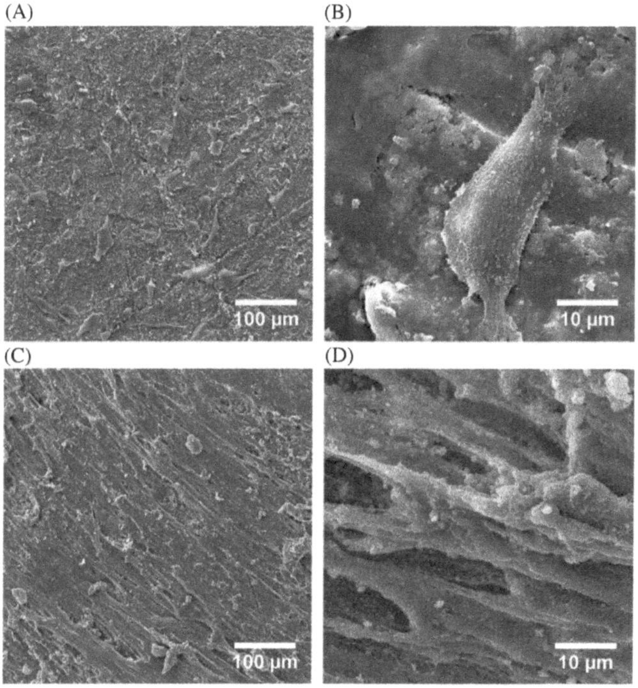

FIGURE 2.19 Scanning electron miscroscpy observations of MG-63 cells on the surface of the dense mineralized collagen: (A) 8 h after seeding under low magnification; (B) 8 h after seeding under high magnification; (C) cultured for 48 h under low magnification; (D) cultured for 48 h under high magnification.

in vitro biocompatibility evaluation. SEM observations of attachment and growth of MG-63 cells on the surface of the dense MC are shown in Fig. 2.19. Cells were well spread in triangle or polygonal shape and flattened on the surface after 8-hour culturing (Fig. 2.19A). Filopodia of the cells could be observed under higher magnification, and the cells anchored to the dense MC tightly via such filopodia (Fig. 2.19B). After being cultured for 48 hours, the cells spread all over the visual field and became fused with each other (Fig. 2.19C), and the secretion of extracellular matrix (ECM) is apparent in magnified micrograph (Fig. 2.19D). As a result, cell behaviors such as attachment, migration, and ECM secretion are evident in SEM observations, thus providing positive evidence for cytocompatibility of the dense MC material.

Cell proliferations on the dense MC are shown by histogram in Fig. 2.20. MG-63 cells proliferated very well on both dense MC samples and bovine cortical bone. The control group had higher cell counts than the dense MC at the early stage, and cell counts on the dense MC exceed that on the control group at the later stage. At the seventh day of the cell proliferation

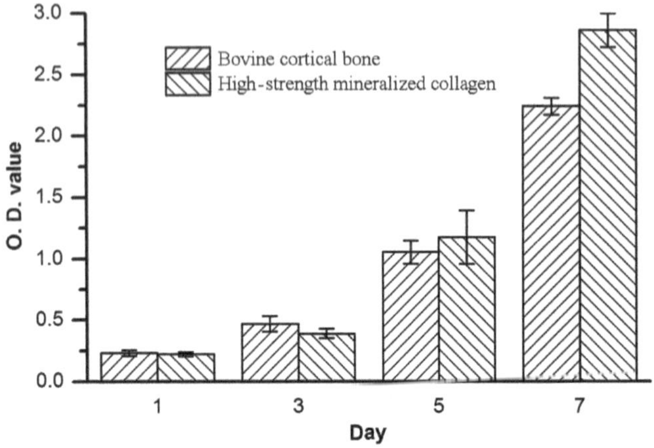

FIGURE 2.20 Cell proliferations on the dense mineralized collagen and the bovine cortical bone.

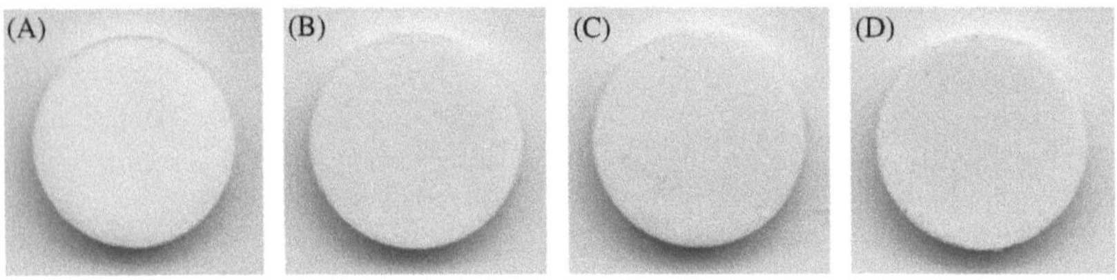

FIGURE 2.21 Newly prepared high-strength mineralized collagen discs and samples taken from the femur of the sheep (A) New preparation materials. (B) 2 months. (C) 4 months. (D) 6 months.

experiment, the amount of the cells was significantly higher than the control group of bovine cortical bone.

2.5.7 In Vivo Biocompatibility and Stability Evaluations

The biocompatibility of high-strength MC is carried out by animal experiments in sheep. After the material was implanted into the femur, the sheep in the experiment did not have any adverse reactions, such as rejection and fever, and no redness was seen in the implanted site. During the 2–6 months after operation, the animals' diet and activity were normal. All animals survived until the time at which samples were taken.

Fig. 2.21 shows the newly prepared high-strength MC discs (Fig. 2.21A) and the samples of the materials (Fig. 2.21B–D) that were taken out of the femur after 2, 4, and 6 months. It can be seen that the material was implanted into the animal without collapse, and the overall structure remained intact.

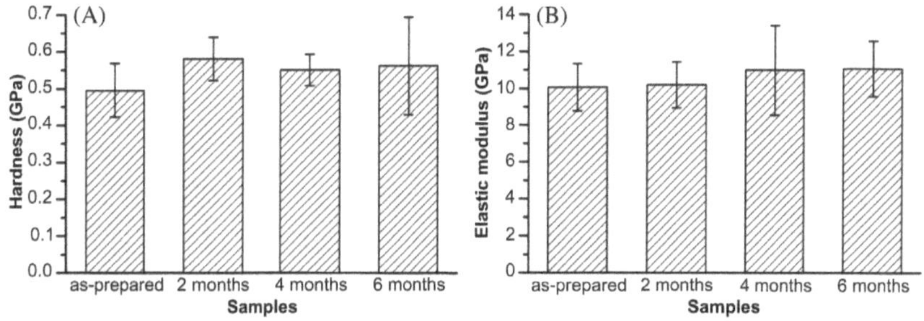

FIGURE 2.22 Mechanical properties of dense mineralized collagen discs retrieved from sheep iliac bone determined by nanoindentation: (A) hardness of the samples; (B) elastic moduli of the samples.

The dense MC discs were carefully taken out from sheep iliac bone at each sampling time point as mentioned above. All the implanted discs were successfully retrieved without crack or crash. Each sample remained intact by visual inspection. Mechanical properties of retrieved dense MC discs were tested via nanoindentation and results are shown in Fig. 2.22. There were no significant changes detected in terms of hardness or elastic modulus for the retrieved dense MC discs. Therefore, mechanical properties of the dense MC could be sustained for a long time, thereby being able to provide long-term effective mechanical support for defect repair at human load-bearing sites.

In this study, a dense MC artificial bone was prepared via in vitro biomimetic mineralization technique and cold compression molding process with a certain pressure. The compressive strength of the material was comparable to human cortical bone, and the compressive modulus as low as that of human cancellous bone can help avoid stress shielding in clinical applications. Both in vitro cell experiments and in vivo implantation assay demonstrated good biocompatibility of the material, and the in vivo stability evaluation indicated that the long-term effective mechanical support could be provided by the dense MC material after being implanted at human load-bearing site. Biodegradation properties and bone remodeling effect of this novel high-strength biomimetic MC artificial bone need to be investigated by further animal experiments.

2.6 COMMON MARKET MINERALIZED COLLAGEN MATERIAL

MC-based artificial bone repair materials have many advantages over traditional metal or ceramic bone graft materials such as biomimetic, biodegradability, good biocompatibility, and excellent biomechanical properties [43,44]. With the increasing acceptance of biomimetic materials, several collagen and hydroxyapatite composite materials have gained market access permits, and more and more doctors are accepting them. Table 2.3 lists

TABLE 2.3 Clinical Commonly Used Mineralized Collagen Artificial Bone Products

Product Name	Manufacturer/ Country	Material Composition	Porosity	Pore Size Distribution	Product Form
Bio-Oss Collagen [45]	Geistlich, Switzerland	10% collagen type I and 90% bovine bone mineral	70%–75%	300–1500 μm	Block
BonGold	Allgens Medical, China	Self-assembled bovine type I collagen and nanohydroxyapatite similar to natural mineralized collagen	70%–88%	50–550 μm	Strips, granules, block, dough-like, spongy
CopiOs [46]	Zimmer, USA	Cattle Type I collagen and 67% minerals	93.39%	N/A	Spongy, dough-like
HEALOS [47]	Johnson & Johnson, USA	70% bovine type I collagen and hydroxyapatite	>95%	4–200 μm	Strips
MOZAIK [48]	Integra, USA	20% collagen type I and 80% beta-tricalcium phosphate	N/A	12–350 μm	Strips, dough-like
MASTERGRAFT Strip/Putty [49,50]	Medtronic, USA	Bovine type I collagen and biphasic bioceramics (15% hydroxyapatite and 85% beta-tricalcium phosphate)	89%	N/A	Strips
OSTEON [51]	Dentium, Korea	8% collagen type I and 92% minerals (30% hydroxyapatite and 70% beta-tricalcium phosphate)	70%	500–1000 μm	Cylinder
OssiMend [52]	Collagen Matrix, USA	45% bovine type I collagen and 55% synthetic calcium phosphate	N/A	N/A	Strip, block, dough-like
Refit	HOYA, Japan	20% bovine type I collagen and 80% hydroxyapatite	95%	100–500 μm	Block
SynOss Putty [53]	Collagen Matrix Dental, USA	Type I collagen and carbonate-containing hydroxyapatite	N/A	N/A	Dough-like
Vitoss FOAM [54]	Stryker, USA	Bovine type I collagen and calcium phosphate	90%	1–1000 μm	Dough-like, strips, injectable, can be arbitrary plastic

commercially available collagen and hydroxyapatite composite materials such as HEALOS (Johnson & Johnson, New Brunswick, New Jersey, United States), Vitoss (Stryker, Kalamazoo, Michigan, United States), OSTEON (Dentium, Suwon, Korea), etc. These products are generally suitable for the repair of bone defects caused by trauma, tumors, and surgical trauma. Although these composites consist of collagen and calcium phosphate ceramics, their pore size, porosity, indications, and material properties are all different.

HEALOS bone repair materials are MC-based materials that have been freeze-dried into strips or flakes for surgical implantation. Its basic ingredient is bovine-derived type I collagen and hydroxyapatite, with a mineral content of nearly 30%. Before mineralization, purified water, organic reagents, etc. are needed to remove lipids, salts, and sugars. Hydroxyapatite is coated on the surface of collagen fibers by controlling the ratio of calcium chloride, sodium phosphate and sodium hydroxide. MC fibers are made into a three-dimensional, open-cell matrix with a porosity greater than 95% and pore size of about 4–200 μm, which can be completely absorbed during the formation and reconstruction of new bone.

Vitoss bone implants consist of calcium phosphate and bovine-derived type I collagen. Products can be prepared into different forms, such as cylindrical, strip, bone, etc. Similar to the human body it has cancellous microstructure, with internal interpenetrating holes with a diameter of 1–1000 μm. It is biodegradable and can guide bone regeneration.

CopiOs bone-filled sponges (Zimmer, Warsaw, Indiana, United States) are synthesized by calcium phosphate and bovine collagen type I collagen by vacuum freeze drying, with a specific gravity of about 67% for minerals. The material claims that its proper acidic environment favors the secretion of osteogenic growth factors, such as bone morphogenetic proteins. The material has a porosity of 93.39% and the scaffold is biodegradable and therefore has good osteoconductivity.

MASTERGRAFT Bar and Bone Bone Implants (Medtronic, Minneapolis, Minnesota, United States) have absorbency, a certain degree of toughness, and good conductivity. They consist of biphasic calcium phosphate (15% hydroxyapatite and 85% beta-tricalcium phosphate) ceramic particles and purified bovine-derived type I collagen, and have porosity up to 89%.

OSTEON II second-generation bone meal consists of 92% synthetic calcium phosphate (30% hydroxyapatite and 70% β-TCP mixed) and 8% collagen type I. Due to its high content of β-TCP, it degrades rapidly and can be completely degraded and absorbed within a few weeks after implantation. It is expected to be used for alveolar crest augmentation, tooth socket fills and osteotomy filling, bone cyst treatment, maxillary sinus lift, and alveolar bone defects.

BonGold bone graft materials, from Beijing Allgnes Medical Science Technology Co. Ltd. are nanohydroxyapatite and collagen I in vitro biomineralized. The mineral content of about 45%, the microstructure, and composition are similar to that of natural bone tissue. BonGold has a variety of forms, such as the strips, particles, block, putty, and spongy, with porosity of more than 70% and pore size of $300 \pm 250\ \mu m$, which provide a good environment for cell adhesion and proliferation. This MC material is the first biomimetic mineralization in the world to prepare a biomimetic synthetic material with natural bone tissue chemical composition and microstructure. This achievement has been extensively reported and positively evaluated by top international academic journals such as *Science* and *Nature Materials*, and the American Chemical Society (ACS) website. International authoritative materials expert and professor at Northwestern University, Samuel I. Stupp, has reported professor Cui' work in detail in his review paper as well as their research on multilevel structure new composite material design, optimization of the organic–inorganic collaborative assembly, and shape and control of implants [55]. *Science* [56] commented in a paper titled

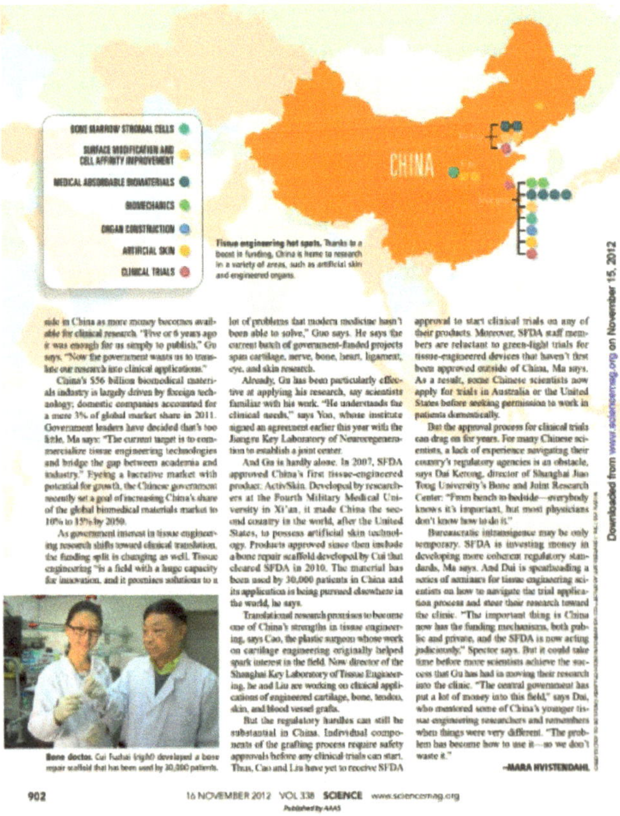
BONE MARROW STROMAL CELLS
SURFACE MODIFICATION AND CELL AFFINITY IMPROVEMENT
MEDICAL ABSORBABLE BIOMATERIALS
BIOMECHANICS
ORGAN CONSTRUCTION
ARTIFICIAL SKIN
CLINICAL TRIALS
CHINA

Tissue engineering hot spots. Thanks to a boost in funding, China is home to research in a variety of areas, such as artificial skin and engineered organs.

side in China as more money becomes available for clinical research. "Five or 6 years ago it was enough for us simply to publish," Gu says. "Now the government wants us to translate our research into clinical applications."

China's $56 billion biomedical materials industry is largely driven by foreign technology; domestic companies accounted for a mere 3% of global market share in 2011. Government leaders have decided that's too little, Ma says: "The current target is to commercialize tissue engineering technologies and bridge the gap between academia and industry." Eyeing a lucrative market with potential for growth, the Chinese government recently set a goal of increasing China's share of the global biomedical materials market to 10% to 15% by 2050.

As government interest in tissue engineering research shifts toward clinical translation, the funding split is changing as well. Tissue engineering "is a field with a huge capacity for innovation, and it promises solutions to a lot of problems that modern medicine hasn't been able to solve," Guo says. He says the current batch of government-funded projects span cartilage, nerve, bone, heart, ligament, eye, and skin research.

Already, Gu has been particularly effective at applying his research, say scientists familiar with his work. "He understands the clinical needs," says Yao, whose institute signed an agreement earlier this year with the Jiangsu Key Laboratory of Neuroregeneration to establish a joint center.

And Gu is hardly alone. In 2007, SFDA approved China's first tissue-engineered product: ActivSkin. Developed by researchers at the Fourth Military Medical University in Xi'an, it made China the second country in the world, after the United States, to possess artificial skin technology. Products approved since then include a bone repair scaffold developed by Cui that cleared SFDA in 2010. The material has been used by 30,000 patients in China and its application is being pursued elsewhere in the world, he says.

Translational research promises to become one of China's strengths in tissue engineering, says Cao, the plastic surgeon whose work on cartilage engineering originally helped spark interest in the field. Now director of the Shanghai Key Laboratory of Tissue Engineering, he and Liu are working on clinical applications of engineered cartilage, bone, tendon, skin, and blood vessel grafts.

But the regulatory hurdles can still be substantial in China. Individual components of the grafting process require safety approvals before any clinical trials can start. Thus, Cao and Liu have yet to receive SFDA approval to start clinical trials on any of their products. Moreover, SFDA staff members are reluctant to green-light trials for tissue-engineered devices that haven't first been approved outside of China, Ma says. As a result, some Chinese scientists now apply for trials in Australia or the United States before seeking permission to work in patients domestically.

But the approval process for clinical trials can drag on for years. For many Chinese scientists, a lack of experience navigating their country's regulatory agencies is an obstacle, says Dai Kerong, director of Shanghai Jiao Tong University's Bone and Joint Research Center: "From bench to bedside—everybody knows it's important, but most physicians don't know how to do it."

Bureaucratic intransigence may be only temporary. SFDA is investing money in developing more coherent regulatory standards, Ma says. And Dai is spearheading a series of seminars for tissue engineering scientists on how to navigate the trial application process and steer their research toward the clinic. "The important thing is China now has the funding mechanisms, both public and private, and the SFDA is now acting judiciously," Spector says. But it could take time before more scientists achieve the success that Gu has had in moving their research into the clinic. "The central government has put a lot of money into this field," says Dai, who mentored some of China's younger tissue engineering researchers and remembers when things were very different. "The problem has become how to use it—so we don't waste it."

–MARA HVISTENDAHL

Bone doctor. Cui Fuzhai (right) developed a bone repair scaffold that has been used by 30,000 patients.

902 16 NOVEMBER 2012 VOL 338 SCIENCE www.sciencemag.org

Published by AAAS

Downloaded from www.sciencemag.org on November 15, 2012

FIGURE 2.23 Science.

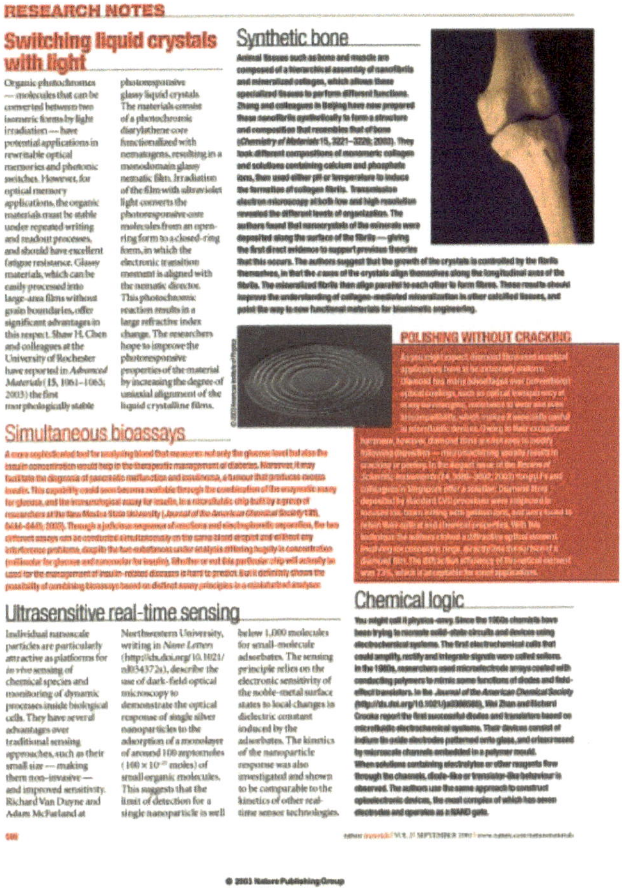

RESEARCH NOTES

Switching liquid crystals with light

Organic photochromes — molecules that can be converted between two isomeric forms by light irradiation — have potential applications in rewritable optical memories and photonic switches. However, for optical memory applications, the organic materials must be stable under repeated writing and readout processes, and should have excellent fatigue resistance. Glassy materials, which can be easily processed into large-area films without grain boundaries, offer significant advantages in this respect. Shaw H. Chen and colleagues at the University of Rochester have reported in *Advanced Materials* (15, 1061–1065; 2003) the first morphologically stable photoresponsive glassy liquid crystals. The materials consist of a photochromic diarylethene core functionalized with nematogens, resulting in a monodomain glassy nematic film. Irradiation of the film with ultraviolet light converts the photoresponsive core molecules from an open-ring form to a closed-ring form, in which the electronic transition moment is aligned with the nematic director. This photochromic reaction results in a large refractive index change. The researchers hope to improve the photoresponsive properties of the material by increasing the degree of uniaxial alignment of the liquid crystalline films.

Synthetic bone

Animal tissues such as bone and muscle are composed of a hierarchical assembly of nanofibrils and mineralized collagen, which allows these specialized tissues to perform different functions. Zhang and colleagues in Beijing have now prepared these nanofibrils synthetically to form a structure and composition that resembles that of bone (*Chemistry of Materials* 15, 3221–3226; 2003). They took different compositions of monomeric collagen and solutions containing calcium and phosphate ions, then used either pH or temperature to induce the formation of collagen fibrils. Transmission electron microscopy at both low and high resolution revealed the different levels of organization. The authors found that nanocrystals of the minerals were deposited along the surface of the fibrils — giving the first direct evidence to support previous theories that this occurs. The authors suggest that the growth of the crystals is controlled by the fibrils themselves, in that the *c* axes of the crystals align themselves along the longitudinal axis of the fibrils. The mineralized fibrils then align parallel to each other to form fibres. These results should improve the understanding of collagen-mediated mineralization in other calcified tissues, and point the way to new functional materials for biomimetic engineering.

POLISHING WITHOUT CRACKING

Simultaneous bioassays

Ultrasensitive real-time sensing

Individual nanoscale particles are particularly attractive as platforms for *in vivo* sensing of chemical species and monitoring of dynamic processes inside biological cells. They have several advantages over traditional sensing approaches, such as their small size — making them non-invasive — and improved sensitivity. Richard Van Duyne and Adam McFarland at Northwestern University, writing in *Nano Letters* (http://dx.doi.org/10.1021/nl034372s), describe the use of dark-field optical microscopy to demonstrate the optical response of single silver nanoparticles to the adsorption of a monolayer of around 100 zeptomoles (100×10^{-21} moles) of small organic molecules. This suggests that the limit of detection for a single nanoparticle is well below 1,000 molecules for small-molecule adsorbates. The sensing principle relies on the electronic sensitivity of the noble-metal surface states to local changes in dielectric constant induced by the adsorbates. The kinetics of the nanoparticle response was also investigated and shown to be comparable to the kinetics of other real-time sensor technologies.

Chemical logic

FIGURE 2.24 Nature Materials.

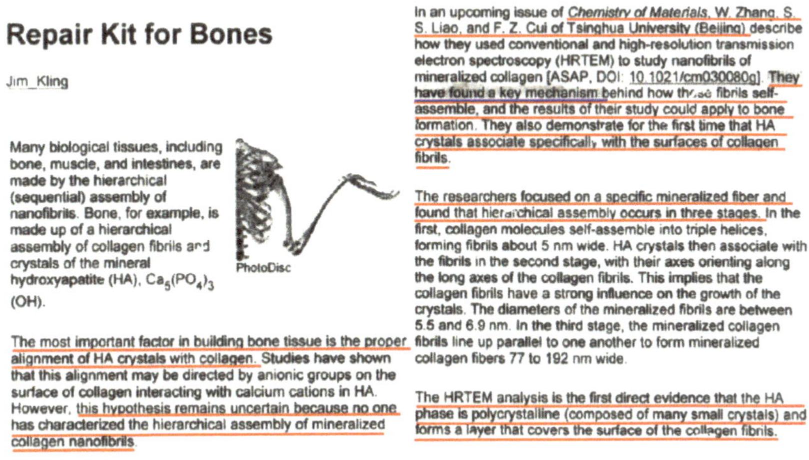

Repair Kit for Bones

Jim_Kling

Many biological tissues, including bone, muscle, and intestines, are made by the hierarchical (sequential) assembly of nanofibrils. Bone, for example, is made up of a hierarchical assembly of collagen fibrils and crystals of the mineral hydroxyapatite (HA), $Ca_5(PO_4)_3(OH)$.

PhotoDisc

The most important factor in building bone tissue is the proper alignment of HA crystals with collagen. Studies have shown that this alignment may be directed by anionic groups on the surface of collagen interacting with calcium cations in HA. However, this hypothesis remains uncertain because no one has characterized the hierarchical assembly of mineralized collagen nanofibrils.

In an upcoming issue of *Chemistry of Materials*, W. Zhang, S. S. Liao, and F. Z. Cui of Tsinghua University (Beijing) describe how they used conventional and high-resolution transmission electron spectroscopy (HRTEM) to study nanofibrils of mineralized collagen [ASAP, DOI: 10.1021/cm030080g]. They have found a key mechanism behind how these fibrils self-assemble, and the results of their study could apply to bone formation. They also demonstrate for the first time that HA crystals associate specifically with the surfaces of collagen fibrils.

The researchers focused on a specific mineralized fiber and found that hierarchical assembly occurs in three stages. In the first, collagen molecules self-assemble into triple helices, forming fibrils about 5 nm wide. HA crystals then associate with the fibrils in the second stage, with their axes orienting along the long axes of the collagen fibrils. This implies that the collagen fibrils have a strong influence on the growth of the crystals. The diameters of the mineralized fibrils are between 5.5 and 6.9 nm. In the third stage, the mineralized collagen fibrils line up parallel to one another to form mineralized collagen fibers 77 to 192 nm wide.

The HRTEM analysis is the first direct evidence that the HA phase is polycrystalline (composed of many small crystals) and forms a layer that covers the surface of the collagen fibrils.

FIGURE 2.25 American Chemical Society.

Biomaterials and Tissue Engineering, citing professor Cui Fuzhai's summary of the recent advances in tissue engineering in China, and accompanied the report on the conversion of medical device products of professor Cui Fuzhai's MC artificial bone repair material work and clinical use (Fig. 2.23). *Nature Materials* [57] also commented specifically for the findings of the study, pointing out that the discovery of collagenous fibers that regulate the surface deposition of inorganic nanocrystals gave the first direct evidence to support the classical hypothesis of biomineralization, arguing that the findings "will raise people's understanding of the mechanism of collagen modulation and mineralization in other mineralization organizations and point the way for the preparation of new functional materials for imitation works"

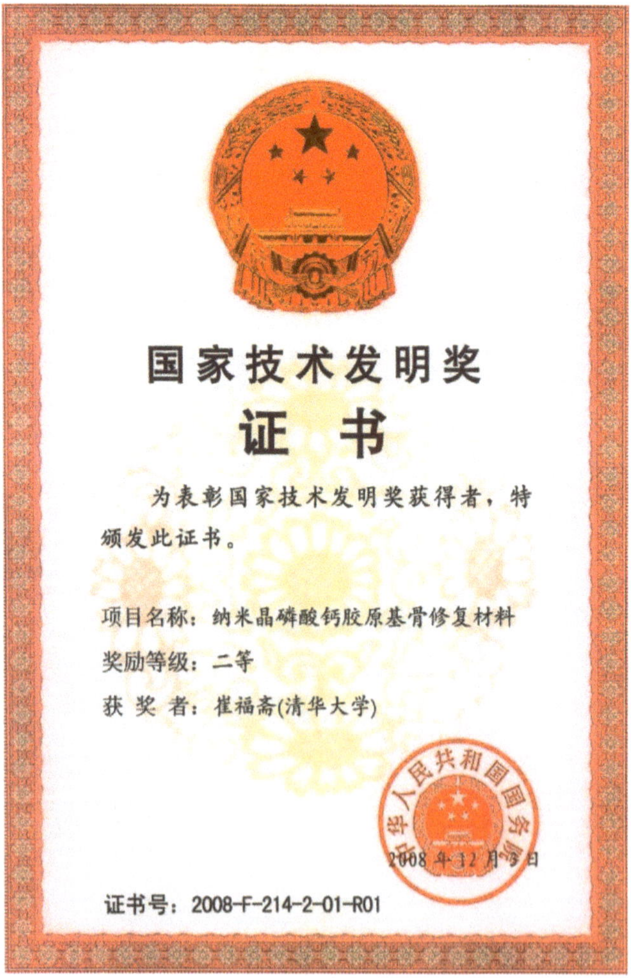

FIGURE 2.26 National Technology Invention.

(Fig. 2.24). The signature article of the ACS' website (www.chemistry.org) has devoted its research work to the project team and spoke highly of it. They pointed out that professor Cui's team discovered the key mechanism of self-assembly of MC fibers. It can be applied to the bone formation process, and for the first time, they have demonstrated the specific binding of hydroxyapatite crystals to the fiber surface (Fig. 2.25). This achievement has extremely important academic significance and scientific value. Professor Cui won the second prize of National Technology Invention in 2008, as shown in Fig. 2.26. The study on the related mineralization mechanism won the National Natural Second Prize of Science as shown in Fig. 2.27.

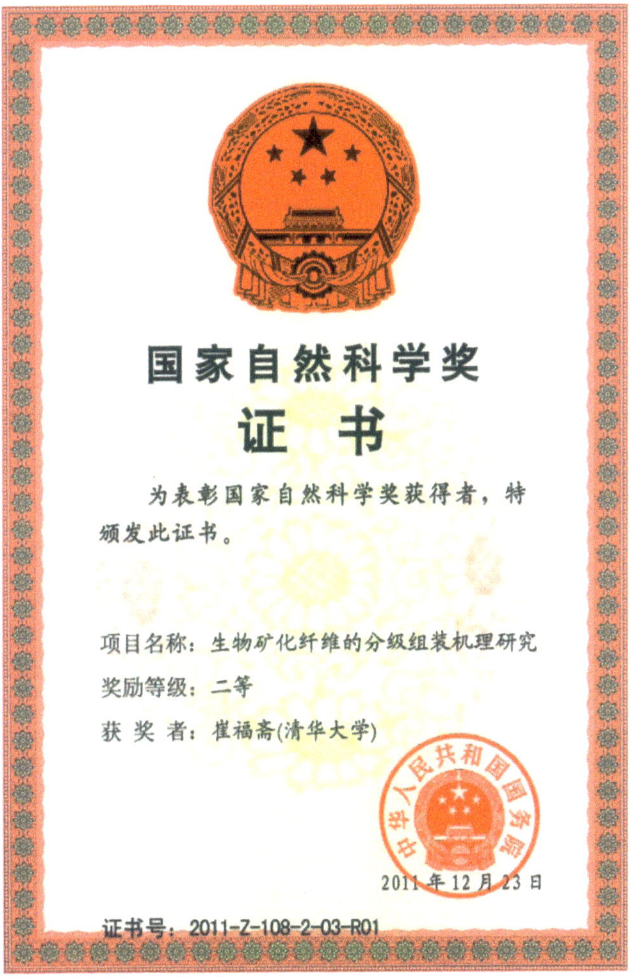

FIGURE 2.27 The National Natural Science Award.

REFERENCES

[1] S. Mann, Molecular recognition in biomineralization, Nature 332 (6160) (1988) 119–124.

[2] G.A. Rodan, T.J. Martin, Therapeutic approaches to bone diseases, Science 289 (5484) (2000) 1508.

[3] L. Yue, G. Sethuraman, W. Wu, et al., The crystallization of fluorapatite in the presence of hydroxyapatite seeds and of hydroxyapatite in the presence of fluorapatite seeds, J. Colloid Interface Sci. 186 (1) (1997) 102–109.

[4] W. Wu, G.H. Nancollas, Interfacial free energies and crystallization in aqueous media, J. Colloid Interface Sci. 182 (2) (1996). 365–373(9).

[5] A.P. Alivisatos, Biomineralization. Naturally aligned nanocrystals, Science 289 (5480) (2000) 736–737.

[6] A.W.I. Wan, S.A. Warno, H.Y. Aboul-Enein, et al., Aggregation-based crystal growth and microstructure development in natural iron oxyhydroxide biomineralization products, Science 289 (5480) (2000) 751–754.

[7] W. Shenton, D. Pum, U.B. Sleytr, et al., Synthesis of cadmium sulphide superlattices using self-assembled bacterial S-layers, Nat. Int. Wkly. J. Sci. 389 (6651) (1997) 585–587.

[8] A.L. Arsenault, A comparative electron microscopic study of apatite crystals in collagen fibrils of rat bone, dentin and calcified Turkey leg tendons, Bone Miner. 6 (2) (1989) 165.

[9] W.J. Landis, K.J. Hodgens, J. Arena, et al., Structural relations between collagen and mineral in bone as determined by high voltage electron microscopic tomography, Microsc. Res. Tech. 33 (2) (1996) 192.

[10] L.M. Siperko, W.J. Landis, Aspects of mineral structure in normally calcifying avian tendon, J. Struct. Biol. 135 (3) (2001) 313–320.

[11] E.P. Katz, S.T. Li, Structure and function of bone collagen fibrils, J. Mol. Biol. 80 (1) (1973) 1–15.

[12] M.J. Olszta, X. Cheng, S.J. Sang, et al., Bone structure and formation: a new perspective, Mater. Sci. Eng. R Rep. 58 (3) (2007) 77–116.

[13] X. Su, K. Sun, F.Z. Cui, et al., Organization of apatite crystals in human woven bone, Bone 32 (2) (2003) 150–162.

[14] E.A. Mcnally, H.P. Schwarcz, G.A. Botton, et al., A model for the ultrastructure of bone based on electron microscopy of ion-milled sections, PLoS One 46 (1) (2015) 44–50.

[15] G. Liu, D. Zhao, A.P. Tomsia, et al., Three-dimensional biomimetic mineralization of dense hydrogel templates, J. Am. Chem. Soc. 131 (29) (2009) 9937–9939.

[16] J.H. Bradt, M. Mertig, A. Angelika Teresiak, et al., Biomimetic mineralization of collagen by combined fibril assembly and calcium phosphate formation, Chem. Mater. 11 (10) (1999) 2694–2701.

[17] W. Zhang, S.S. Liao, F.Z. Cui, Hierarchical self-assembly of nano-fibrils in mineralized collagen, Chem. Mater. 15 (16) (2003) 3221–3226.

[18] T.T. Thula, F. Svedlund, D.E. Rodriguez, et al., Mimicking the nanostructure of bone: comparison of polymeric process-directing agents, Polymers 3 (1) (2010) 10–35.

[19] C.G. Bellows, J.E. Aubin, J.N.M. Heersche, et al., Mineralized bone nodules formed in vitro from enzymatically released rat calvaria cell populations, Calcif. Tissue Int. 38 (3) (1986) 143–154.

[20] N.B.P.D. Jon, S.E. Graves, C.A. Smoothy, Formation of mineralized nodules by bone derived cells in vitro: a model of bone formation? Am. J. Med. Genet. 45 (2) (1993) 163.

[21] Y. Liu, D. Luo, X.X. Kou, et al., Hierarchical intrafibrillar nanocarbonated apatite assembly improves the nanomechanics and cytocompatibility of mineralized collagen, Adv. Funct. Mater. 23 (11) (2013).

[22] V. Uskoković, W. Li, S. Habelitz, Amelogenin as a promoter of nucleation and crystal growth of apatite, J. Cryst. Growth 316 (1) (2011) 106–117.

[23] J. Ge, F.Z. Cui, X.M. Wang, et al., Property variations in the prism and the organic sheath within enamel by nanoindentation, Biomaterials 26 (16) (2005) 3333–3339.

[24] J. Ge, F.Z. Cui, N. Ji, et al., New observation of hierarchical structure of human enamel, Chin. J. Conserv. Dent. 16 (2) (2006) 61–66.

[25] X.M. Wang, F.Z. Cui, J. Ge, et al., Hierarchical structural comparisons of bones from wild-type and liliput(dtc232) gene-mutated Zebrafish, J. Struct. Biol. 145 (3) (2004) 236–245.

[26] X.M. Wang, F.Z. Cui, J. Ge, et al., Alterations in mineral properties of zebrafish skeletal bone induced by liliput dtc232 gene mutation, J. Cryst. Growth 258 (3–4) (2003) 394–401.

[27] Dopping-Hepenstal P., Ali S., Stamp T. Matrix vesicles in the osteoid of human bone, in: A. Ascenzi, E. Bonucci, B. deBernard (Eds.) Proceedings of the Thirty Second International Conference on Matrix Vesicles, Milano, Italy, Wichtig Editore, 1981, pp. 229–234.

[28] C. Hemleben, R.O. Anderson, W. Berthold, et al., Calcification and chamber formation in Foraminifera—a brief overview, in: B.S.C. Leadbeater, R. Riding (Eds.), Biomineralization in Lower Plants and Animals, Clarendon Press, Oxford, 1986.

[29] D.S. Young JR, P.R. Bown, S. Mann, Coccolith ultrastructure and biominerali-sation, J. Struct. Biol. 126 (3) (1999) 195–215.

[30] W.J. Landis, M.J. Song, A. Leith, et al., Mineral and organic matrix interaction in normally calcifying tendon visualized in three dimensions by high-voltage electron microscopic tomography and graphic image reconstruction, J. Struct. Biol. 110 (1) (1993) 39–54.

[31] J.R. Young, J.M. Didymus, P.R. Brown, et al., Crystal assembly and phylogenetic evolution in heterococcoliths, Nature 356 (6369) (1992) 516–518.

[32] N.C. Blumenthal, V. Cosma, E. Gomes, Regulation of hydroxyapatite formation by gelatin and type I collagen gels, Calcif. Tissue Int. 48 (6) (1991) 440–442.

[33] K.S. Tenhuisen, R.I. Martin, M. Klimkiewicz, et al., Formation and properties of a synthetic bone composite: hydroxyapatite-collagen, J. Biomed. Mater. Res. 29 (7) (1995).

[34] A. Bigi, E. Boanini, A. Silvia Panzavolta, et al., Biomimetic growth of hydroxyapatite on gelatin films doped with sodium polyacrylate, Biomacromolecules 1 (4) (2000) 752–756.

[35] C. Du, F.Z. Cui, Q.L. Feng, et al., Tissue response to nano-hydroxyapatite/collagen composite implants in marrow cavity, J. Biomed. Mater. Res. A. 42 (4) (2015) 540–548.

[36] S.H. Rhee, J.D. Lee, J. Tanaka, Nucleation of hydroxyapatite crystal through chemical interaction with collagen, J. Am. Ceram. Soc. 83 (11) (2000) 2890–2892.

[37] Z. Wei, Z.L. Huang, S.S. Liao, et al., Nucleation sites of calcium phosphate crystals during collagen mineralization, J. Am. Ceram. Soc. 86 (6) (2003) 1052–1054.

[38] B. Yang, F.Z. Cui, Molecular modeling and mechanics studies on the initial stage of the collagen-mineralization process, Curr. Appl. Phys. 7 (2007) e2–e5.

[39] F.Z. Cui, Y. Wang, Q. Cai, et al., Conformation change of collagen during the initial stage of biomineralization of calcium phosphate, J. Mater. Chem. 18 (32) (2008) 3835–3840.

[40] F.Z. Cui, W. Zhang, Y.U. Xing, Biomimetic self-assembly of nano-fibrils of mineralized collagen, J. Dalian Univ. (2004).

[41] B.O. Fowler, ChemInform abstract: infrared studies of apatites part 2. Preparation of normal and isotopically substituted calcium, strontium and barium hydroxyapatites and spectra-structure-composition correlations, Inorg. Chem. 13 (1) (1974) 207–214.

[42] Y. Leung, M.A. Walters, R.Z. Legeros, Second derivative infrared spectra of hydroxyapatite, Spectrochim. Acta 46 (10) (1990) 1453–1459.

[43] Z.Y. Qiu, C.S. Tao, H. Cui, et al., High-strength mineralized collagen artificial bone, Front. Mater. Sci. 8 (1) (2014) 53–62.

[44] E. Ling-Ling, L. Feng, H.C. Liu, et al., The effect of calcium phosphate composite scaffolds on the osteogenic differentiation of rabbit dental pulp stem cells, J. Biomed. Mater. Res. A 103 (5) (2014) 1732–1745.

[45] 510(k) Summary of K122894. [cited 2018 3.23]. Available from: <https://www.accessdata.fda.gov/cdrh_docs/pdf12/k122894.pdf>.

[46] 510(k) Summary of K033679. [cited 2018 3.23]. Available from: <http://www.accessdata.fda.gov/cdrh_docs/pdf3/>.

[47] 510(k) Summary of K012751. [cited 2018 3.23]. Available from: <http://www.accessdata.fda.gov/cdrh_docs/pdf/>.

[48] 510(k) Summary of K063124. [cited 2018 3.23]. Available from: <https://www.accessdata.fda.gov/cdrh_docs/pdf6/k063124.pdf>.

[49] 510(k) Summary of K082166. [cited 2018 3.23]. Available from: <http://www.accessdata.fda.gov/cdrh_docs/pdf8/>.

[50] 510(k) Summary of K081784. [cited 2018 3.23]. Available from: <http://www.accessdata.fda.gov/cdrh_docs/pdf8/>.

[51] Indication for use of OSTEON III. [cited 2018 3.23]. Available from: <https://www.accessdata.fda.gov/cdrh_docs/pdf15/k153676.pdf>.

[52] Indications for use OssiMend. [cited 2018 3.23]. Available from: <https://www.accessdata.fda.gov/cdrh_docs/pdf5/k052812.pdf>.

[53] Indications for use SynOss. [cited 2018 3.23]. Available from: <https://www.accessdata.fda.gov/cdrh_docs/pdf8/k083742.pdf>.

[54] 510(k) summary of K032288. [cited 2018 3.23]. Available from: <http://www.accessdata.fda.gov/cdrh_docs/pdf3/>.

[55] L.C. Palmer, C.J. Newcomb, S.R. Kaltz, et al., Biomimetic systems for hydroxyapatite mineralization inspired by bone and enamel, ChemRev 108 (2008) 4754–4783.

[56] M. Hvistendahl, China's push in tissue engineering, Science 338 (6109) (2012) 900.

[57] Polishing, sensing, switching and synthesizing. Nat. Mater. 2 (2003).

Chapter 3

Biomimetic Mineralized Collagen Biocompatibility

Zi-Rui Wang, Yun Cui and Zhi-Ye Qiu
Beijing Allgens Medical Science and Technology Co., Ltd., Beijing, P.R. China

Biocompatibility refers to the property of biological tissue of living organisms to react to nonliving materials [1]. Generally, it refers to the compatibility between the material and the host, including histocompatibility and blood compatibility. In recent years, the viewpoint of biocompatibility has also undergone major changes, not only for nonliving materials but also for active materials (tissue engineering materials). At the same time, it is generally accepted that biocompatibility includes two major principles: one is biosafety, and the other is biofunctionality (or the promotion of body function) [2]. Ideal bone graft materials require good biocompatibility. The so-called biocompatibility refers to the body reaction to the implanted material [3].

In recent years, tissue engineering has developed rapidly. In bone engineering, the main function of scaffold material is to provide three-dimensional space for cell growth and metabolism, which has a large impact on the seed cell biological phenotype and culture [4]. A good scaffold material should have such features as no cytotoxicity, good biocompatibility, little effect on the phenotypic characteristics of cells, and suitability for three-dimensional spatial structure [5]. Biomimetic mineralized collagen (MC) material has good affinity with osteoblasts, and the cells are easy to attach to the material. The porous structure of the material also makes cells easy to grow in, while the nutrients are easy to transport [6]. In vitro cell culture experiments show that the MC material has excellent biocompatibility, biodegradability, good bone compatibility, and high bone conduction [7].

3.1 CELL RESPONSE TO THE MATERIAL

In general, in vitro cell culture methods are used to evaluate the cell–polymer interface response by placing cells on the surface of the material and measuring cell adhesion, proliferation, survival, function, and death under culture conditions [8].

Mineralized Collagen Bone Graft Substitutes. DOI: https://doi.org/10.1016/B978-0-08-102717-2.00003-5

3.1.1 Cell Adhesion

In both in vivo and in vitro culture, the surface of the medical material quickly adsorbs the surrounding protein or extracellular matrix (ECM), and the adjacent cells can adhere to the surface of the material. Receptors on the cell membrane recognize the proteins of these ligands then bind tightly to make cell adhesion. Usually cells start to spread, migrate, divide or differentiate, secrete, grow or perform other behaviors after cell adhesion [9].

1. In the cell adhesion process, the majority of cells cultured in vitro have adherent growth characteristics. Cells adhere in the material surface for a long period of time. The process can be generally divided into several steps: (1) adsorption; (2) contact; (3) adherence; (4) expansion.
2. In terms of cell adhesion mechanisms, cells adhere to other cells and the ECM through adhesion receptors that bind to specific polypeptide sequences of other proteins. Cells involved in the material surface adhesion, in essence, are the cell membrane protein, ECM proteins, and cytoskeletal proteins. Biological studies have shown that there is a receptor called the integrin family on the cell membrane surface of adherent cells. These receptors specifically recognize growth factors, adherent factors, and hormones in serum and ECM [9].

3.1.2 Cell Migration

Cell migration is an important phenomenon in tissue engineering. The migration of a single cell is a very important factor in reconstructing the tissues and organs that form. In the early stages of cell migration, similar to cell spreading, pseudopods on the cell membrane stretch through the assembly of actin microfibrils at the leading edge of the cell. The cell membrane then attaches to the substrate via integrin receptors. Pseudo-rigid and material firmly adhered to produce contractile force, the receptor is released, and the cells move forward. Eventually, the cell's integrin receptor circulates forward, continuing the process [9].

3.1.3 Cell Proliferation and Differentiation

After cells adhere to the material, they will evolve according to their own natural cycle. ECM or cell-contacted material has a significant effect on cell proliferation. All cells are produced by other cell division; the cells go through a series of orderly processes to complete the breeding. The result of a cell going through this orderly process is the duplication of its chromosomes into two daughter cells. The process of replication and division is referred to as the cell cycle [9].

3.1.4 Cell Aggregation

Cell aggregation is an important means of generating tissues and organs. In normal tissue structure, cells are aggregated and interact with each other. This force is closely related to cell activity, cell differentiation, migration, and tissue formation. In the process of cell culture, only the aggregation can reconstruct the interaction between the cells. Experiments show that the cells cultured in the aggregated state have generally improved cell function and survival rate. Even though the cells are dispersed by agitation, cells are still aggregated in suspension culture. The addition of serum and serum proteins can promote the cell aggregation and control the detachment of cells from the surface of the material and promote cell aggregation. The degree of aggregation is determined by measuring the size of the cells aggregated.

3.1.5 Cell Function

In tissue engineering, it is generally hoped that special functions of cells will be obtained, such as improving the detoxification and protein secretion of hepatocytes and generating ECM proteins in fibroblasts, osteoblasts, and chondrocytes, which is an important physiological phenomenon [10]. Improving cellular function is a topic of great concern in tissue engineering and medical materials. Since cell function is closely related to the material, cell function can be evaluated for the cell–material interface response.

3.2 BIOMINERALIZED COLLAGEN CELL EXPERIMENTS

3.2.1 The Effect of Mineralized Collagen Material and Bone Marrow Mesenchymal Stem Cells Cultured on the Cell Phenotype

3.2.1.1 Material

Biomineralized collagen material (Beijing Allgens Medical Science & Technology Co., Ltd.) was used. Disinfection of the surgical field was carried out with 1% iodophor. The bone marrow was extracted with a syringe anticoagulant and 16 g needle on the rabbit dorsal side of the iliac crest (containing heparin solution 3 mL, 1000U/mL); 3 mL of bone marrow was extracted on each side (6 mL each rabbit). After the cells were centrifuged, the cells were separated by Ficoll, washed, and counted. The cells were inoculated into two culture flasks (25 cm) at a concentration of 1 × 105/mL and cultured in a CO_2 incubator at 37°C with a humidity of 5%. The main components of the culture medium included sodium glycerophosphate 10 mmol/L, 1640, 10% fetal calf serum, penicillin and streptomycin each 100 IU/mL, pH = 7.2. Inverted phase contrast microscope was used to observe the growth of cells. Five days after the first liquid change, the bottle was gently shaken after the supernatant was drained, and cell growth observed. Liquid was changed every 2–3 days. On day 10, cells will cover the bottom of the bottle. Passage cells were rinsed with 0.9% saline, digested with 0.05% trypsin + 0.01% EDTA, and centrifuged after beating at 1500 r for 7 minutes, with centrifugal radius of 11.18 cm. The supernatant was added to a small amount of culture solution after shaking to prepare a cell suspension, having a concentration of 1 × 106/mL. Next was added 1 mL cell suspension on the surface of the material; the material size was 1 cm^3, with pore size of 100–400 μm. Material and cells were put into the incubator for 4 hours, then another 1 mL of culture medium was added. The growth of the cells was observed by inverted phase contrast microscope. The cells were analyzed by flow cytometry (CD34, CD68, CD105) after being stained with alkaline phosphatase (ALP) before and after culture.

3.2.1.2 Method: Mesenchymal Stem Cell Phenotype

ALP staining: after suspending the cells in the culture medium, the cells are added to the cell culture flasks to cover the slide. After adherent cells were stained with naphthol AS-BI ALP, they were compared with mesenchymal stem cell (MSC) digested after 2 weeks of culture. The procedures are as follows: Remove the cover glass from the culture flask, washed with D-Hanks and fixed with 4% paraformaldehyde, then rinsed with distilled water; take naphthol stock solution 10 mL, red TR10mg reinforcing mix made of naphthol AS-BI application solution. Drop naphthol AS-BI solution on the coverslip, and let it sit for 5–20 minutes, wash with water and stain with hematoxylin, wash with distilled water again, then seal with glycerol–gelatin. The cells were observed with an ordinary optical microscope.

Flow cytometry: for the second generation of MSC culture flask, drain the old culture liquid of the MSC and MC complex, digest the cells with 3 mL of 0.25% trypsin at room temperature for about 1 minute (microscopic control of time), until the cells are slightly rounded, stop trypsin digestion and discard the trypsin solution. D-Hanks solution is added; gently blow the cells repeatedly, making them into single cell suspension, then transfer the cell suspension to a centrifuge tube, centrifuge for 10 minutes (at 1500 r/min speed). Discard most of the supernatant, leaving about 0.5 mL of supernatant to suspend the cells, vertex the cell suspension. The cells were rapidly injected into cold ethanol at 4°C with a dropper (final concentration of ethanol was 70%) and placed in a refrigerator at 4°C until use. Preheat flow cytometry for 30 minutes; follow the protocol to operate the flow cytometry. Add a good fluorescent microsphere fluid to see whether the light path and flow path is normal or not. Add 100 μL cell suspension and CD34, CD68, Laminin, CD44, CD105, CD166 monoclonal antibody, incubate for 30 minutes, then the machine will automatically detect cells (collected cells 15,000–20,000).

3.2.1.3 Results

MSC isolation and purification and MC coculture with MSCs: 24h after seeding in culture flask, a little adhesions can be observed. The early adherent cells were irregular or short-spin type, and then the adherent cells were divided and added, and the morphology gradually changed into a long fusiform shape. After MSCs is full, it is passaged or cultured with mineralized collagen MSCs. MSCs and mineralized collagen are well complexed, attached, grown, propagated and differentiated on mineralized collagen.

ALP staining results: After induction of passaged MSC and digestion and staining with ALP, the staining was positive with little difference (Fig. 3.1).

Flow cytometry results: test sample results showed that after induction of culture of MSC and the passage of material from the digestion of MSC, CD34, CD68, Laminin were negative. This proves that this type of cells are not Hematopoietic cells, mononuclear (macrophages) or fibroblasts. CD44, CD105, CD166 positive expression. The percentage of MSC positive cells before the combined culture was 97.8% for CD44, 94.59% for CD105, and 97.72% for CD166. From nano-hydroxyapatite/collagen (nHAC) digestion down to MSC, it was as follows: CD44 98.3%, CD105 95.71%, and CD166 95.6% (Fig. 3.2).

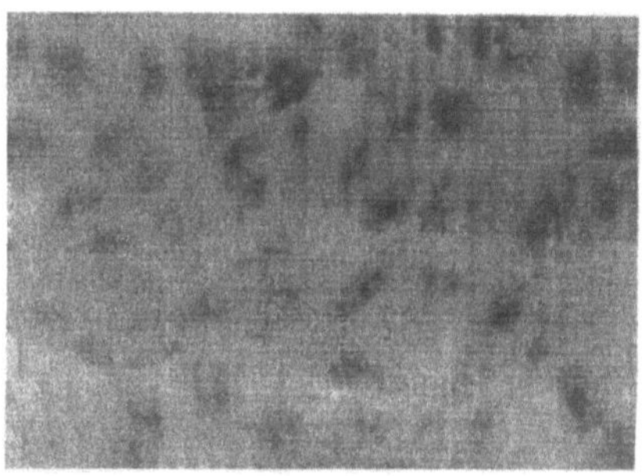

FIGURE 3.1 Mesenchymal stem cell mineralized collagen cocultured alkaline phosphatase (AKP) staining.

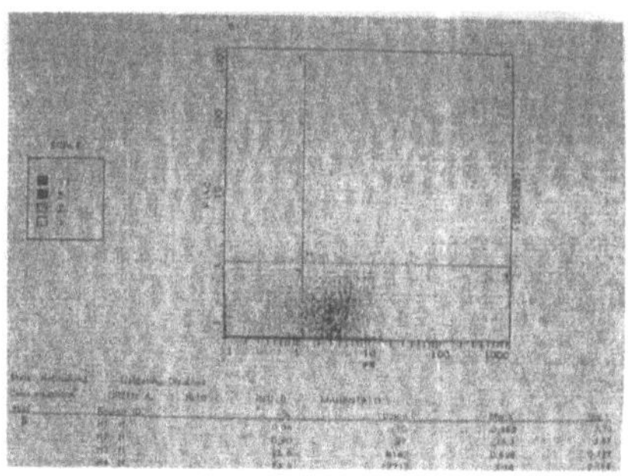

FIGURE 3.2 Flow cytometry mesenchymal stem cell CD34 negative CD105 positive.

3.2.1.4 Conclusion

Natural bone matrix is a combination of inorganic components and organic molecules of macromolecules. The main inorganic component is nanohydroxyapatite, with organic components being mainly collagen and a small amount of polysaccharides, glycoproteins, and so on. Therefore, it is the key to obtain nanohydroxyapatite in the study of bone implants and to make it uniformly mixed with collagen. In the past, the study of bionic bone was either on the coarse inorganic mineral particles, or the organic/inorganic compound was inhomogeneous, thus affecting its performance. The MC material in this study is a novel nanocomposite material prepared on the basis of bionics and previous collagen–calcium phosphate composite materials. The material is similar to natural bone in both microstructure and composition and is expected to be one of the preferred materials in bone tissue engineering [11].

Seed cells are very important raw materials in tissue engineering research. Because autologous cells do not have immune rejection, they are the most studied seed cells. Minimally invasive techniques extracted from somatic tissue, isolated and cultured cells, and then transplanted into the recipient for the repair of tissue defects is a development trend. It was first reported in the 1960s that some of the attached cells in bone marrow samples differentiated into similar bone and cartilage colonies during culture. Later it was confirmed that these colonies are stem cells that exist in the marrow stromal system and have multiple differentiation potential. It can be induced by different inducing factors to differentiate into bone, cartilage, muscle, and fat; these cells are called MSCs. The main feature of stem cells is that they are simple in structure and belong to primitive cells that do not have specific functions. They can proliferate in a self-replicating manner and can differentiate into specific directions under specific conditions, producing several precursor cells of the subline [5,12,13]. Bone marrow MSCs in bone marrow stromal cells have a very strong differentiation potential and proliferation ability, which in recent years in the field of tissue engineering has been widely attention.

MSCs cultured in this experiment have the following features: adherence, spreading, increasing value and aggregating on MC porous materials, and are entangled by pseudopodia, indicating that the mineralized materials exhibit good cell affinity and biocompatibility. Cells can absorb and utilize MC materials well. The nanohydroxyapatite and collagen from MC material are similar in composition and microstructure to the natural bone in vivo environment, completing the biomimetic process from nanometer to micron level. This technique is currently used for the repair of osteonecrosis and perforation of the medullary cavity [14,15]. This experiment confirmed that MC is a good tissue scaffold material; is easily complexed with MSC; is suitable for seed cell attachment, growth, proliferation, and differentiation; and has no effect on the cell phenotype [11].

3.2.2 Genetic Toxicity of Mineralized Collagen and its Effect on Cultured Cells In Vitro

In vitro cell transformation assay is a genotoxic test of the transformation of mammalian cells cultured in vitro. It is a technique for detecting carcinogens by exposing cells to carcinogens and simulating the effect of carcinogens in the body in an in vitro culture environment. This method can be effectively used for in vitro screening of carcinogenic activity, as not only can it detect genotoxic potential carcinogens, but also nongenotoxic carcinogens.

3.2.2.1 Materials and Methods

1. The main equipment and materials: ultraclean bench; phase contrast microscope; enzyme-linked immunosorbent assay; DMEM; fetal bovine serum; Methylthiazol tetrazolium (MTT), dimethylformamide sulfoxide (DMSO), trypsin, dexamethasone, vitamin C (Sigma); ALP assay kit; phenol; histidine auxotrophic; *Salmonella typhimurium* strain TA98, TAl00; azide sodium (SA); 2-Aminofluorene (2-AF) (Sigma).
2. Preparation of extract: preparation of leaching solution for Ames mutagenicity test: take 4 discs of round nHAC, 8 mm in diameter and 0.5 mm in thickness in a small beaker, add 20 mL of normal saline, and seal with tin foil. Placed in 37°C constant temperature water bath for 72 hours for preparation of material leachate. Test within 24 hours.

   Preparation of leachates for cytological assays: Cell culture medium (freshly prepared, pH = 7.2) is the extraction medium. According to nHAC weight/extraction medium = 1 g/10 mL ratio preparation, 37°C, 5% CO_2 saturated humidity extraction incubator for 48 hours.
3. Ames mutagenicity test: the material leaching solution was diluted with saline to make a stock solution. The serial dilutions of 1/2, 1/4, and 1/8 were prepared; *S. typhimurium* histidine auxotrophic TA98 and TAl00 were used as indicator strains; Rat hepatic microsomal enzyme (S9) was induced by polyamino biphenyl, made into liver homogenate and stored in refrigerator at −80°C. The activity was measured by 2-aminofluorene when using it. Daphnomycin 25 μg/0.1 mL; 2-aminofluorene (2-AF) 50 μg/0.1 mL; sodium azide (SA) 5 μg/0.1 mL for positive control;

   Among them, daunorubicin and SA were indicated as direct mutagenic activity of TA98 and TAl00 respectively (without S9). 2-AF was indicated as an indirect mutagenic activity of TA98 and TAl00 (plus S9), and the same volume of physiological saline as a negative control. Positive control, negative control, and test solution of each dose group were set up in three parallel dishes. Adopting plate incorporation method, under the condition of adding S9 and not adding S9, the result was observed after culturing at 37°C for 48 hours. Average number of colonies restore mutation from each of three parallel plates in each group. The results of the test led to the mutation ratio (*MR* = number of colonies restoring mutation in the experimental group R_t/number of colonies restoring mutation in the negative control group R_c).

4. Cell culture: two types of cells were selected. One is primary culture of human periodontal ligament fibroblast (PDLF): healthy orthodontic teeth (18–28 years old), under sterile conditions, washed with Hanks solution three times, curettage of root one-third of the periodontal ligament tissue was separated into 1-mm^3-sized tissue pieces. Placed flat on the bottom of the flask, the tissue blocks were separated by a distance of about 0.5 cm. Inverted and incubated at 37°C in a 5% CO_2 incubator for 2 hours. After the tissue pieces were dried up slightly, 2 mL of the culture medium was added for further incubation. After cell growth, liquid was changed every 3 days. When the cells are confluent, they are digested with trypsin and passaged. Take the fifth generation of cells for experiment. The second type of cells were rabbit osteoblasts: 1 New Zealand rabbit (born 1 month) was killed by decapitation and the long bones of the extremities were aseptically removed and longitudinally incised. Rinse the bone marrow cavity with DMEM culture solution, collect the rinse solution, and gently blow it. Let stand for 1 minute to allow the large tissue to settle and take the supernatant for culture. The culture medium was a DMEM culture fluid containing 10% fetal bovine serum. After confluent monolayers were collected, they were routinely digested and passaged with 0.25% trypsin. The passaged cells were added to conditioned medium (DMEM complete medium supplemented with dexamethasone 1×10^{-8} mol/L, β-glycerophosphate sodium 10 mmol/L, and vitamin C 50 mg/L) to continue culture, and the bone marrow stromal cells were transformed into osteogenesis cell.
5. The effect of MC material on proliferation rate of human PDLF-like cells: Periodontal fibroblast-like cells were prepared as a cell suspension of 5×10^4 cells/mL and seeded in 96-well plates. Plates were incubated in an incubator for 24 hours to allow cells to attach to the wall. The original culture medium was discarded, and the nHAC material extract was diluted with the cell maintenance solution at the concentration of the stock solution, 1/2, 1/4, 1/8 into the experimental group, and the negative control group was treated with the fresh cell maintenance solution, 100 μL/mL per well. Set up 8 parallel samples, continue to incubate for 2, 4, and 7 days. Add 50 μL/well of MTT (5 mg/mL) continue to culture for another 2 hours. Then stop, rinse with Phosphate Buffered Saline (PBS) twice, discard the fluid in the well, add DMSO 150 μL/well, gently shaking 10–15 minutes, measure absorbance value (A) at the test wavelength 490 nm. Calculate relative growth ratio (RGR) of cells: RGR of nHAC = mean of experimental group A/mean of negative control group × 100%.
6. The effect of MC on ALP activity in rabbit osteoblasts: Rabbit osteoblasts were seeded into 96-well plates at a concentration of 1×10^6/mL,

and 200 μL of cell suspension was seeded into each well. The positive control was 6.4 mL/L phenol and the negative control was cell culture medium. After the cells were incubated for 24 hours, the supernatant was removed. In the above experimental groups was added 200 μL to each well, incubated at 37°C, 5% CO_2 environment. 5 μL of the extract solution was added to assay wells, standard wells, and blank wells. 5 μL of 0.1 mg/mL phenol standard solution was added to the standard wells, and 5 μL of double distilled water was added to the blank wells. Add 50 μL of buffer solution and 50 μL of matrix solution. Mix well and then put in 37°C water bath for 15 minutes. Add 150 μL of color reagent and mix immediately. The absorbance value of each well (Optical density (OD) value, zeroed with a blank tube) was measured at 520 nm wavelength by an enzyme-linked immunosorbent assay, and the detection was repeated 3 times. 100 mL of serum was incubated with the substrate for 15 minutes at 37°C to produce 1 mg of phenol as a gold unit. Calculation formula:

$$\text{Alkaline phosphatase}\left(\text{gold units}/100\ \text{mL}\right) = \frac{\text{absorbance of test well}}{\text{absorbance of standard well}} \times \frac{\text{phenol amount in standard well}}{0.005\ \text{mg}} \times \frac{100\ \text{mL}}{0.05\ \text{mL}}$$

7. Statistical methods: Use SPSS10.0 software for data analysis.

3.2.2.2 Results

1. See Table 3.1 for the number of recovered colonies in each group. The MR1, 1/2, 1/4, 1/8 = Rt1, 1/2, 1/4, 1/8/R_c were less than 2 in each concentration of test solution in the experimental group. $MR_p = R_p/R_c$ in each positive control group. Both are greater than two.
2. RGR values of PDLF-like cells in the experimental group and the negative control group are shown in Table 3.2.
3. The ALP activity values of osteoblasts in the experimental group and the negative control group are shown in Table 3.3.
4. With the extension of culture time, the ALP content in both groups increased. there was no statistically significant difference ($P > .05$) of the ALP levels between the two groups at the same time point.

3.2.2.3 Conclusion

The Ames mutagenesis experiment used a histidine auxotrophic mutant strain (TAhis-) of *S. typhimurium*. In this strain lacking histidine, only a few colonies that undergo spontaneous reversion mutations can grow. After mutagenesis of the test substance, the reversion mutations increased, so that the number of colonies growing on the medium lacking histidine greatly increased. Based on this characteristic of the strain, the nHAC extract was

TABLE 3.1 Ames Mutagenicity Test Results $X \pm S$

Strains	TA98 (S9 −)	TA98 (S9 +)	TA100 (S9 −)	TA100 (S9 −)
Negative control Rc[a]	36 ± 8.1	35 ± 7.3	35 ± 7.3	181 ± 10.4
Material extract Rt1	36 ± 7.3	36 ± 5.7	36 ± 5.7	180 ± 6.5
1/2 dilute Rt1/2	35 ± 6.9	36 ± 6.1	36 ± 6.1	185 ± 9.1
1/4 dilute Rt1/4	38 ± 8.4	36 ± 9.1	36 ± 9.1	178 ± 10.3
1/8 dilute Rt1/8	37 ± 3.2	36 ± 7.2	36 ± 7.2	182 ± 4.1
Positive control R_p	624 ± 81.1[b]	2276 ± 283.5[c]	2276 ± 283.5[d]	3047 ± 341.6[c]
S9 No strain test	–	–	–	–

[a]Negative control is normal saline.
[b]Positive control is daunomycin (25 μg/0.1 mL).
[c]Positive control is 2-aminofluorene (50 μg/0.1 mL).
[d]Positive control is stack sodium azide (5 μg/0.1 mL).

TABLE 3.2 Relative Growth Ratio 0/0 $X \pm S$ of Human Periodontal Ligament Fibroblasts in nHAC

Material	Material Extract	RGR		
		2 Days	4 Days	7 Days
nHAC	1	109.1 ± 29	106.3 ± 9.2	110.8 ± 8.4
	1/2	103.1 ± 4.6	106.8 ± 5.4	112.8 ± 9.0
	1/4	101.6 ± 3.9	105.8 ± 6.4	105.4 ± 7.3
	1/8	96.7 ± 7.5	103.5 ± 6.4	97.4 ± 5.3
Negative control	–	100	100	100

TABLE 3.3 Determination of Alkaline Phosphatase Activity Xlk

Grouping	1 Days	3 Days	5 Days
100% nHAC Extract	1.419 ± 0.187	2.812 ± 0.116	4.783 ± 0.472
Negative control	1.335 ± 0.092	2.798 ± 0.093	4.520 ± 0.539

mixed with each standard broth and cultured in a minimal medium, and whether or not mutagenic material was present in the composite artificial bone was judged based on the number of reverted colonies. Since the nHACs explored in this experiment are used for implantation in humans, the human hepatocyte microsomal enzyme system may initiate the mutagenesis (indirect mutagenesis) of the material, but no such enzyme is present in the bacteria. To make the experimental conditions closer to the in vivo environment and to make the experimental results more practical, we added the rat hepatocyte microsomal enzyme system S9 to the material extraction solution after the nonactivation experiment to perform an activation test, and observed the reversion of mutant colonies after induction. In addition, when observing the results, we first observed the growth of the background lawn, only the background colonies are similar to the negative control, and after the contamination of the bacteria is eliminated, the colonies seen are the restored mutant colonies, thereby ensuring the reliability of the test results. The results of this experiment showed that the average number of reversion mutant colonies in each positive control group was more than twice as high as the average number of that in the corresponding negative control group ($MR_p > 2$). It was confirmed that the histidine auxotrophic mutant strain of *S. typhimurium* tested the test substance; and the fact that the average number of reversion mutant colonies per strain did not exceed two times the average number of that in its corresponding negative control group ($MR < 2$) shows that the material has no mutagenic activity in the presence or absence of S9, demonstrating that the use of nHAC for in vivo implantation is safe in terms of genotoxicity.

The effect of the extract on the main functional cells (periodontal fibroblast-like cells, osteoblasts) at the implantation site can not only reflect the cytotoxicity of the material, but also can reflect the effects of materials on the proliferation of periodontal ligament fibroblast-like cells; osteoblast proliferation and differentiation. ALP is one of the main characteristic enzymes for osteoblast differentiation. Detection of ALP activity is one of the important indicators for identifying osteoblasts and evaluating their functional activity. Because the detection index is more material specific, the experimental results have more real and reliable reference value for the clinical application of the material. The results of this experiment showed that the proliferation rate of PDLF-like cells after treatment with different concentrations of nHAC extracts did not decrease. From a numerical point of view, the proliferation rate seems to have risen. The reason may be that the collagen component of nHAC has a certain role in promoting cell adhesion and proliferation, and its specific mechanism needs further study. At the same time, the extract of nHAC did not affect the functional expression of rabbit osteoblasts. It can be seen from this experiment that nanohydroxyapatite composite collagen material has no potential genotoxicity and no inhibitory effect on PDLFs, osteoblast proliferation and differentiation. It could be used in oral and maxillofacial surgery as a good bone graft and bone tissue engineering scaffold material [16].

3.3 THE EXPERIMENTAL EVALUATION OF THE OSTEOCLASTS OF MINERALIZED COLLAGEN

3.3.1 Osteogenic Differentiation Gene Expression Profiling of Human Mesenchymal Stem Cells on Hydroxyapatite and Mineralized Collagen

In this study, the human mesenchymal stem cells (hMSCs) were cultured using hydroxyapatite and MC, and their proliferation, adhesion, and differentiation, especially the molecular mechanism of gene level were investigated. Proliferation and morphological responses of hMSCs and their osteogenic differentiation were detected by quantitative detection of ALP. Analysis was done through microarray gene expression, and gene expression data with gene ontology and path analysis were studied. The results showed that MC promoted cell proliferation and osteogenic differentiation of hMSCs. Microarray analysis showed that MC was beneficial to the expression of genes related to osteoblasts, such as bmp-2, COL1A1, CTSK, and stimulated osteogenic differentiation, such as osteoblast differentiation pathway and bone system development pathway.

3.3.1.1 Experimental

1. Materials and methods

   MC is provided by Beijing Allgens Medical Science and Technology Co., Ltd, China. hydroxyapatite is provided by Institute of Nuclear and New Energy Technology, Tsinghua University, China. Elastic modulus test using universal material testing machine and 10 kn load cell test was conducted, with the lateral speed set to 0.5 mm/min and loaded until the sample is compressed to about 30% of the original length. The phase composition of the samples were identified by X-ray diffraction (XRD) using monochrome CuK α radiation ($\lambda = 1.5405$ Å, 120 mA, 40 kV) in a continuous scan mode with a scanning speed of 8°/min, and the 2θ range from 10 degrees to 60 degrees was used to determine the phase composition. The molecular structure of the samples was characterized by Fourier transform infrared spectroscopy at a resolution of 0.35 cm^{-1} and 32 scans with wavenumber from 250 to 2500 cm^{-1}.

2. Cell culture on MC and hydroxyapatite

   Cells were cultured in 29-cell proliferation medium including DMEM, 10% fetal bovine serum, 2 mm L-glutamine, 100 u/mL penicillin, streptomycin and 100 mg/mL, with humidifying in 5% CO_2 incubator. HMSCs increased the initial seeding density per cm^2 in the medium by 1000 and updated every 2 days. The cells were collected by about

80%–90% of the common population. The MC and hydroxyapatite were incubated in the PBS and culture medium before the cell was sown for 4 hours, with the best infiltration medium entering the material. The disks were placed on the edge of each hole and a cell suspension was placed at the top of each disk. To avoid cell waste, the plates were tilted and the cells suspended in each disk. The culture medium was updated every 2 days.

3. Morphology observation of hMSCs

   The morphology of hMSCs was observed by scanning electron microscope (SEM) and confocal microscope. During the 24 hours incubation process, the cells were washed by PBS. At room temperature, the cells were fixed for 20 minutes, and the samples observed by SEM were dehydrated by alcohol gradient. After the sample was coated with gold, the sample was observed by SEM. For a confocal microscope sample, the cells were treated with Triton x-100 for 5 minutes, then stained with rhodamine for the cytoskeleton and 4,6-diamino -2- phenyl indole (DAPI) of the nucleus.

4. Quantitative detection of hMSCs proliferation

   Cell proliferation is carried out by the cell count of the kit-8 test ($n = 3$). Cells are cultured in MC and hydroxyapatite and cultured in 24-orifice plates. The blank panel group, as a control group, cultured cells in the proliferation medium, as mentioned above. In the time point (4 hours, 2, 4, 6 days), 50 mL of CCK 8 was added in sample solution, after incubating at 37°C for 4 hours, enzyme linked immunosorbent assay (ELISA) plate reader (490 nm) was used to estimate cell survival rate.

5. Osteogenic differentiation detection of hMSCs

   ALP is a key enzyme in the process of osteogenesis differentiation, and its activity increases with the enhancement of cell osteogenesis differentiation. Therefore, ALP activity is an important index of cell differentiation. To demonstrate the difference of hMSCs osteogenic differentiation on MC and hydroxyapatite, ALP activity was measured by ALP in the sample, which was quantified according to the instruction time (5, 10, 15 days). The blank panel group was also treated as a control group and cultured cells in the proliferation medium.

6. RNA isolation and microarray hybridization

   Total RNA was extracted from hMSCs on MC and hydroxyapatite using TRIzol reagent (Thermo Fisher Scientific Inc., United States) according to the protocol. The RNA quality was detected by Agilent 2100 Bioanalyzer and RNA LabChip kits (Agilent Technologies, United States). The sample pools of three independent biological replicates were mixed for gene expression analysis. Next, 100 ng of total RNA was used for transcriptional profiling with Affymetrix 3'IVT microarray analysis (Affymetrix Inc., United States) using the Affymetrix 3'IVT Express Kit to generate biotin-labeled antisense cRNA. The labeled cRNA was used for hybridization. After an automated process of washing and staining by the AGCC software (Affymetrix Inc., United States), absolute values of expression were calculated from the scanned array using the Affymetrix Command Console software.

7. The microarray analysis

To identify differentially expressed genes, pairwise comparison analyses were performed with analysis system using functions in R-package in R-software and NCBI Entrez gene database. The genes of hMSCs on experimental MC and hydroxyapatite were compared with those on the control group. The gene expression differences were identified with a stringent cutoff, the genes of at least one probe signal in the treatment and the control chip for the same gene showed parent, and only those up- or downregulated genes exceeding the threshold of threefold change were selected for further analysis.

8. Statistical analysis

All data were expressed as means ± standard deviation. Single factor analysis of variance technique was used to assess the statistical significance of the results between the groups. The statistical assessment was done by the software SPSS 13.0 at a confidence level of 95%.

3.3.1.2 Results

1. Characterization of MC and hydroxyapatite

The finished samples of MC and hydroxyapatite are shown in Fig. 3.3A. Experimental samples are discs with 1 cm in diameter and 2 mm in thickness. The elastic modulus of MC and hydroxyapatite are shown in Fig. 3.3B. The compressive elastic modulus of MC was close to human cortical bone, while that of hydroxyapatite is much higher than human cortical bone. According to Wolff's law, stress is a key factor to the growth of bone tissue. However, an implant with excessively higher modulus would lead to stress shielding that is unfavorable to bone regeneration. Therefore, stress shielding is inevitable by using a block of hydroxyapatite ceramic with such high modulus, while the biomimetic

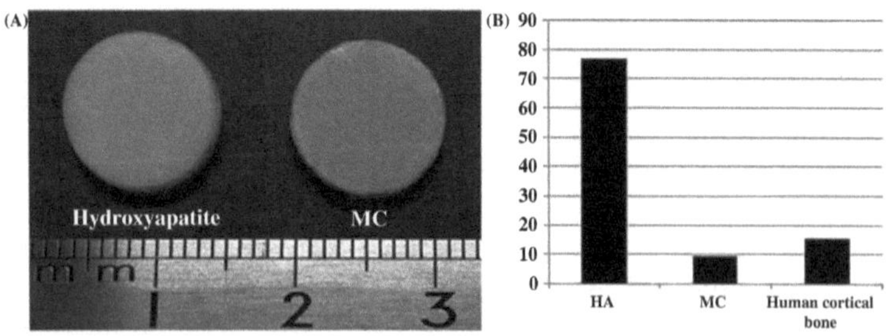

FIGURE 3.3 (A) The morphology and (B) the elastic modulus of hydroxyapatite and mineralized collagen samples.

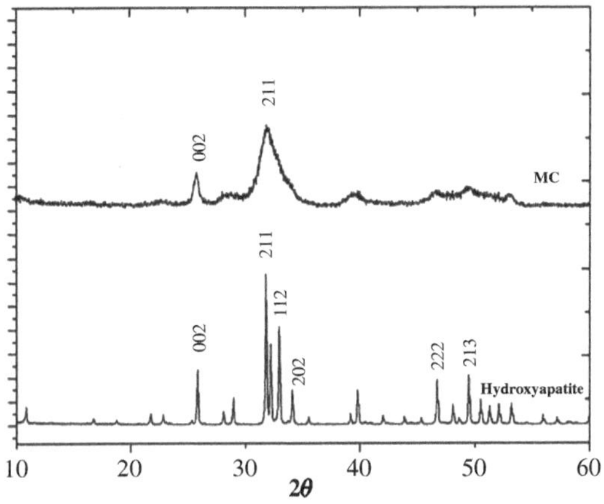

FIGURE 3.4 X-ray diffraction patterns of materials.

MC with similar compressive modulus to human cortical bone could avoid disadvantageous stress shielding in biomedical applications.

The phase composition of MC and hydroxyapatite were identified by XRD. Fig. 3.4 shows that the hydroxyapatite group had the typical XRD pattern of standard hydroxyapatite and all the diffraction peaks could be assigned to the standard card of hydroxyapatite (ICDD PDF card #9-432). Otherwise, in the MC group, according to above standard card of hydroxyapatite, all the reflections can be readily indexed to hydroxyapatite conforming to a space group, whose crystallinity was inferior to that of samples hydroxyapatite. The XRD patterns demonstrated that the mineral composition formed during the biomimetic mineralization was poor crystalline hydroxyapatite within nanoscale size, which is in conformity with our previous studies on MC.

The FTIR spectra of MC and hydroxyapatite are shown in Fig. 3.5, and they accord with our previous studies. hydroxyapatite showed PO_4^{3-} stretching band at 1045, 960, 602, and 571 cm^{-1}. The absorption band located at 631 cm^{-1} was the characteristic peak of O–H. MC showed characteristic peaks of type-I collagen are probed at 1653 (amide I), 1550 (amide II), and 1032 cm^{-1} (C–OH). Another two bands at 1471 and 1417 cm^{-1} were assignable to the $-CH_3$ and $=CH_2$ bending vibrations.

2. Morphology of hMSCs

As SEM micrographs show in Fig. 3.6, adhesion and growth of hMSCs onto the test materials exhibited changed cell morphology and viability. After 48 hours of culture, the adhesion and morphology of cells analysis further confirmed the differences of cells cultured on different groups. In the MC group, cells grew normally and regularly in parallel. On the edge of cell contact area, some tiny fibrils were observed. On the hydroxyapatite surface, cells had larger spreading areas and this spread

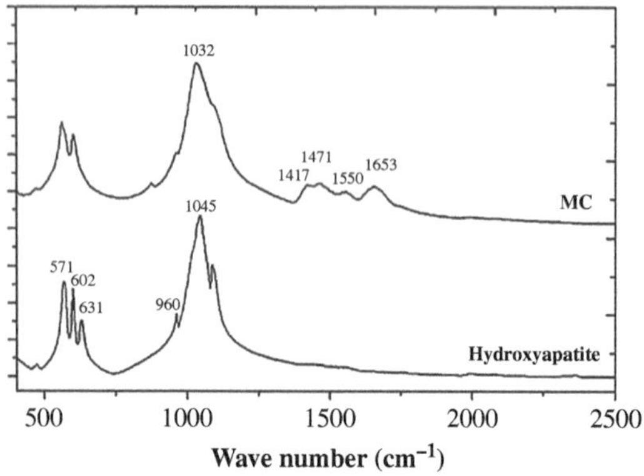

FIGURE 3.5 Fourier transform infrared spectroscopy of the mineralized collagen and hydroxyapatite samples.

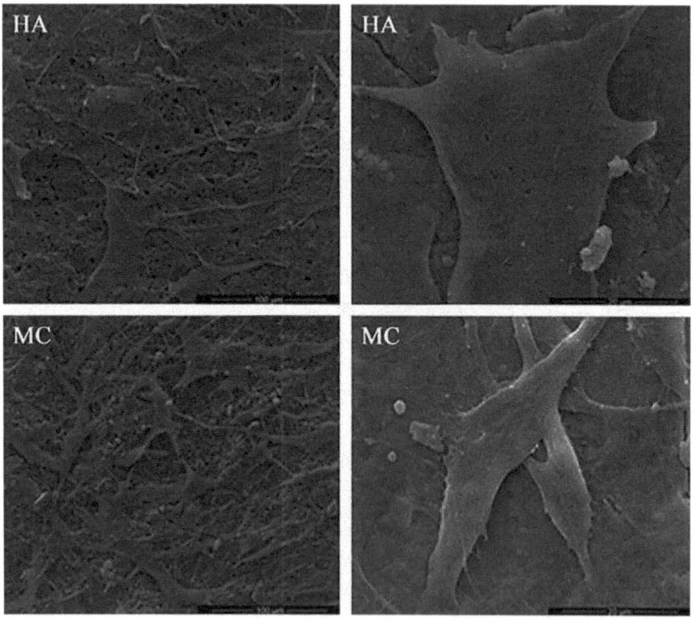

FIGURE 3.6 The scanning electron microscope micrographs of cells cultured on hydroxyapatite and mineralized collagen surfaces with serum-free conditions after 24 h.

flattened, and there were hardly any membranous "pseudopods" from the cell body. As shown by confocal images in Fig. 3.7, the number of bMSCs on the MC was also greater than that on the hydroxyapatite substrate. Such phenomenon indicated that hMSCs adhered and grew better on the MC than on the hydroxyapatite substrate.

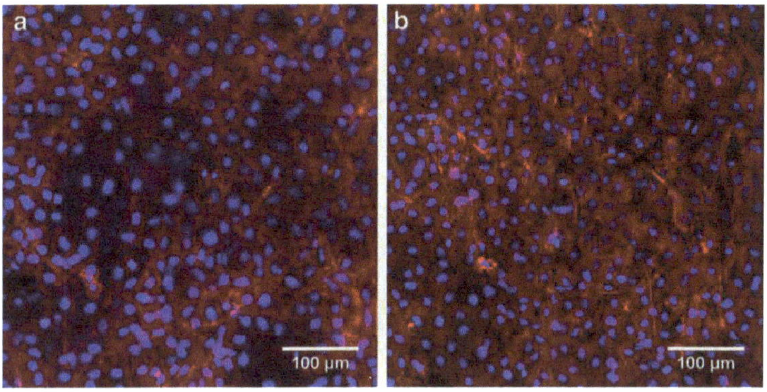

FIGURE 3.7 The confocal images of bMSCs on (A) hydroxyapatite and (B) mineralized collagen surfaces cultured for 24 h.

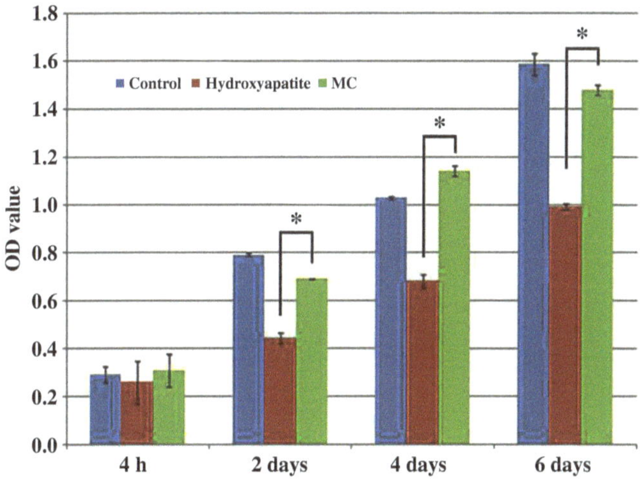

FIGURE 3.8 The proliferation of cells cultured on different substrates for 4 h and 2, 4, and 6 days by the MTT assay ($n = 6$). *Significant difference ($P < .05$).

3. Proliferation of hMSCs

From the SEM results, we found different materials had impact on hMSCs. Further quantitative detection was carried out by cell proliferation assay, as shown in Fig. 3.8. At 4 hours, there was a small but not significant difference among different groups. Two days later, the cells in the control group and MC group increased remarkably. Different from the case of the first day, the quantity of hMSCs hydroxyapatite group was less than the control group apparently. From day 4 and day 6, the growth of cells in the control group and MC group was similar. While the hydroxyapatite group had an inhibitory effect on cell proliferation and the cells remained at a very low level. Hence, MC has better biocompatibility than hydroxyapatite and can keep the cell proliferation in a longer culture period.

4. Differentiation of hMSCs

High ALP levels can occur if active bone formation is occurring, as ALP is a byproduct of osteoblast activity. ALP detection results showed that MC had the ability to induce hMSCs to differentiate into osteoblasts. After 15 days, the ALP activity of the cells on the MC surface was significantly greater than that on hydroxyapatite (Fig. 3.9). This result is in conformity with those previously published by our group. Such previous study indicated that not only the ALP, but also the expressions of many other osteogenic markers (osteocalcin, Col1a1, cbfa1, etc.) were upregulated by the biomimetic MC.

5. The gene expression differences analysis

The hMSCs cultured on MC, hydroxyapatite, and control groups showed different gene expression profiles by gene chip analysis, which may reflect the cellular mechanisms of osteogenic differentiation. To understand the mechanisms, the different genes that met the selection conditions and expressed more than twofold changes were selected for further analysis. There were in total 922 upregulated and 1417 downregulated genes for hMSCs in the hydroxyapatite group compared with the control; whereas there were 289 and 2166 genes for hMSCs in the MC group compared with the control. By comparing the hMSCs on the hydroxyapatite to those on the MC, there were 1504 upregulated and 139 downregulated genes. These differently expressed genes were applied to further pathway and gene ontology (GO) term analyses.

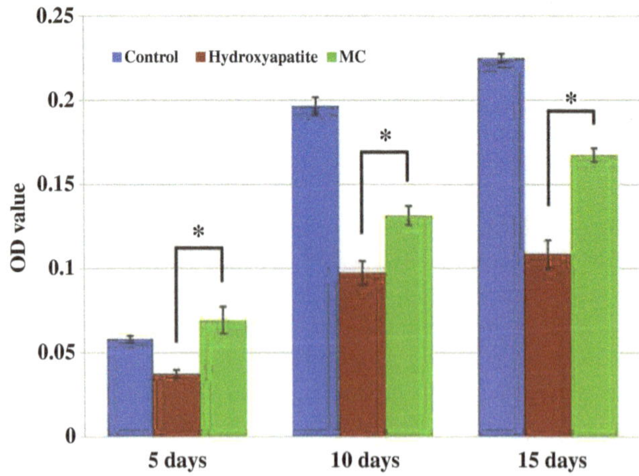

FIGURE 3.9 Alkaline phosphatase detection results showed that mineralized collagen had the ability to induce human mesenchymal stem cells to differentiate into osteoblasts. *Significant difference ($P < .05$).

a. GO term analysis

To categorize transcripts by putative function, we have utilized the GO classification scheme. GO provides a dynamic controlled vocabulary and hierarchy that unifies descriptions of cellular, biological, and molecular functions across genomes (Fig. 3.10A–C). It helped to analyze the functions of genes. The up- and downregulated genes of every chemical group were analyzed separately, and $P < .05$ was considered significant. For those much more enriched genes in a GO term, only the top 10 genes were listed in relevant tables.

For cells on the MC group, many genes were upregulated in the catalog "biological process" associated with "cell differentiation" function (Table 3.4). For example, in terms of "positive regulation of cell proliferation," "CYR61" can induce cysteine-rich angiogenesis; "DDR2" functions as cell surface receptor for fibrillar collagen and regulates cell differentiation, remodeling of the ECM; "BMP2" is an important bone morphogenetic protein. In the "molecular function,"

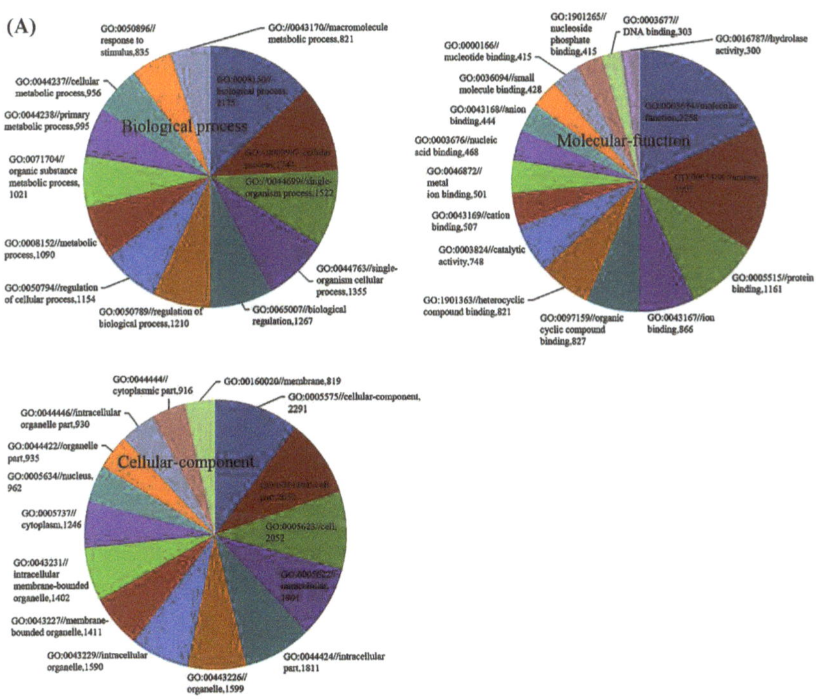

FIGURE 3.10 Percentage representation of gene ontology mappings for differential gene clusters (A) in the mineralized collagen (MC) group compared with the control group, (B) in the hydroxyapatite group compared with the control group, and (C) in the MC group compared with hydroxyapatite group. In molecular function category, the function referring to the largest number of differential gene was molecular function, followed by binding.

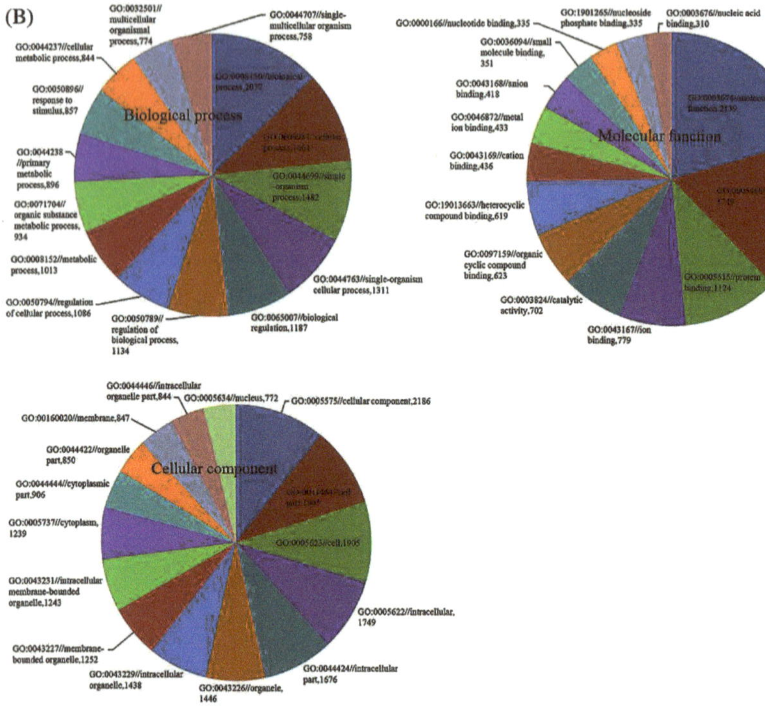

FIGURE 3.10 (Continued).

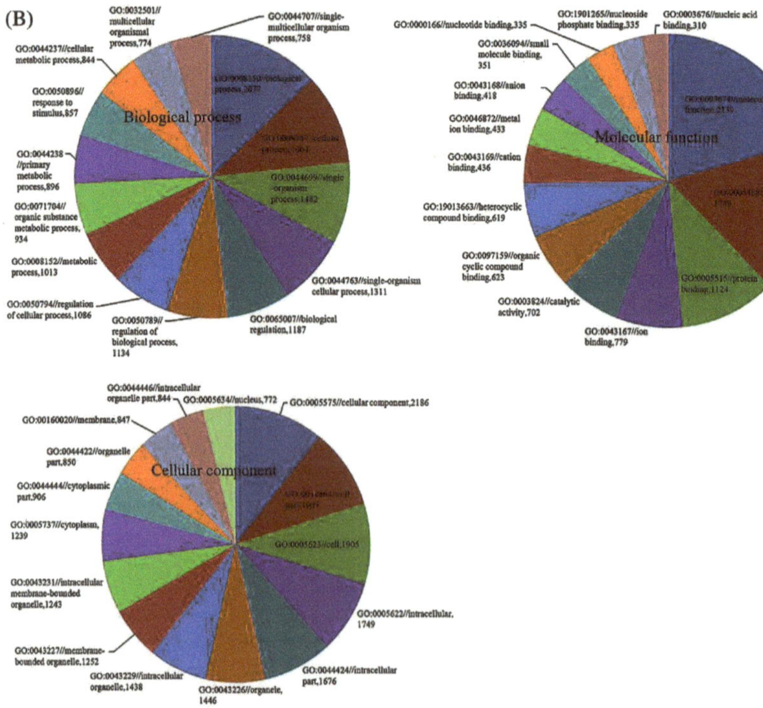

FIGURE 3.10 (Continued).

TABLE 3.4 Gene Ontology Term Analysis of Upregulated Genes on Mineralized Collagen Group

GO Terms	Hits	Gene Symbol	Percent	*P*
Biological process positive regulation of cell differentiation	93	COL1A1; CTGF; CYR61; RCOR1; HIF1A; LOXL2; ETV5; PDE5A; MED1; NCOA1	8.53	1.9143E-05
Ossification	30	COL1A1; CTGF; EGFR; LRRC17; TGFB3; COL13A1; CDH11; BMP2; GLI2; CBS	8.20	0.0201
Skeletal system development	101	COL1A1; COL1A2; CTGF; CYR61; SETD2; MGP; GLG1; HIF1A; PBX1; RDH10	12.52	1.3545E-14
Bone development	30	COL1A1; GLG1; THBS1; DDR2; PAPSS2; ANKRD11; SKI; WHSC1; GLG1; SULF1	15.38	3.5079E-07
Cellular component Cell surface	102	COL1A1; COL1A2; FKBP1A; PDIA6; COL4A2; DHCR24; MLEC; SCD; CLSTN1; RPN2	8.81	7.2187E-07
Molecular function Collagen binding	17	ABI3BP; THBS1; NID2; DDR2; SMAD4; PCOLCE2; ADAM9; NID1; SERPINH1; ADAM9	21.79	8.2127E-07

most associated genes contributed to the cellular response to the osteogenic differentiation. Apart from this, some other genes were also enriched in catalog "cellular component," such as "COL1A1" and "COL1A2," involving in fibrillar collagen. In addition, some genes of cell proliferation also enriched, such as IL6ST and CTGF.

Comparing the hydroxyapatite group with the MC group, among the significant GO terms were several enriched terms associated with cell differentiation, ossification, skeletal system development, bone development, and correspondingly the signal transduction in "biological process," "molecular functions," and "cellular component" categories (Table 3.5).

b. KEGG term analysis

Kyoto encyclopedia of Genes and Genomes (KEGG) pathways analyses were used to evaluate the statistically significant pathways associated

TABLE 3.5 Gene Ontology Term Analysis of Upregulated Genes on Comparing the Hydroxyapatite Group With the Mineralized Collagen Group

GO Terms	Hits	Gene Symbol	Percent	*P*
Biological process positive regulation of cell differentiation	75	SERPINF1; HES1; C13orf15; JUN; ACVR1; FOXO3; SPAG9; MED1; NCOA1	6.88	8.3740E-08
Ossification	34	CTSK; SLC26A2; HIRA; SMO; SMAD1; GPNMB; EGFR; RUNX2; MMP14; TGFB3	9.29	2.3301E-05
Skeletal system development	23	SETD2; PRRX1; WDR19; SULF2; SMO; GLI3; SIX1; PCSK5; RUNX2; SATB2	11.06	7.0880E-05
Bone development	15	LRP6; SULF2; SMAD1; GLI3; RUNX2; PTGER4; ANKRD11; GHR; SKI; SULF2	7.69	0.0470
Cellular component extracellular matrix	91	COL1A2; COL3A1; COL4A2; IGFBP7; SERPINE1; LUM; SERPINF1; TNC; COL18A1	10.64	0
Molecular functionCollagen binding	75	SERPINF1; HES1; C13orf15; JUN; ACVR1; FOXO3; SPAG9; MED1; NCOA1	6.88	8.3740E-08

with differentially expressed genes. The up- and downregulated genes of hMSCs in the three chemical groups were analyzed, respectively. Probes were mapped to gene identifiers, and gene identifiers were used as the input in the statistical analysis; $P < .05$ was considered significant. For cells in the MC group, the enrichment analysis revealed that 28 pathways were associated with upregulated and downregulated genes, as listed in Table 3.6. Comparing the hydroxyapatite group with the MC group, the enrichment analysis revealed that 8 pathways were associated with upregulated and downregulated genes, as listed in Table 3.7.

Analysis of microarray data indicated that some genes involved in osteoblast differentiation and function were significantly upregulated in the hydroxyapatite and MC groups (Fig. 3.11), including FGF2, EDNRA, growth hormone receptor (GHR), FOSL2, IL1R, CTSK, CREB1, and so on.

TABLE 3.6 Pathway Analysis of Up- and Downregulated Genes on Mineralized Collagen

Pathway	Hits	Percent	*P*
Focal adhesion	125	13.2556	0
ECM-receptor interaction	66	19.2983	0
Pathways in cancer	122	9.5987	6.36E-09
Bacterial invasion of epithelial cells	53	12.045	1.96E-07
Amoebiasis	52	12.0930	2.25E-07
Cell cycle—yeast	37	13.3093	1.28E-06
Spliceosome	61	10.6087	1.97E-06
Regulation of actin cytoskeleton	85	9.3715	3.64E-06
Protein processing in endoplasmic reticulum	65	10.0154	6.35E-06
Small-cell lung cancer	40	11.7994	9.88E-06
Cell cycle	47	10.9813	1.19E-05
Thiamine metabolism	7	35	7.52E-05
Colorectal cancer	33	11.1111	0.000182
Progesterone-mediated oocyte maturation	36	10.4046	0.000346
Meiosis—yeast	29	11.1969	0.000383
Prion diseases	18	13.4328	0.000581
Malaria	22	12.1547	0.000623
Leukocyte transendothelial migration	52	8.9041	0.000905
Cell adhesion molecules	47	8.96946	0.001343
Pathogenic *Escherichia coli* infection	25	10.7758	0.00161
TGF-beta signaling pathway	28	10.1449	0.002168
Axon guidance	49	8.5069	0.003169
Phagosome	56	8.2111	0.003614
Ubiquitin-mediated proteolysis	48	8.4656	0.003808
Melanoma	25	10.0401	0.004152
Oocyte meiosis	41	8.6864	0.004612
Sulfur metabolism	9	15.5172	0.005122
Renal cell carcinoma	27	9.6428	0.005145

TABLE 3.7 Pathway Analysis of Up- and Downregulated Genes in the Mineralized Collagen Group Compared With the Hydroxyapatite Group

Pathway	Hits	Percent	*P*
TGF-beta signaling pathway	28	10.1449	7.46E-08
ECM-receptor interaction	29	8.4795	1.89E-06
Pathways in cancer	70	5.5074	5.67E-06
Wnt signaling pathway	43	6.3328	1.65E-05
Focal adhesion	53	5.6203	4.77E-05
Complement and coagulation cascades	23	7.5657	0.000124
Protein digestion and absorption	26	6.7885	0.000264
Prostate cancer	25	10.1449	0.000951

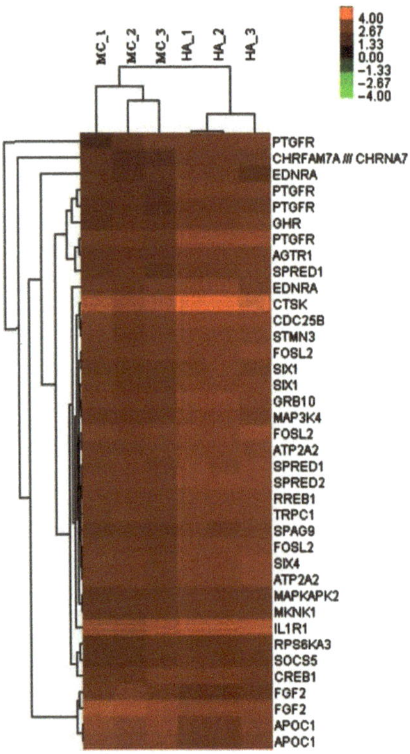

FIGURE 3.11 Visual display of the cluster analysis for the mineralized collagen group compared with the hydroxyapatite group.

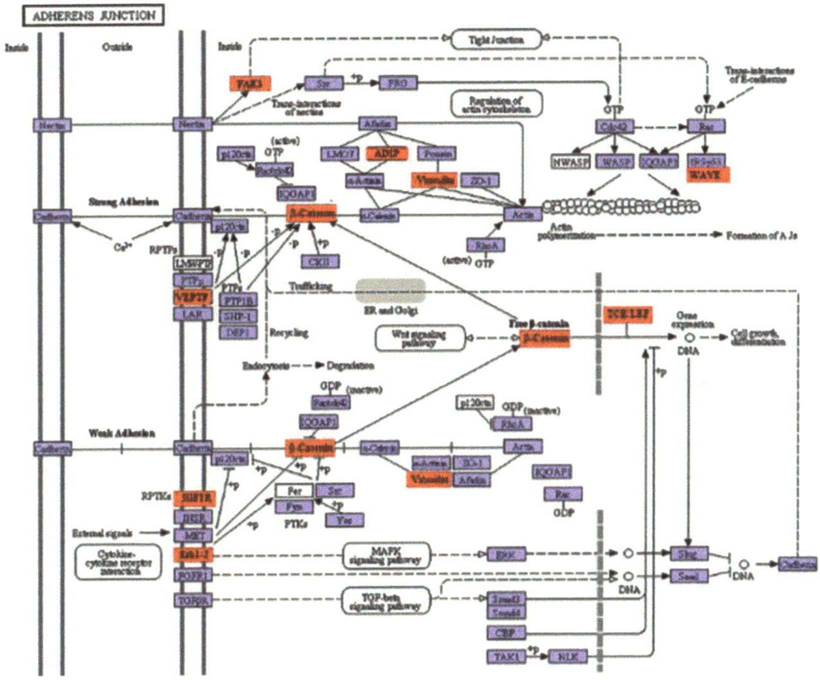

FIGURE 3.12 Upregulated expression in osteoblast differentiation pathway was assigned as red in the figure. The change of expression quantity refers to the mineralized collagen group compared with the hydroxyapatite group.

FGF2, a signal molecule of the fibroblast growth factor (FGF) family, was significantly increased (Fig. 3.12). FGF2 has been shown to accelerate fracture healing in mice. Similarly, EDNRA, the endothelin receptor type A, was induced in the MC and hydroxyapatite groups. Endothelin-1 (ET-1) signaling is important for postnatal bone formation. ET-1 promotes osteoblast proliferation, survival, and differentiation in vitro. Moreover, deletion of endothelin receptor type A in osteoblast resulted in impaired osteoblast differentiation and bone formation.

Growth hormone (GH) is known to promote anabolic bone formation. The effect of GH on bones partly works through GHR expressed in osteoblasts. Indeed, GHR is critical to mediate proproliferation and antiapoptotic functions of IGF-1 signals. Interestingly, GHR is significantly upregulated in the MC and hydroxyapatite groups, implying a role of local GH signaling in MC-induced osteoblast differentiation.

FOSL2, a Fos-related transcriptional factor of the AP-1 family, is a positive regulator of osteoblast differentiation and collagen synthesis. FOSL2 was significantly upregulated in the MC group, suggesting that FOSL2 plays an important role in MC-induced osteoblastogenesis and matrix synthesis.

In summary, MC promoted osteoblast differentiation and function through regulating a network of osteogenic factors. Moreover, signaling pathways associated with cell adhesion were also triggered, for example, the adherence junction pathway (Fig. 3.14).

3.3.1.3 Conclusion

The major finding of this study was that MC could promote osteogenic differentiation of hMSCs. Microarray analysis detected that MC was conducive to express bone gene, such as BMP-2, COL1A1, CTSK, and stimulate a pathway of osteogenic differentiation, for example, osteoblast differentiation pathway, skeletal system development pathway. Meanwhile, hMSCs could exhibit changed cell behaviors, including cell proliferation, adhesion, and apoptosis on different materials. This is helpful to know the molecular mechanism of cellular chemistry controlling and should be useful for the development of biomaterials to regulate the preservation, proliferation, and differentiation of hMSCs.

3.3.2 Effects of Mineralized Collagen on Osteoblastic Differentiation of Bone Marrow Stromal Stem Cells Induced by Platelet-Rich Plasma

3.3.2.1 Materials and Methods

1. The main reagents and instruments: osteocalcin radioimmunoassay kit, RT-PCR kit, S-450 SEM, FACScan flow cytometry, ALP kit, Polymerase Chain Reaction (PCR) thermal cycler, FQD-33A fluorescence quantitative PCR instrument.
2. The MC material has a mineral content of about 50% and a collagen content of about 40%, and the material has a degradation time of 3–6 months in vivo. The material has a porous structure, the pore size is 50–400 μm, the average porosity 70%–80%. According to the requirements of the experiment, the material should be cut into 8 mm × 8 mm × 3 mm in size, undergo 60Co radiation sterilization, ethanol soaking for 1 hour before use; then wash away the ethanol with water.
3. Experimental method:

   Isolation and culture of rBMSCs: A large white rabbit of 2 months (body weight: 1.5 kg). Take 4–6 mL bone marrow from rabbit bilateral tibia and femur. Anticoagulation with heparin is carried out, the slowly add bone marrow into the previously added 4 mL lymphocyte stratification tube. Centrifugation at 2000 r/min speed for 20 minutes, then take the middle of the mononuclear cell layer, washed twice with PBS. Add complete DMEM (containing 100 mL/L bovine serum) medium and seeded in 25 mL plastic flasks at a density of 5 × 109/L. Place in 37°C, 50 mL/L CO_2 incubator. The first fluid change is on day 3, after that, change fluid every 2–3 days. After 80% confluence, cells are harvested by trypsin digestion at 2.5 g/L and subcultured at a 1:2 ratio.

Identification of rabbit bone marrow stromal cells by flow cytometry: The second generation of rBM-SCs was made into a single-cell suspension and centrifuged at 1000 r/min for 5 minutes. The supernatant was discarded, rinsed with PBS, and incubated with fluorescently labeled CD90 (purchased from BD-PharM ingen), CD45, and CD11b (purchased from Serotec) antibody for 90 minutes at 4°C in the dark. Then it was centrifuged at 1000 r/min for 5 minutes, supernatant discarded, and rinsed with PBS. Flow cytometry screening CD11b and CD45 antibody negative, and CD90 antibody positive cell population was used in this experiment.

Preparation of platelet-rich plasma (PRP): 10 mL of whole blood was taken from the same rabbit ear central artery (10% sodium citrate anticoagulant added in advance), and centrifuged at 1500 r/min for 10 minutes. The upper plasma and platelets were extracted, and centrifuged again at 3000 r/min for 10 minutes; the precipitation is PRP. Platelets are counted for whole blood and PRP to ensure that the number of platelets in the PRP is more than four times that of whole blood. One milliliter of PRP was added to 98 mL of DMEM medium and 1 mL of a 100 g/L $CaCl_2$ solution containing 5000 U of bovine thrombin was added to obtain DMEM-conditioned medium containing 10 mL/L of PRP.

4. Experimental grouping

Experimental group: the treated nHAC was infiltrated with DMEM containing 10 mL/L PRP for 24 hours and then placed in the wells of a 24-well culture plate. Then rBMSCs cell suspension 100 μL (concentration of 1 × 109/L) was added dropwise to the nHAC surface, 37°C, 50 mL/L CO_2 incubator for 2 hours. The nHAC is flipped to the other side with the same concentration of rBMSCs cell suspension 100 μL, and continued to culture for 2 hours. Discard the old medium in the wells and add 200 μL of DMEM conditioned medium containing 10 mL/L PRP to prevent it from passing through the surface of the material. Place in a 37°C, 50 mL/L CO_2 incubator. The DMEM conditioned medium containing 10 mL/L PRP should be changed every 3 days.

Control group: take 200 μL (concentration of 1 × 109/L) suspension of rBMSCs and inoculate in 24-well culture plates and incubate at 37°C in 50 mL/L CO_2 incubator for 4 hours. Discard the depleted medium in the wells, add 200 μL of DMEM conditioned medium containing 10 mL/L PRP and continue to culture in a 37°C, 50 mL/L CO_2 incubator. The DMEM conditioned medium containing 10 mL/L PRP was changed every 3 days.

5. SEM: the experimental group with nHAC attached to cells was observed under electron microscope.

ALP activity and osteocalcin content determination: digestion and collection cells of experimental group and control group. Test ALP activity and osteocalcin content according to kit instructions.

Real-time RT-PCR was used to detect the relative expression of osteopontin mRNA. The cells in the experimental group and the control group were collected after 2 weeks' incubation, and the relative expression of osteopontin mRNA was detected.

3.3.2.2 Results

1. Flow cytometry results are shown in Fig. 3.13. The positive rate of CD90 expression in this experimental group was (89.25 ± 2.71)%, while the positive rates of CD45 and CD11b were (4.13 ± 1.61)% and (6.51 ± 2.38)%, respectively.
2. Cell/scaffold composite SEM

   SEM nHAC showed three-dimensional porous network structure, with a large number of pores and a wide range of traffic; see Fig. 3.14A and B. Hydroxyapatite grains are evenly distributed on the pore walls formed by the collagen matrix, with grain sizes on the nanometer scale; see Fig. 3.14C. In the early stage of composite culture, spherical bone marrow stromal cells were seen to grow in the nHAC pores, as shown in Fig. 3.14D. Cells became flattened, multiprotuberant, and extended into the pores with pseudopodia, which became firm on binding with nHAC; see Fig. 3.14E. ECM was secreted around the cells, and some of the pseudopodia made contact and fused; see Fig. 3.14F.
3. ALP activity, osteocalcin content results

   The activity of ALP increased with the prolongation of culture time and reached the peak at 14 days, after which ALP decreased. From the seventh day, the ALP content in the experimental group increased significantly ($P < .05$) compared with the control group (289.0 ± 26.7) U/L and (20.67 ± 2.54) U/L, respectively. The content of osteocalcin increased with the prolongation of culture time. The content of osteocalcin in the

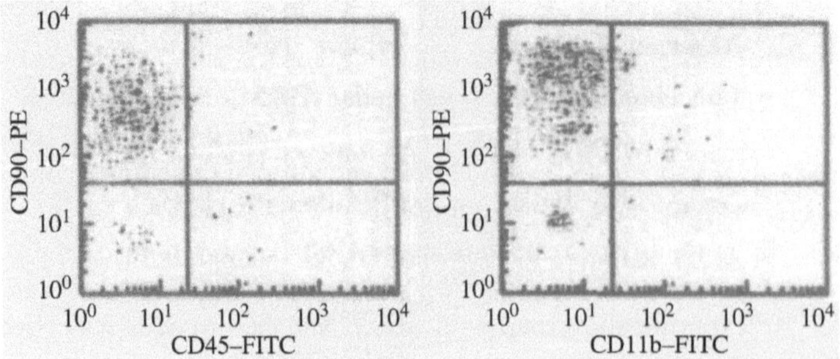

FIGURE 3.13 rBMSCs surface antigen characteristics.

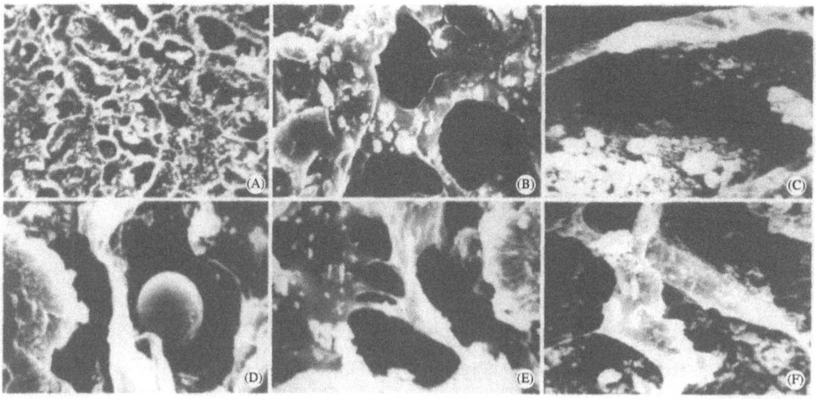

FIGURE 3.14 Scanning electron microscopy observation: nHAC and platelet-rich plasma cocultured with nHAC bone marrow stromal cells (A–F).

TABLE 3.8 Relative Gene Expression (Osteopontin)

Group	Housekeeping Gene GAPDH		Target Gene Osteopontin		
	Quantitative Results Mean	Relative	Quantitative Results Mean	Corrected Result	Relative Expression
Control	9610	1.00	2160	2160	1.00
Experimental	5960	0.62	6400	10,322	4.78

experimental group increased significantly from day 14 ($P < .05$), and it was (0.67 ± 0.02) μg/L and (0.59 ± 0.03) μg/L.

4. Osteopontin gene mRNA relative expression

The results showed that the C_t value of the housekeeping gene and the target gene of the test sample was good (mean: GAPDH 18.84, osteopontin 27.79 for experimental group; GAPDH 19.59, osteopontin 26.13 for control group respectively), and the repeatability among the parallel samples was good. The standard curve was used to quantify the housekeeping gene and the target gene respectively. After the housekeeping gene was corrected, the mRNA expression levels of the two comparative samples were correctly analyzed. The experimental group was 4.78 times that of the control group (Table 3.8).

3.3.2.3 Conclusion

The results of this experiment showed that rBMSCs adhere, spread, proliferate and entangle with each other by pseudopodia, indicating MC material has good biocompatibility and cell affinity. In addition, the nanohydroxyapatite contained in nHAC has a surface effect, and there are many dangling bonds in the surface atoms of the nanohydroxyapatite and the chemical activity with high unsaturation. These can increase the biological activity of the material and osteoinduction ability, and may also affect the signaling pathways, which is conducive to the adhesion of rBMSCs and thus promotes their differentiation. nHAC as a scaffold provides a good static stereotactic condition for rBMSCs and further enhances PRP-induced ability of rBMSCs to differentiate into osteoblasts compared with two-dimensional culture conditions. This provides a new feasible way for the construction of tissue-engineered bone in vitro. However, the optimization of its construction method and the osteogenic effect in vivo still need further study [17].

3.3.3 The Observed Difference of RAW264.7 Macrophage Phenotype on Mineralized Collagen and Hydroxyapatite

Understanding the interaction between biomaterials and the immune system has become more and more important. MC has the same chemical components and microstructures as natural bone tissue, and is considered as a better biomaterial for bone prostheses compared with hydroxyapatite. However, there is little information about how MC affects inflammatory responses. In this study, we investigate the inflammatory responses to MC and hydroxyapatite by culturing RAW264.7 cells on their surfaces. We observed that MC increases CD206 + staining and IL-10 (M2 macrophages), whereas hydroxyapatite shows cells expressing more CD86 and secreting more TNF-α. This result indicates that MC may attenuate inflammatory responses to implanted bone prostheses.

3.3.3.1 Materials and Methods

Murine monocyte macrophages RAW264.7 were purchased from the Type Culture Collection of the Chinese Academy of Sciences (Shanghai, China) and cultured in DMEM (HyClone) supplemented with 10% fetal bovine serum (Every Green), penicillin (100 units/mL) and streptomycin (100 μg/mL) (HyClone) at 37°C in a humidified atmosphere of 5% CO_2. Cells were cultured on the surface of MC and hydroxyapatite, and culture glasses were set as control group. After 24 hours, The samples were examined with a fluorescence microscope. After 1 and 3 days, the samples were examined with a fluorescence microscope. The immunofluorescence results can be divided into the following: CD86 + (M1), CD206 + (M2), CD86 + /CD206 + (M1/M2), and CD86-/CD206-(M0) cells. We selected five random areas per slide at × 10 magnification and captured digital images for each treatment group at each time point. Then we manually counted the number of each phenotype based on the positive staining of the cell present in the selected fields. The mean ($n = 15$) for each cell phenotype was calculated for each group. RAW264.7 cells were seeded on the surface of MC, hydroxyapatite, and culture glass as previously mentioned. Culture media supernatants were collected at 1 and 3 days. Mouse TNF-α and IL-10 ELISA Kit were used to detect levels of proinflammatory cytokine TNF-α and antiinflammatory cytokine IL-10 separately.

3.3.3.2 Results

1. Morphology of macrophages grown on MC and hydroxyapatite

   RAW264.7 cells were seeded on the MC and hydroxyapatite and culture glass. The macrophages on the hydroxyapatite surface had more amoeboid-like protrusions compared with those grown on MC and culture glass (Fig. 3.15).
2. Macrophage phenotypic response to MC and hydroxyapatite

   Three color immunofluorescence staining images of each treatment group at their corresponding time points demonstrated that MC increases CD206+ staining (M2 macrophages), whereas hydroxyapatite showed cells expressing more CD86 (M1 macrophages). Moreover, cells cultured on glass did not express high amounts of either CD86 or CD206 (Figs. 3.16 and 3.17).
3. Macrophage TNF-α and IL-10 secretion

   Cytokines produced in the MC group had a significant shift toward increasing levels of IL-10 with time, as well as low levels of TNF-α, and the hydroxyapatite group had the opposite phenomenon, namely that levels of TNF-α were much higher than the MC group and levels of IL-10 were low. Levels of both TNF-α and IL-10 were low in the control group (Fig. 3.18).

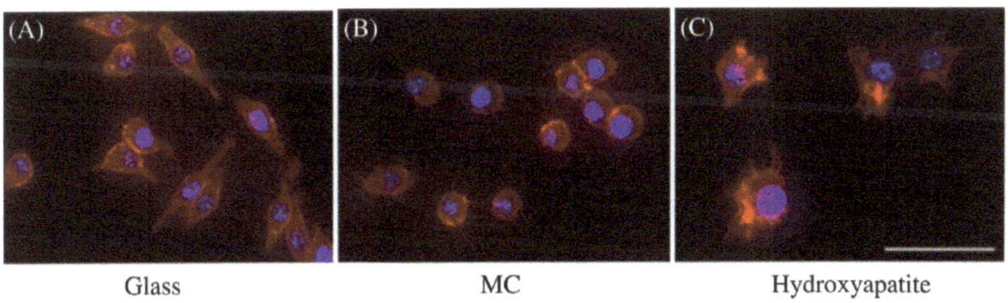

FIGURE 3.15 Morphology of RAW264.7 macrophages cultured on glass (A), mineralized collagen (MC) (B), and hydroxyapatite (C). Fluorescence images of RAW264.7 cells grown on glass, MC, and hydroxyapatite were stained with rhodamine-phalloidin and DAPI. Scale bar = 50 μm.

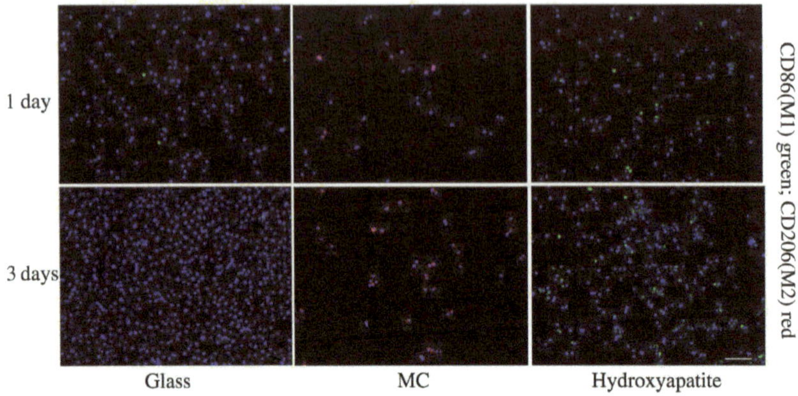

FIGURE 3.16 Representative fluorescent images of glass, mineralized collagen, and hydroxyapatite at different time points. M1 phenotype is indicated in green, M2 phenotype is indicated in red, mixed M1/M2 phenotype is shown as yellow, and M0 phenotype are cells without staining. The nuclei were stained with DAPI in blue. Scale bar = 100 μm.

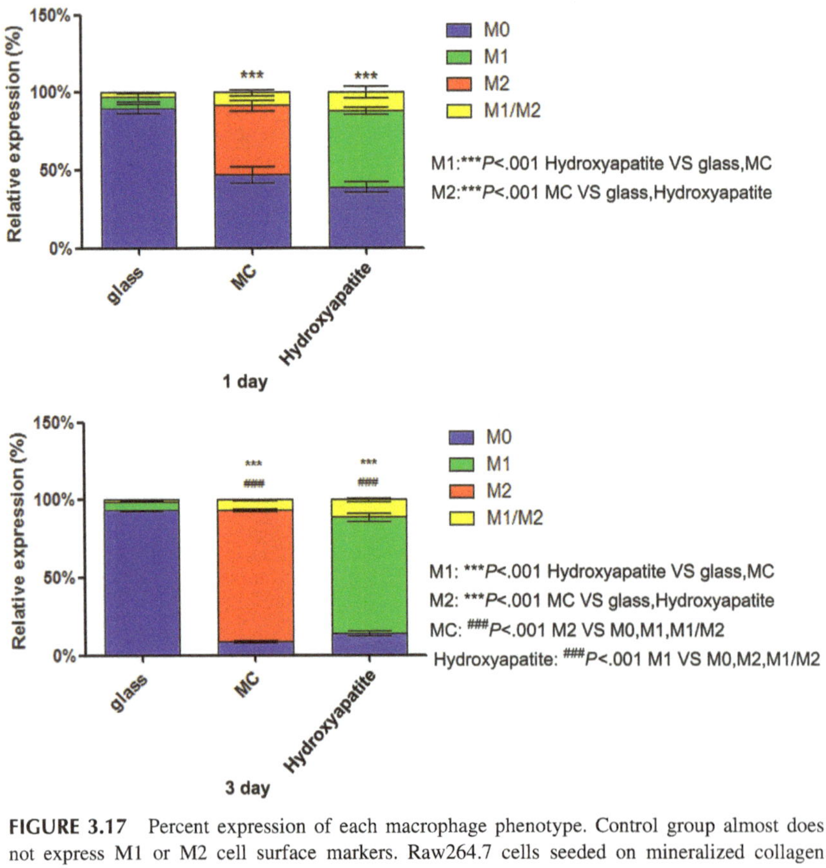

FIGURE 3.17 Percent expression of each macrophage phenotype. Control group almost does not express M1 or M2 cell surface markers. Raw264.7 cells seeded on mineralized collagen express significantly more M2 macrophage phenotype at 3 days. hydroxyapatite express mostly M1 macrophage phenotype at 3 days.

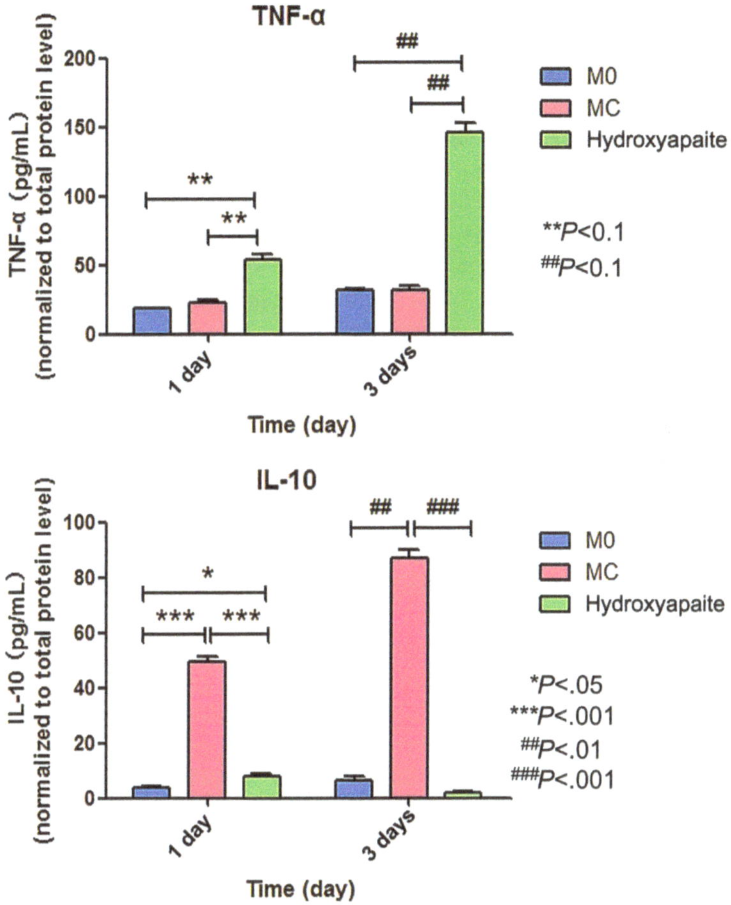

FIGURE 3.18 Cytokines secreted in mineralized collagen, hydroxyapatite, and control groups.

3.3.3.3 Discussion

Macrophages, derived from monocytes, play a key role in the immune system [18,19]. Recently, macrophages have attracted wide attention as an important regulator that controls disease progression and damaged tissue reconstruction. The function of macrophages is just like a switch that controls the body's inflammatory response and maintains the balance of the proinflammatory and antiinflammatory response [20]. As a kind of multifunctional cell, macrophages can manifest different phenotypes under the influence of different microenvironments [21–23]. Two terms have been used to describe macrophage phenotypes, classically activated macrophages (M1) and alternatively activated macrophages (M2). The proinflammatory macrophage phenotype, signified as M1, mainly secrets some proinflammatory cytokine and plays a role in the host immune status at the beginning of the inflammatory response as well as leads to inflammatory lesions of the body's normal tissues [23–25]. The antiinflammatory macrophage phenotype, signified as M2, downregulates the immune response, promoting wound healing and fibrosis through the secretion of antiinflammatory cytokines. M2 macrophage plays an important role in the late stage of inflammation [6–8]. M1 and M2 macrophages' polarization phenotypes exhibit strong dynamics and plasticity and they can differentiate to opposing phenotype when exposed to the opposing phenotype's induction signals. The infiltrated macrophages in tissues have a successive form from M1 to M2 phenotype and the different proportion of M1 and M2 can indicate the direction of inflammation, healing, and reconstruction [23].

With the development of tissue engineering and regenerative medicine, an increasing number of people have begun to realize that biomaterials can be used to regulate inflammation. Understanding the interaction between biomaterials and the immune system has become more and more important. If an implanted biomaterial can support the normal M1/M2 transformation, there will be better tissue reconstruction and downstream effects, as well as less fibrosis and scar tissue formation [20,26].

In our study, obvious differences of the phenotype cells cultured on the two biomaterials had been observed just after 1 day of the test. In this study, we found that morphology of macrophages grown on the surfaces of both MC and hydroxyapatite are different from the control group. Previous studies have shown that the morphology of macrophages cultured on different biomaterials was associated with cellular activation and polarization phenotype [27]. Previous studies have shown that M1 macrophages have bigger cell surface area and distinct lamelliopodial extension as well as amoeboid morphology, whereas M2 macrophages have elongated morphology. Those cells were grown on MC and culture glass and they are similar with M1 macrophages. Meanwhile, macrophages adhering to MCs had a rounder morphology than those grown on hydroxyapatite and culture glass. There are also studies indicating that the morphological changes of adherent macrophages are associated with their secretion of inflammatory cytokines and spherical or hemispherical macrophages secreted fewer proinflammatory cytokines [28]. And in our study, the results of cytokines measurement were consistent with the theory of morphology.

When we observed the different morphology of macrophages cultured on MC and hydroxyapatite, we further stained CD86 and CD206, which are the characteristic surface markers for M1 and M2 macrophages respectively. The immunofluorescence results showed that MC produced a significantly greater population of M2-staining cells compared with the control group and hydroxyapatite. In contrast, hydroxyapatite produced significantly more M1 macrophages compared with the control group and MC at all time points. In addition, the particle degree between MC and hydroxyapatite is different. The size of hydroxyapatite powder will become bigger after sintering and its diameter is around 10 μm. However, the MC powder is nanoparticles. The difference of particle degree between the two biomaterials may be a reason leading to the different experiment results and we will discuss this issue in our future studies.

It is generally known that the tissue reconstruction and wound healing after biomaterials are implanted into body depends on the balance of M1/M2 macrophages. M2 macrophages could promote the formation of functional tissue and support for healing of wounds, whereas M1 macrophages are against this regeneration process. These data suggested that MC could induce macrophages' polarization toward M2 and that may be a potential mechanism by which MC promotes bone tissue regeneration.

In conclusion, the current study showed the obvious difference of adherent macrophages morphology on MC and hydroxyapatite biomaterials surfaces and this is probably correlated with macrophages' activation state. Furthermore, we also observed that MC-induced macrophages' polarization toward the M2 phenotype. This finding provides important information for the use of MC in regard to immune responses.

3.4 BIOLOGICAL EVALUATION

In recent years, the field of biomaterials has developed rapidly, and ensuring the safety of medical materials in the human body is the most basic concern in the development process. On the basis of understanding the biocompatibility of materials, biological evaluation of biomaterials is an important step for achieving its safety. Biological evaluation mainly refers to the qualitative analysis of materials (natural or synthetic) that is expected to be applied to the human body, before entering the clinic, and the analysis of existing materials or information, followed by simulation of in vitro biological experiments and animal experiment if needed. After comprehensive information and data analysis and safety assessment, it is necessary to make a relatively scientific evaluation on the risk of the material application to the human body. The significance of the evaluation lies in predicting the potential hazards of the material during its use in contact with humans, ensuring the safety of the application of the material and minimizing the risk of insecurity.

The material should have good biocompatibility and can be integrated into the host tissue without causing any immune rejection. This is mainly reflected in two aspects: surface properties and degradation products. The surface properties directly affect the short-term behavior on the cells and tissues that have just been contacted at the time of implantation; the degradation products affect the long-term effects on the surrounding tissues and their response to the degradation product. The surface properties of materials, including chemical and topological structures, can affect cell adhesion and proliferation. The surface chemical properties of the material affects the function of protein adsorption and thus affects the cell's activity, while its topological structure mainly affects the osteoconductivity [29].

1. Cytotoxicity test

   Cytotoxicity assays use cell culture techniques to determine cytostatic, cell lysis (cell death), colony formation, and other cellular effects of cells, materials, and/or their extracts using cytotoxicity assays [30].
2. Irritation test or intradermal reaction

   Stimulation tests are used to determine the potential stimulatory effects of medical devices, materials, and/or their extracts on corresponding parts of a suitable model (e.g., skin, eye, and mucous membranes). The tests should be conducted in accordance with the route of use or contact (skin, eye, mucosa) and time [31].

   An intradermal reaction test was used to evaluate the tissue's local response to the medical device extract. Intradermal reaction assays can also be used in medical devices that are not suitable for stimulating skin or mucous membrane tests (e.g., medical devices that are implanted or in contact with blood). The intradermal reaction test also applies to hydrophobic extracts. The MC material has no stimulatory effect and no intradermal reaction.
3. Acute toxicity test

   An acute systemic toxicity test was used to assess the potential hazards of one or more exposures to medical devices, materials, and/or their extracts within 24 hours in an animal model. This type of test includes a pyrogen test used to detect the material-heating reaction of a medical device or material extract. The individual experiments cannot distinguish between the pyrogen-generating reactions due to the material itself or endotoxin contamination [32]. MC material has no acutely toxic effect.
4. Genetic toxicity test

   This involves using a panel of in vitro genetic toxicity tests, testing mammalian or nonmammalian cell culture or other techniques to determine genetic mutations, changes in chromosome structure and quantity, and other DNA caused by medical devices, materials, and/or their extracts or genotoxicity. If in vitro tests are positive, in vivo mutagenicity tests should be performed; otherwise materials should be inferred to be mutagenic [33]. MC material is not genetically toxic.
5. Implantation test

   The local pathological effect on living tissue was evaluated using an implantation test under visual observation and microscopy. Surgical methods are used to implant or place a sample of a material or end product into the intended application site or tissue (such as a special dental application test). These tests should be adapted to the device and the material's route of exposure and time [34]. There was no significant difference in the local tissue reaction between the MC material and the control group.

6. Chronic toxicity test

Chronic toxicity tests are used to contact medical devices, materials, and/or their extracts for a period of time that is not less than the life span of the experimental animals (typically 6 months for rats). These tests should be commensurate with the role of the device or material or the route and timing of exposure. MC material has no chronic toxicity.

7. Sensitization reaction

This test uses a suitable model to evaluate the potential contact sensitization of materials and/or their extracts. These tests are very important, because even a small amount of the use or contact of solution may lead to abnormal or sensitization reactions. MC material has no sensitization reaction.

REFERENCES

[1] J.Q. Liu, X.Y. Liu, C.B. Deng, et al., Progress of the biocompatibility of bone graft substitute, Biomed. Eng. Clin. Med. 15 (3) (2011) 291–297.

[2] H. Zhou, Y. Liang, Biosafety and biocompatibility of a variety of biological materials, J. Clin. Rehab. Tissue Eng. Res. 13 (38) (2009) 7559–7562.

[3] Y. Niu, X. He, L.H. Zhang, et al., Preparation of bio-derived bone and its histocompatibility, Clin. Rehabil. Tissue Eng. Res. 12 (7) (2008) 1385–1389.

[4] H. Ssh, M.A. Shokrgozar, A. Khavandi, et al., In vitro biological evaluation of beta-TCP/HDPE—A novel orthopedic composite: a survey using human osteoblast and fibroblast bone cells, J. Biomed. Mater. Res. Part A 84A (2) (2008) 491–499.

[5] M.A. Knight, G.R. Evans, Tissue engineering: progress and challenges, Plastic Reconstr. Surg. 114 (114) (2004) 26E–37E.

[6] Y. Liu, Y. Fu, S. Liu, et al., Effects of microstructure of mineralized collagen scaffolds on cell morphology of MG 63, J. Peking Univ. (Health Sci.) 46 (1) (2014) 19–24.

[7] T.C. Shen, Q. Xia, Y.H. Huang, et al., Application of nano-hydroxyapatite/collagen in orthopaedics, J. Clin. Rehabil. Tissue Eng. Res. 11 (1) (2007) 48–51.

[8] J.H. Ning, H.C. Liu, Cells in ecology and the next generation of bone repair materials, Chin. J. Prosthodont. 1 (2) (2000) 108–110.

[9] Administration PDotSFaD, Passive Medical Devices and Medical Materials, Medical Science and Technology Press, China, 2010.

[10] J.B. Dong, Biological properties of bone morphogenetic proteins and basic fibroblast growth factor in biological materials for repair of articular cartilage defect, Chin. J. Tissue Eng. Res. 20 (20) (2016) 2915–2920.

[11] W. Sun, Z.R. Li, L. Zhang, et al., Effects of nano-hydrixyapatite/collagen to bone marrow mesenchymal stem cell on phenotype change, Chin. J. Misdiagn. 6 (8) (2006) 1419–1421.

[12] H.F. Bian, Current status and progress of cord blood hematopoietic stem cell transplantation, Chin. J. Misdiagn. 4 (4) (2004) 524–526.

[13] X.Y. Hong, B. Wang, J. Du, et al., In vitro isolation and culture of human umbilical cord blood mesenchymal stem cells, Chin. J. Misdiagn. 5 (17) (2005) 3218–3220.

[14] W. Sun, Z.R. Li, Z.C. Shi, et al., Effect of nano-hydroxyapatite collagen bone and marrow mesenchymal stem cell on treatment of rabbit osteonectosis of the femoral head defect, Chin. J. Rep. Reconstr. Surg. 19 (9) (2005) 703–706.

[15] W. Huang, Y. Liu, P.F. Gao, Clinical observation of collagen-based nano-bone repair of perforation of pulp floor, Chin. J. Misdiagn. 5 (18) (2005) 3457–3458.
[16] P. Chen, T.Q. Mao, B. Liu, et al., Genetoxicity of clooagen based composite and its influence on cultured cell in vitro, J. Oral Sci. Res. 21 (4) (2005) 353–356.
[17] C.Y. Wang, Y.S. Yao, H.J. Ai, et al., Effects of nano-hydroxyapatite/collagen on differentiation of bone marrow stromal cell into osteoblasts in-duced by platelet-rich plasma in vitro, J. Oral Sci. Res. 23 (3) (2007) 241–244.
[18] J.L. Shepard, L.I. Zon, Developmental derivation of embryonic and adult macrophages, Curr. Opin. Hematol. 7 (1) (2000) 3–8.
[19] S. Gordon, P.R. Taylor, Monocyte and macrophage heterogeneity, Nat. Rev. Immunol. 5 (12) (2005) 953–964.
[20] B.N. Brown, B.D. Ratner, S.B. Goodman, et al., Macrophage polarization: an opportunity for improved outcomes in biomaterials and regenerative medicine, Biomaterials 33 (15) (2012) 3792.
[21] A. Mantovani, A. Sica, S. Sozzani, et al., The chemokine system in diverse forms of macrophage activation and polarization, Trends Immunol. 25 (12) (2004) 677–686.
[22] P.J. Murray, J.E. Allen, S.K. Biswas, et al., Macrophage activation and polarization: nomenclature and experimental guidelines, Immunity 41 (1) (2014) 14.
[23] D.M. Mosser, J.P. Edwards, Exploring the full spectrum of macrophage activation, Nat. Rev. Immunol. 8 (12) (2008) 958.
[24] S. Gordon, Alternative activation of macrophages, Nat. Rev. Immunol. 3 (1) (2003) 23.
[25] P.R. Taylor, L. Martinez-Pomares, M. Stacey, et al., Macrophage receptors and immune recognition, Annu. Rev. Immunol. 23 (1) (2005) 901.
[26] B.N. Brown, R. Londono, S. Tottey, et al., Macrophage phenotype as a predictor of constructive remodeling following the implantation of biologically derived surgical mesh materials, Acta Biomater. 8 (3) (2012) 978.
[27] F.Y. Mcwhorter, T. Wang, P. Nguyen, et al., Modulation of macrophage phenotype by cell shape, Proc. Natl. Acad. Sci. USA 110 (43) (2013) 17253.
[28] H.S. Lee, S.J. Stachelek, N. Tomczyk, et al., Correlating macrophage morphology and cytokine production resulting from biomaterial contact, J. Biomed. Mater. Res. Part A 101A (1) (2013) 203–212.
[29] J.E. Davies, Mechanisms of endosseous integration, Int. J. Prosthodont. 11 (5) (1998) 391.
[30] GB/T 16886.5, Biological evaluation of medical devices. Part 5: In vitro cytotoxicity tests, National standards of the People's Republic of China: General Administration of Quality Supervision, Inspection and Quarantine, 2003.
[31] GB/T 16886.10, Biological evaluation of medical devices. Part 10: Stimulation and delayed type hypersensitivity tests, National standards of the People's Republic of China: General Administration of Quality Supervision, Inspection and Quarantine, 2005.
[32] GB/T 16886.3, Biological evaluation of medical devices, Part 11: Systemic toxicity tes, National standards of the People's Republic of China: Quality Inspection Center for Medical Polymer Products of the State Administration of Pharmaceuticals, 2011.
[33] GB/T 16886.3, Biological evaluation of medical devices, Part 3: Genetic toxicity, carcinogenicity and reproductive toxicity tests, National standards of the People's Republic of China: General Administration of Quality Supervision, Inspection and Quarantine, 2008.
[34] GB/T 16886.6, Biological evaluation of medical devices. Part 6: Local response test after implantation, National standards of the People's Republic of China: General Administration of Quality Supervision, Inspection and Quarantine, 2015.

Chapter 4

Assessing the Effect of Mineralized Collagen Based Materials by Animal Experimentation

Wei Ai, Yan-Li Hu, Zhi-Min He, Tian-Xi Song and Zi-Rui Wang
Beijing Allgens Medical Science and Technology Co., Ltd., Beijing, P.R. China

Animal experimentation is use of nonhuman animals in experiments to help ensure safety and effect of drugs and treatment to improve human health. With development of modern medical science and technology, it is well known that besides the social problems as food shortage, population and aging, there are also public health hazards that are a threat to human health. Animal testing is the use of nonhuman animals in experiments for applied research against these problems, including testing disease treatments and toxicology. These may involve the use of animal models of diseases or conditions. Almost every medical discovery in the 20th century used animals in some ways. Even complex computers cannot model connections between molecules, cells tissues, organs, organisms, and the environment. Hence the technique of animal testing has been wildly developed in developed countries. After succeeding in developing mineralized collagen (MC) based materials, a series of animal tests were performed to investigate their osteogenic and bone repair effects.

4.1 SEGMENTAL BONE DEFECTS REPAIR IN RABBIT RADIUS MODEL [1]

4.1.1 Objective

To examine the repair capability of MC based materials in a rabbit segmental defects radius model.

Mineralized Collagen Bone Graft Substitutes. DOI: https://doi.org/10.1016/B978-0-08-102717-2.00004-7

4.1.2 Experimental Method

4.1.2.1 Study Plan

Twelve New Zealand rabbit (weight 2.5–3 kg) with 15-mm segmental defects in radius were investigated.

4.1.2.2 Study Design

All rabbits were divided into two groups. In the experiment group MC based materials were implanted; meanwhile there was no treatment in the negative control group. The animals were killed at the 4th, 8th, and 12th week.

4.1.2.3 Study Materials

MC based materials 15 mm × 5 mm × 5 mm.

4.1.2.4 Study Method

Animals were anesthetized with 3% pentobarbital sodium intramuscular injection as 0.3 mg/kg weight. Hair removal, fastening, disinfection, spreadsheet were prepared as routinely. Anterolateral incision in right side forelimb of rabbit was operated and skin, hypoderm, deep fascia were incised in order. Separation was operated along intramuscular space to exposure radius. The junction in the middle and upper 1/3 of radius was cut off by handheld dental grinding machine so as to cause 15-mm bone segmental defects. BonGold (BM) bone graft material was implanted in experiment groups, and nothing implanted in the blank control group. The surgery was stitched layer by layer without fixation. Animals were sacrificed and samples were taken at week 4, 8, 12, 16, 24 after operation respectively.

4.1.2.5 Study Observations

1. Clinical gross observations: observe the condition of animal diet, activity, and wound healing after operation. Observe the change of defect site after sample taken out. The sample was cut longitudinally after decalcification to observe interior structure change.
2. Image analysis: X-ray on the forelimb was taken under anesthesia at week 4, 8, 12, 16, 24 after operation to observe repair condition in every group animal. The X-ray was taken at 55 kv, 50 mA, for 0.2 seconds.
3. Histological observation: the specimens were processed for resin embedding and slicing used for hematoxylin-eosin (H&E) and Masson staining. New bone formation and material degradation was observed.

4.1.3 Experiment Result (Figs. 4.1–4.6)

All wounds healed well in animals without infection or swelling. At week 12 after operation, there was no repair in bone defects in the blank control group without bone graft material. However for the BonGold bone graft

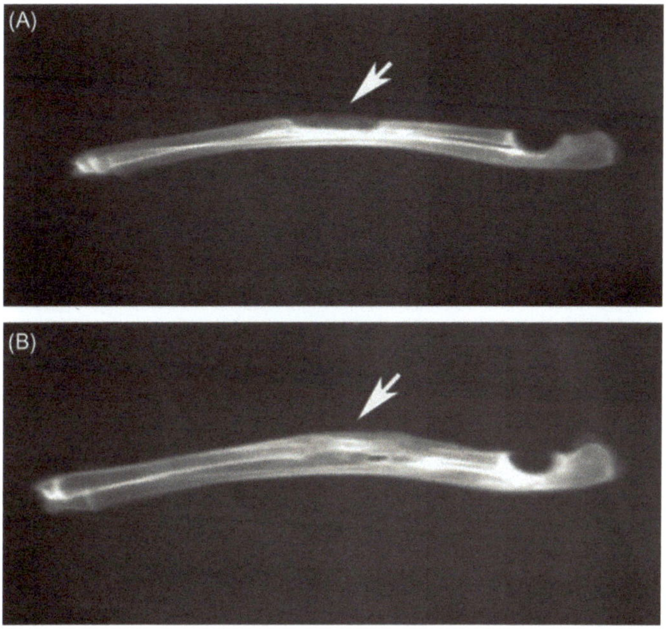

FIGURE 4.1 Twelve weeks after implantation (A: negative control, B: experiment group).

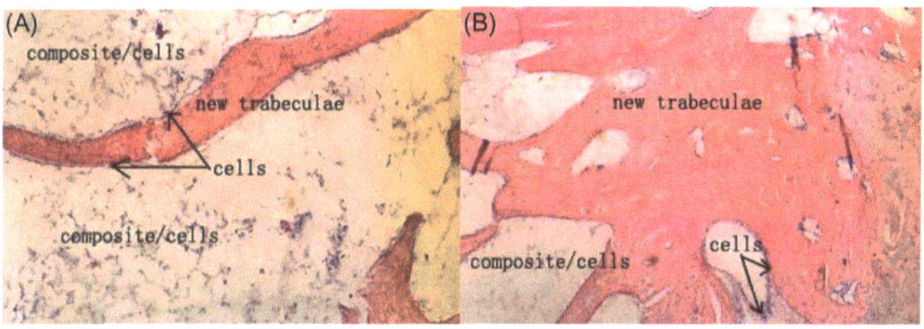

FIGURE 4.2 Tissue section observation of mineralized collagen material involved in bone defect reconstruction in rabbit tibia defect repair experiment, Week 12 after implantation: HE staining (hematoxylin-eosin staining) (A: 8 weeks postsurgery, B: 12 weeks postsurgery).

material implanted group, at week 12, two sides cortical bones connected fully, and defects healed (Fig. 4.4). The BonGold bone graft material implanted group bone repair was further demonstrated by Figs. 4.5 and 4.6. Fig. 4.5 showed the longitudinal section of specimen at week 12 after operation. The material profile was obscure and there was new bone formation observed. Tissue section showed that there was not only elementary bone connection at material edge but also newly formed trabeculae increased with time. Fig. 4.6 showed that both side cortical bones connected fully in defects at week 12 after operation and myelopoiesis had formed. There were newly formed trabeculae, which demonstrated new bone regeneration.

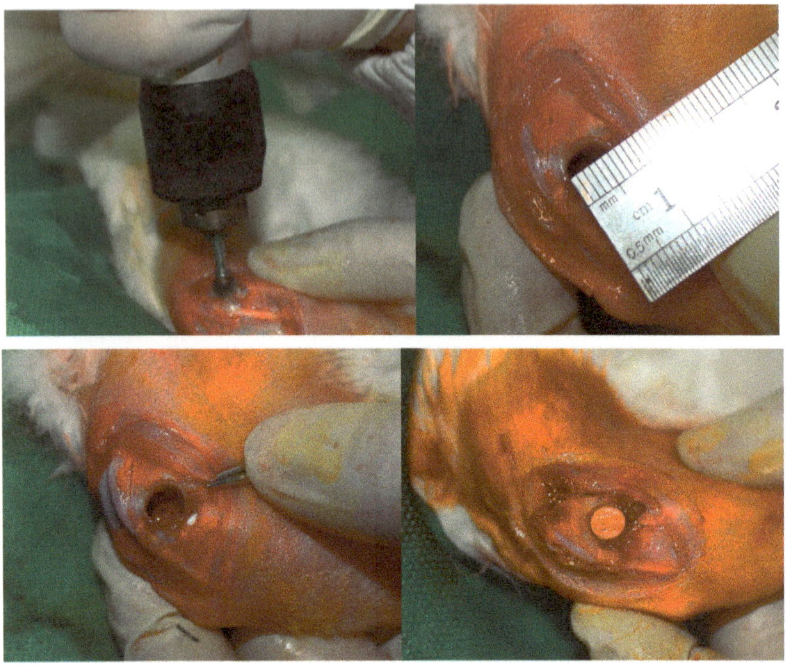

FIGURE 4.3 Photos for surgery.

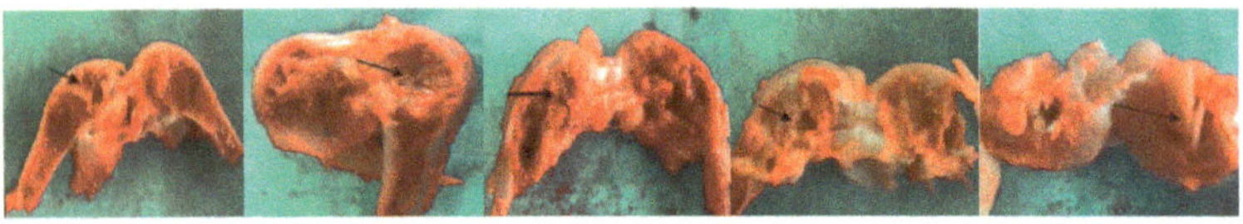

AGB BGM BGM + AGB BGM + BM Empty

FIGURE 4.4 Gross observation at 12 weeks postsurgery.

4.1.4 Discussion

The time of material degradation in vivo would last 3–6 months, depending on the implant site. MC based materials are active for bone regeneration and repairing the bone defect. During the healing process the material was fit together with trabecula and replaced step by step by new bone. MC based materials are active in the bone replacement process [2].

4.1.5 Conclusion

Implantation experiment showed that BonGold bone graft material is osteoconductive and can aid in bone repair by facilitating new bone regeneration.

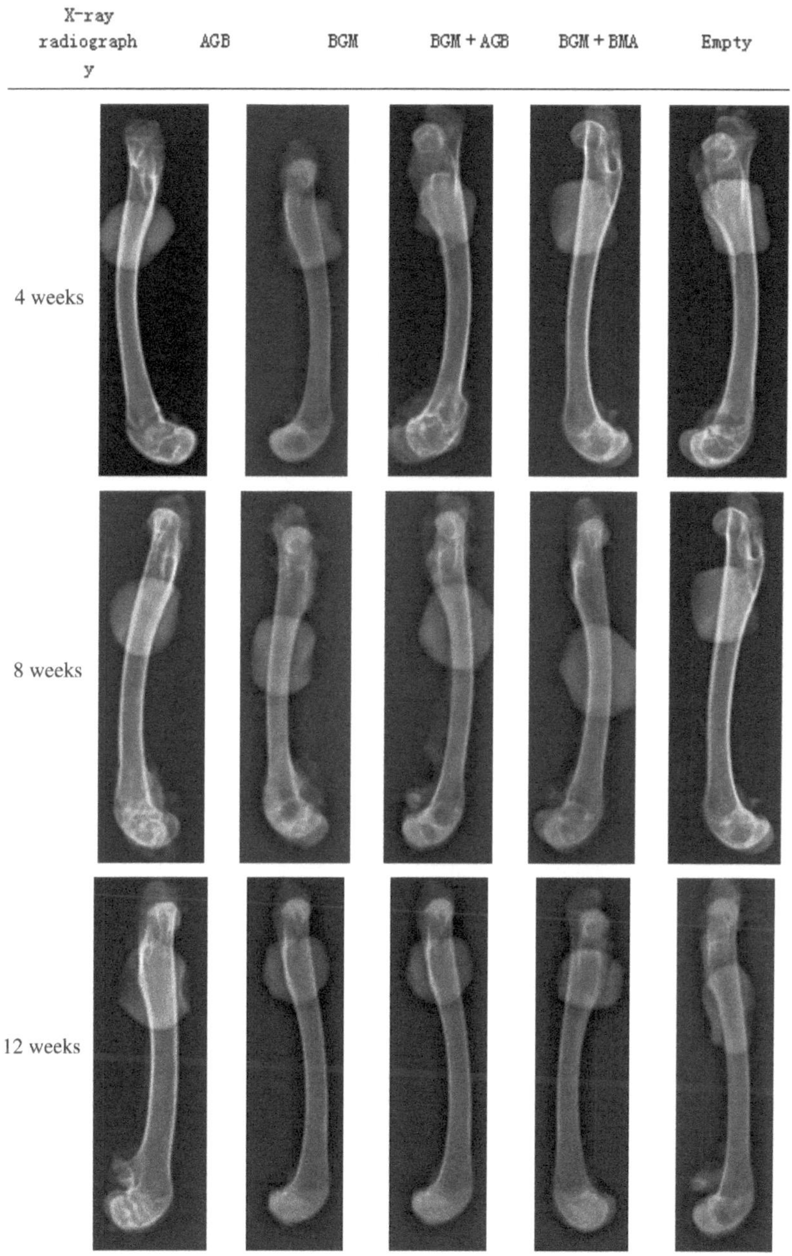

FIGURE 4.5 X-ray radiography demonstrated bone repair at 4, 8, and 12 weeks AGB (Autograft); BGM (Bongold™ Material); BMA (Bone Marrow).

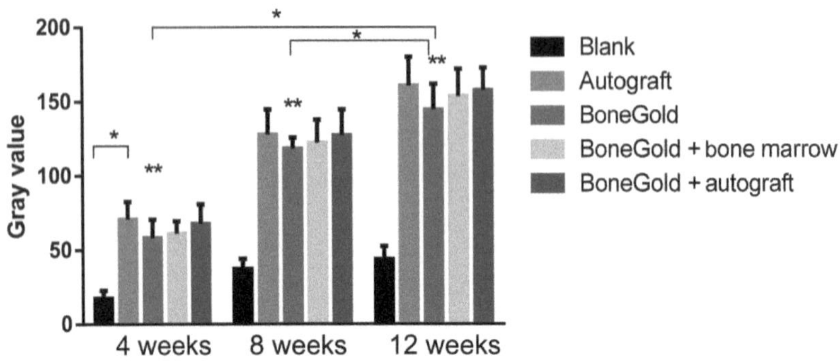

FIGURE 4.6 X-ray radiography gray values at 4, 8, and 12 weeks.
(Remark: *Gray value analysis, each group compared with their own by previous time point, $P < .01$ indicates statistically significant, **BGM group is not significantly different from other groups (e.g., AGB, BMG + BMA and BMG + AGB) $P > .05$).

4.2 BONE VOID FILLING ON FEMORAL CONDYLE DEFECT MODEL IN NEW ZEALAND WHITE RABBIT

4.2.1 Objective

To evaluate MC based materials filling properties on femoral condyle defect.

4.2.2 Study Method

4.2.2.1 Study Design

Sixty New Zealand rabbits (weight 2.5 kg, 3 months old) were taken for experiment. For each animal a cancellous bone defect (6 mm in diameter and 10 mm in depth) was created in the medial femoral condyles perpendicular to femur orientation using a dental drill with the condition of irrigation.

4.2.2.2 Grouping

All animals were divided randomly into experiment and control groups. For the control group, autograft bone (AGB) material was used in the positive group and no treatment for the negative control. There were three experiment groups; each group used BonGold (BG), BGM/BMA composites, and BGM/AGB composites respectively (Tables 4.1 and 4.2).

4.2.2.3 Study Materials

MC based materials was kept at room temperature. First they were soaked with bone marrow aspirate on the ratio of 1:1, and then mixed with autologous bone chips at a 2:1 ratio (e.g., 2 g MC based materials mixed with 1 g autologous bone chips).

TABLE 4.1 Study Design: Study Grouping

Group No.	Implants	Number of Rabbits	Time Point for Evaluation
1	Autograft (AGB)	3 rabbits in each group for each time point, 45 in total; other 15 rabbits for biomechanical tests (only for 12 weeks)	4, 8, 12 weeks
2	Bongold (BGM)		
3	BGM/BMA composites		
4	BGM/AGB composites		
5	Empty		

4.2.2.4 Study Methods

Animals were anesthetized with sumianxin via ear vein and one limb underwent lateral incision in the knee under sterile conditions. After removal of periosteum, the femoral condyle was exposed. A cancellous bone defects (6 mm in diameter and 10 mm in depth) was created in the medial femoral condyles perpendicular to femur orientation using a dental drill with the condition of irrigation. The defect was placed within the epiphysis, avoiding communication with the knee joint cavity and in the probe measurement care was taken to not penetrate opposite cortical bone. After debraiding, each defect was filled with different materials described above by press-fitting into defect site and the incision was subsequently closed. The wounds were bandaged without fixation. To avoid infection, penicillin G sodium salt was injected intramuscularly for 3 days postoperatively.

4.2.2.5 Study Observations

1. Gross observations:

   The gross observation was performed for 14 days postsurgery, and included feeding, wound healing, and limb activities. Gross observation of defect repair at necropsy was performed at the 4th, 8th, and 12th weeks.
2. Radiography imaging analysis:

   The rabbit were anesthetized with an intramuscular injection of sodium pentobarbital at the 4th, 8th, and 12th weeks postsurgery, their limbs were extirpated and examined using three-dimensional (3D) computed tomography (CT) reconstruction scan (GE Lightspeed Ultra 16, Milwaukee, Wisconsin); X-ray images were taken with X-ray machine (Siemens X-ray equipment, Siemens AG, Germany) from a

TABLE 4.2 Study Sites Per Animal and Analysis

Time	Number of Rabbits	Number of Sites Per Article (2 Sites/Per Animal)					Analysis		
		Empty	AGB	BGM	BGM + BMA	BGM + AGB	Histology	CT	Biomechanical
4 weeks	15	6	6	6	6	6	×	×	NA
8 weeks	15	6	6	6	6	6	×	×	NA
12 weeks	15	6	6	6	6	6	×	×	NA
12 weeks (Biomechanical)	15	6	6	6	6	6	NA	NA	×

distance of 100 cm (60 kVp and 300 mA) with an exposure time of 0.03 seconds. The radiographs were observed for the presence of new bone formation.

The radiographic gray value of the implantation area in the bone defect sites was measured using the pathological image analysis software (IPP 6.0).

3. Histological observation:

   The tested bone specimens were collected from the animals sacrificed on the 4th, 8th, and 12th postoperative days and a 1-cm-long piece of the femur including the defect site and normal bone on both sides was cut using a saw. Specimens were further cut into 3–4 mm-thick discs and then dehydrated by a graded series of ethanol (70%, 90%, and 100%). Subsequently the samples were decalcified in 10% formic acid. The specimens were processed for resin embedding and slicing used for H&E and Masson staining. The stained sections and bone formation were viewed under the optical microscope Olympus X71 (Olympus Optical Co. Ltd, Japan).

4. Biomechanical testing:

   By 12 weeks postsurgery, 3 femoral condyles of each group were shaped into cylindrical specimen (10 mm × 15 mm), were washed by physiological saline to help specimen hold in moisture and cooling state, and were frozen at −20°C. After unfreezing the tensile mechanical property was tested with mechanical tester (AG-IC 100kN SHIMADZU) and the crosshead speed was set at 0.5 cm/min. The stress–strain curve, tensile strength, and stiffness were recorded for analysis.

5. Statistical:

   Data analysis was performed by using Statistic Package for Social Science (SPSS). The *t*-test was performed by comparing two groups. *P*-value smaller than 0.05 was considered statistically significant.

4.2.3 Results and Discussions

4.2.3.1 Gross Observations

(1) Empty group: fragmented and was only filled with thin fibrous connective tissue without bone formation and calcification. (2) BG group: good integration of the implanted BG with the host bone tissue and the boundary of the two is obscured. (3) BG + BMA group: fully reunited bone defect in which the callus tissue bridged in the defect is ossified. (4) BG + AGB group: good integration of the implants with the host bone. (5) AGB group: fully repaired bone defect site where the boundary of the implants with the host bone very hard to discern.

4.2.3.2 *Radiography Imaging*

1. X-ray radiography imaging analysis
   a. At the 4th week, the border was well defined in the empty group with low gray value. There are high-density shadows in AGB and AGB + BGM group and the border became blurry. Meanwhile the gray value in BGM and BGM + BMA groups are higher than empty group. During the statistical analysis there is marked difference between empty group and the other four groups ($P < .01$) and no difference among the four groups ($P > .05$).
   b. At the 8th week, the gray value did not change in the empty group compared with the value in the 4th week, and no reduction in defect area. Meantime in the BGM group the gray value increased compared with the 4th week with reduction in the defect area. The other groups show similar results with the BGM group. The details are shown in the table.
   c. At the 12th week, the border of defect area in the AGB group was blurred. Similarly the BGM + BMA and BG + AGB groups showed good amount of new bone in the defect site and the border disappeared. An obvious reduction in defect area of BGM and BGM + BMA group can be seen. The details are shown in the table.
2. 3D-CT imaging analysis
   a. At the 4th week postsurgery, the autograft group had demonstrated greater amount of new bone in the defect site. The defect area in the groups of BGM, BGM + AGB and BGM + BMA are reduced obviously compared with the empty group.
   b. At the 8th week, the defect site in BGM, BGM + BMA, BGM + AGB reduced obviously compared with at 4 weeks. The AGB group had showed the greater advantage in recovery; only a little piece in the middle was covered by hypodense tissue.
   c. At the 12th week, there was a near rehabilitation in BGM, BGM + BMA, and BGM + AGB group, as compared with the empty group. A complete rehabilitation was found in the AGB group (Fig. 4.7, Table 4.3).

4.2.3.3 *Histological Observation*

1. Histological evaluation
   a. At 4th week, BG group demonstrated scattered new bone formation while some materials were still present in the center. There were collagen fibers and formation of trabeculae in porosity of materials. Some bony growth at the edge can be seen. There was predominantly inflammatory tissue and connective formation for empty defects.
   b. At 8th week, the BG group demonstrated mostly mature bone (MB), bone matrix, and connective tissue with little degradation product of materials, which show no difference with AGB group. Meanwhile in

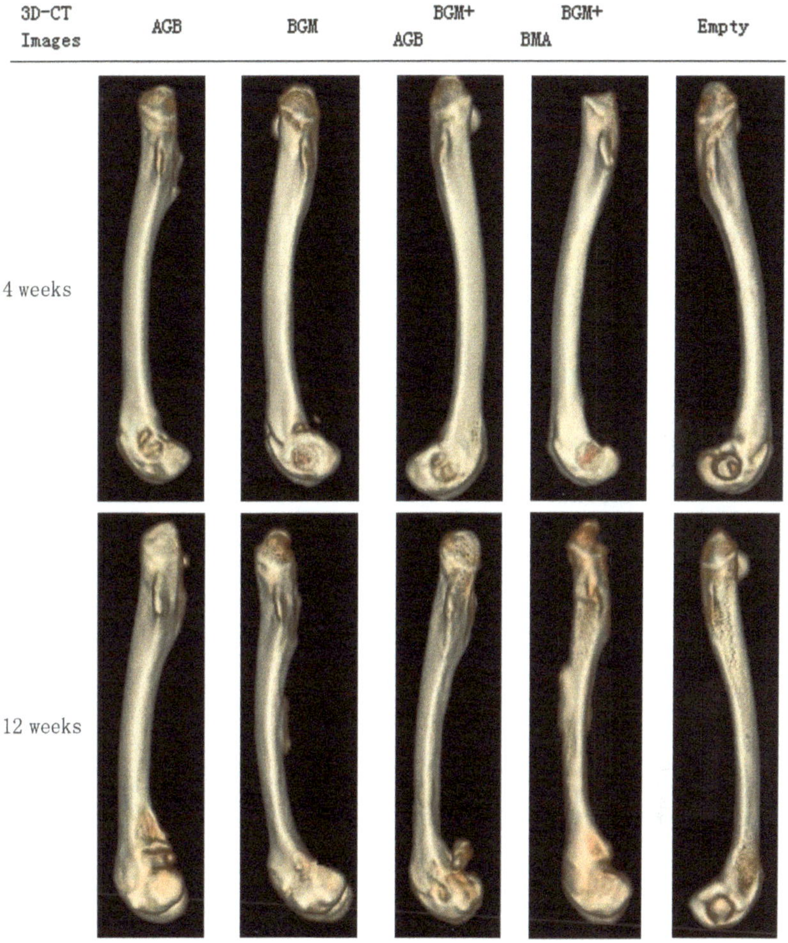

FIGURE 4.7 3D-CT images at 12 weeks.

TABLE 4.3 X-Ray Gray Value of Bone Repair at 4, 8, and 12 Weeks, Showing the Significant Difference ($P<.01$)

	Empty	AGB	BGM	BGM + BMA	BGM + AGB
4 weeks	17.4 ± 5.3	70.8 ± 11.8	58.3 ± 12.2	61.3 ± 8.3	67.5 ± 13.4
8 weeks	37.3 ± 6.7	127.4 ± 17.4	118.0 ± 7.6	122.1 ± 15.8	127 ± 17.8
12 weeks	43.7 ± 8.9	160.7 ± 13.3	144.6 ± 17.3	153.6 ± 14.4	157 ± 15.2

BG + BMA group the filling site was presented with new bone formation with almost total degradation. In the negative control group the void site was filled with collagen connective tissue with limited bone regeneration.

c. At 12th week, the defect sites in BG + AGB, BG and BG + BMA were covered by MB with degradation of void material and a good osseointegration was found with no clear border. By evaluation of new bone area and microvessel density there is no significant difference compared with AGB group. Negative control group presented limited bone regeneration (Figs. 4.8–4.11).

4.2.3.4 Mechanical Testing

In the 12th week postsurgery, mechanical testing was performed and the results are shown in the table. The summarized maximum load on the test group

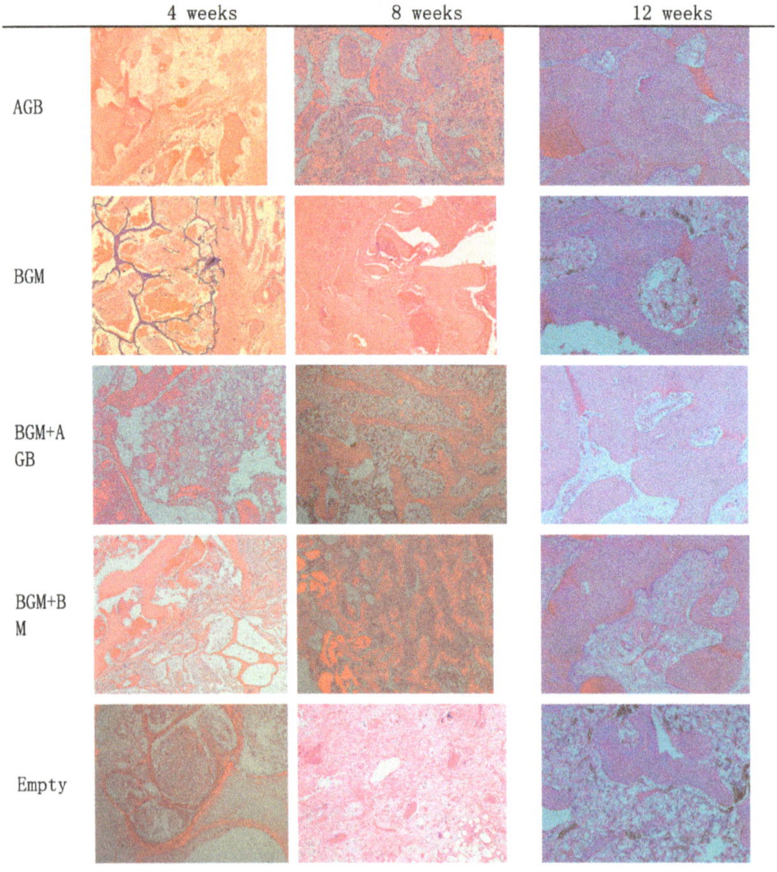

FIGURE 4.8 Histological observation in 4, 8, and 12 weeks postsurgery (HE staining, 40 ×).

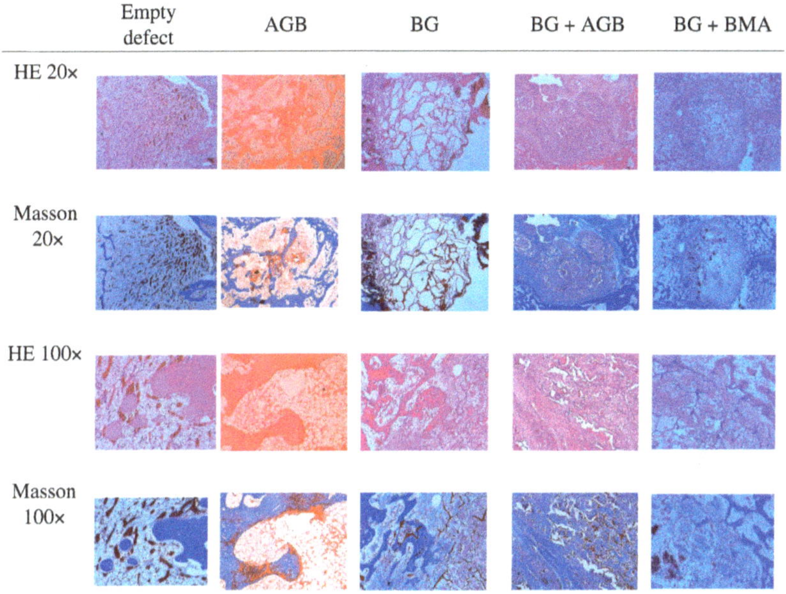

FIGURE 4.9 Histological observation at 12 weeks postsurgery (hematoxylin-eosin and Masson staining, 20 × /100 ×).

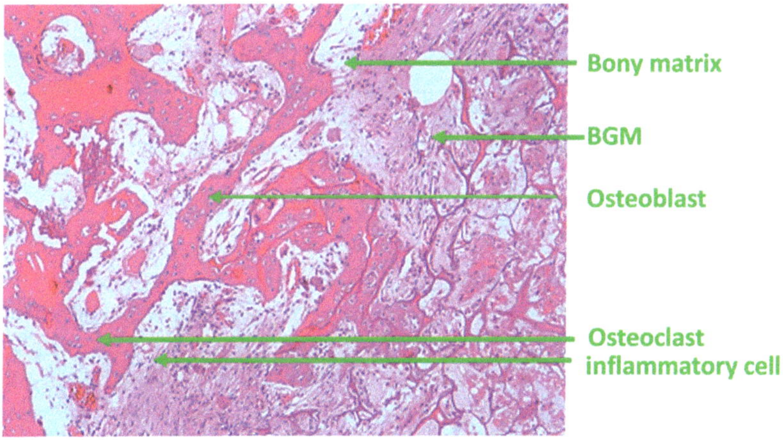

FIGURE 4.10 HE staining for bone repair of BG group (100 ×).

demonstrated that BG, BG + BMA, and BG + AGB group shared similar maximum load, which has significant different against negative control ($P < .05$).

4.2.4 Discussion

Many bone-grafting materials are used to repair bony defects. However each has specific disadvantages. Autogenous bone has been taken as the "gold

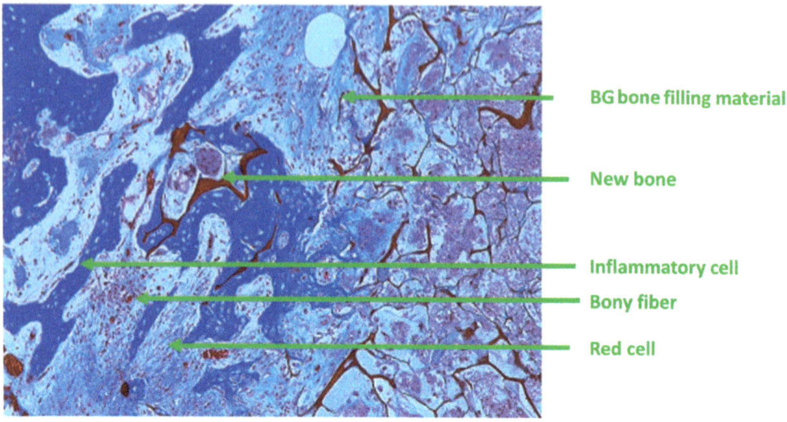

FIGURE 4.11 Masson staining for bone repair of BG group (100 ×).

standard" for filling bone void, but its disadvantages include limited quantity and extra surgery. Allograft can serve as bone grafting materials closer to autogenous bone, but it is controversial and may be associated with complications. These include a risk for disease transmission, and delayed incorporation with host bone.

Artificial bone substitute materials such as metal, ceramic, or polymer can also be used for clinical use. They have some shortcomings, such as lack of biocompatibility, poor efficacy, and not absorbable. MC based materials have similar ingredients and microstructure to human bone, and can serve for bone regeneration, in which it can be replaced by new bone by creeping substitution. In the experiment MC based materials show no difference to autogenous bone when mixed with bone marrow or autogenous bone.

4.2.5 Conclusions

In the New Zealand rabbit critical-size femoral condyle defect model, BG used either alone or in combination with bone marrow aspirate or AGB has shown similar effect compared with the autograft. During the experiment no animal showed metabolic disorder, and there was also no inflammation in the liver. It has demonstrated the safety and effectiveness of MC based materials. MC based materials are also comparable to autogenous bone as bone filling material (BFM). Hence the MC based materials are fit for bone defect repair.

4.3 LUMBAR INTERTRANSVERSE PROCESS SPINAL FUSION IN RABBITS [3]

4.3.1 Objective

To evaluate MC based materials filling properties on lumbar intertransverse fusion.

4.3.2 Study Design

4.3.2.1 Design

Sixty-four rabbits were randomly divided into four groups: autogenous cancellous bone (ACB) group, nanohydroxyapatite/collagen composite (Nano-HAC) group, autogenous bone mixed with Nano-HAC composite (ACB + Nano-HAC) and Nano-HAC composite with recombinant human BMP-2 (Nano-HAC + BMP-2). A transverse process of L5 and L6 was performed. Rabbits were killed at 2, 4, 6, and 10 weeks to qualitatively compare fusions achieved using radiography, manual palpation, and histology. Besides these methods, uniaxial tensile mechanical testing was also performed at 6 and 10 weeks.

4.3.2.2 Study Animals

Sixty-four mature female New Zealand rabbits (1 year old) were randomly divided into four groups: ACB group, Nano-HAC group, autogenous bone mixed with nano-HAC (ACB + Nano-HAC), and Nano-HAC with recombinant human BMP-2 (Nano-HAC + BMP-2). Two rabbits of each group were killed for radiography, manual palpation, and histology, whereas six rabbits of each group were killed at 6 and 10 weeks for radiography and manual palpation. Two of these were performed for histology and the other four rabbits for additional mechanical testing.

4.3.2.3 Materials

MC based materials and recombinant human BMP-2.

4.3.2.4 Methods

Rabbits were anesthetized by intramuscular injection of 0.1 mL/kg of compound ketamine injection. After being placed in the prone position, they were shaved, prepared with povidone-iodine, and draped in sterile fashion. A dorsal midline incision was made through the skin, followed by bilateral paramedian incisions through the lumbodorsal fascia. The intermuscular plane between multifidus and longissimus was developed to expose the transverse processes of L5 and L6. An electric burr was used to decorticate the transverse processes and expose cancellous bone. If the iliac crest bone was required, it was harvested by extending the fascial incisions over the posterior iliac crests. The iliac crest bone was morselized with a rongeur. All graft materials were placed between the decorticated transverse in the paraspinal bed. For ACB group, c.2–2.5 mL iliac crests were implanted for each site. For Nano-HAC group 2.5 mL material for each implant site. For ACB + Nano-HAC group the iliac bone was mixed with Nano-HAC in ratio 1:1, 2.5 mL for each side. For the Nano-HAC + BMP-2 group, the sterilized recombinant human bone morphogenetic protein (rhBMP-2) solution was dripped into the collagen just before implantation surgery. 3 mg thBMP-2 was combined with 2.5 mL Nano-HAC for each site.

4.3.2.5 Observation

1. Manual palpation:

   The fused motion segment and the adjacent nonoperated motion segment (L4-L5, L5-L6, and L6-L7) were manually palpated. Each motion segment was graded as fused or not fused, based on the presence of any motion between the vertebral bodies.

2. Radiographic analysis

   X-ray posterior radiographs were taken shortly before the rabbit was killed. X-ray was taken under anesthesia to observe repair condition in every group animal. The X-ray was taken at 55 kv, 2.8 mA, for 33 ms. To observe the bone trabecular growth at the bone grafting site, continuous bone trabecular growth was considered as fusion, while other cases were considered as non-fusion.

3. Histology

   All of the harvested tissue was radiographed with a radiograph apparatus, fixed with 10% neutral formalin, and embedded in mixture of Grocery Manufacturers Association (GMA) and Butyl Methacrylate (BMA). Sections (5 μm in thickness) were cut, stained with H&E, and modified with Goldner's trichrome. They were then examined under an OLYMPUS light microscope.

4. Biomechanical testing

   Animals were killed and the lumbar spine (L3-L7) was removed intact from the bodies. The soft tissue was removed from the ventral side and from between the spinous processes. The L5-L6 and L3-L4 motion segments were separated from the remainder of the specimen. The intervertebral discs were sectioned. The load was applied to L5-L6 motion segment via two steel rods and drilled from anterior to posterior through the vertebral bodies. The tensile mechanical property was tested with a type CSS-1101 mechanical tester and the crosshead speed was set at 0.5 cm/min. The stress–strain curve was recorded by software CSS-4400. The tensile strength was determined as the maximum point of the stress–strain curve and the elastic modulus was calculated a slope of the initial linear portion of the stress–strain curve. STATA was used to analyze the data for each of the mechanical testing parameters.

4.3.3 Result

4.3.3.1 Manual Palpation

For the ACB group, no fusion was found at 2nd week, 1 fusion at 4th week; 4 fusions at 6th week, and 4 fusions at 10th week. For Nano-HAC group, no fusion at the 2nd, 4th, 6th, and 10th weeks; for ACB + Nano-HAC group, no fusion was found at 2nd and 4th weeks, and3 fusions at 6th week and 10th week. For Nano-HAC + BMP-2 group, no fusion was found at 2nd and 4th weeks, 4 fusions at 6th week and 5 fusions at 10th week.

TABLE 4.4 Maximum Load of the Sample in 12th Week Postsurgery

Group	Maximum Load (KN)
Empty	0.132 ± 0.005
AGB	0.334 ± 0.014
BGM	0.296 ± 0.013
BGM + BMA	0.307 ± 0.016
BGM + AGB	0.311 ± 0.012

All rabbits tolerated the surgical procedure well. Two rabbits in ACB group died on days 9, 10 postsurgery and were replaced with other animals. Three animals had paralysis in left lower limb. One rabbit in ACB + Nano-HAC group suffered paralysis in right lower limb but recovered within 48 hours postsurgery. Possible reasons would be damage to the waist sacral nerve underneath the iliac. After measurement there is no further paralysis in the other rabbits. There were five superficial infections, which caused no effect for the experiment and another infection was found in the left site in an animal in the Nano- hydroxyapatite + BMP-2 group. Two rabbits in the ACB group died from massive hemorrhage or other intraoperative complications while the other animals showed good tolerated to the surgical procedure (Table 4.4).

4.3.3.2 Radiograph Observation

In the ACB group there is some callus at 2 weeks and more discontinuous callus formation at 4 weeks. Continuous callus was found in 4 rabbits at 6 weeks and 5 rabbits at 10 weeks (shown in Fig. 4.12A). For the Nano-HAC group there is no callus among all rabbits at 2, 4, 6 weeks; some callus can be found at 10 weeks. No significant differences were found between ACB + Nano-HAC group and ACB group at 2, 4 weeks (shown in Fig. 4.12B). Continuous callus was found in 3 rabbits at 6 weeks and 4 rabbits at 10 weeks (shown in Fig. 4.12C). In the Nano-HAC + BMP-2 group, more discontinuous callus was found at 2 weeks. Continuous callus was found in 1 rabbit at 4 weeks; 5 animals at 6 weeks, and 6 at 10 weeks (shown in Fig. 4.12D).

4.3.3.3 Histologic Analysis

ACB group: at 2nd week, new bone was formed in the parapophysis but not in central vertebra. A large quantity of new bone was found in the

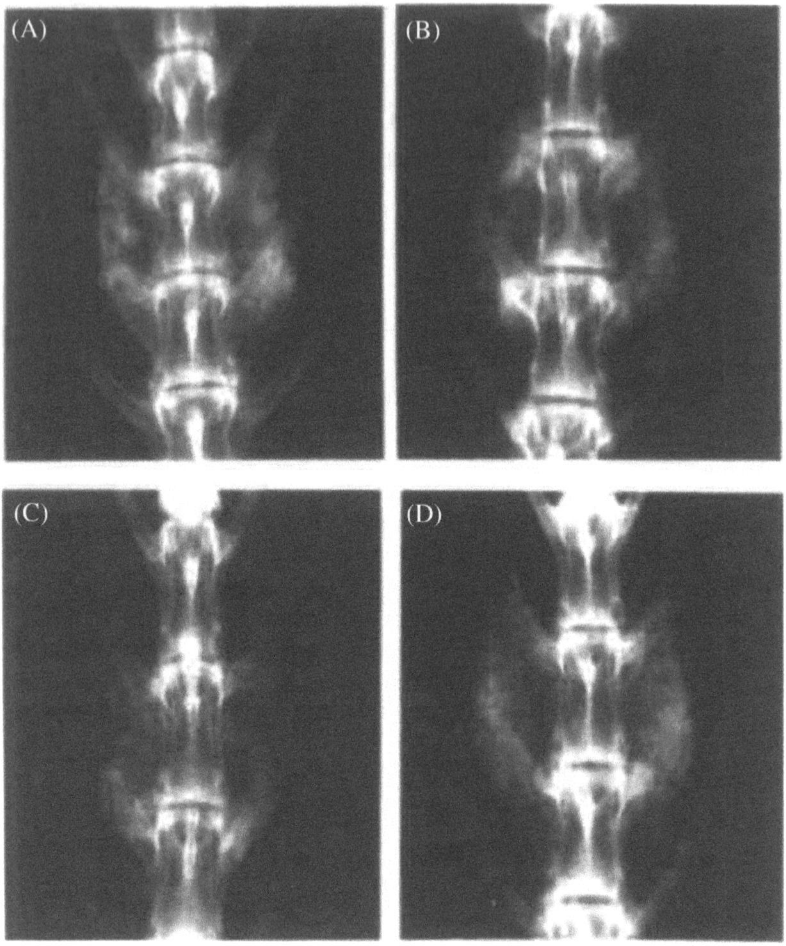

FIGURE 4.12 (A) Autogenous cancellous bone 10 W; (B) nano-hydroapatite/collagen (Nano-HAC) 10 W; (C) ACB + Nano-HAC 10 W; (D) Nano-HAC + rhBMP-2 10 W.

parapophysis at 4th week, mostly by endochondral ossification with some intramembranous ossification. There is new bone with increase in connective tissue in the central vertebra. At 6th weeks higher percentage of new bone matrix appeared and the mature fibrous tissue was formed by fiber collagen. Also there are many collagen fibers found in the central vertebra and obviously bone formation around implant materials. At the 10th week, myelopoiesis with reduced connective tissue was found in parapophysis. Formed mineralized nodules and new osteoid tissue was found in the central vertebra (Fig. 4.13A).

Nano-HAC group: at the 2nd week, new bone was formed in parapophysis and some cells were growing into the pores of Nano-HAC material. New

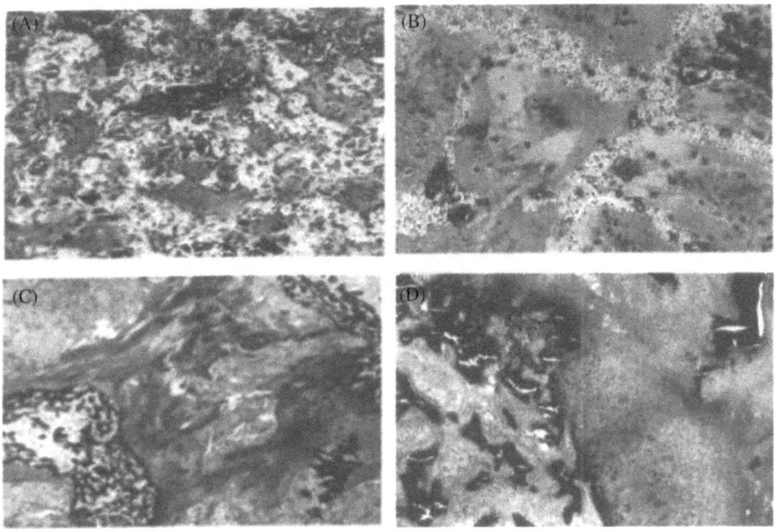

FIGURE 4.13 (A) Autogenous cancellous bone 4 W. (B) nano-hydroapatite/collagen (Nano-HAC) 6 W. (C) ACB + Nano-HAC 6 W. (D) Nano-HAC + rhBMP-2 2 W.

bone was formed around Nano-HAC filling material. At 4th week large quantity of new bone was found in parapophysis, and Nano-HAC material had degraded and was surrounded by fiber tissue. The cells, included polykaryocytes, osteoblasts, and fibroblasts were growing into the pores. They degraded the material and hydroxyapatite crystals were deposited. New bony matrix was formed. A similar result was found in central vertebra besides reduced bony matrix. At 6th week lots of cells like polykaryocytes, osteoblasts, and fibroblasts were found in the pores of materials and the material was degraded further. More hydroxyapatite crystals can be found with more new bony matrix. At 10th week more bony matrix can be found either in central vertebra or edge with mature fiber tissue. More cells can be found in pores. More degradation of material can be found but it is not completely degraded (Fig. 4.13B).

ACB + Nano-HAC group: it showed no significant difference compared with the group ACB and Nano-HAC at 2nd, 4th, 6th, and 10th weeks (Fig. 4.13C).

Nano-HAC + BMP-2 group: at 2nd week, the Nano-HAC material was surrounded by fiber tissue and a quick degradation has been shown with formation of new bony matrix. There were few cells in the pores. At the 4th week, more bony matrix can be found among Nano-HAC material and it has become mature. There are a large number of cells growing into the pores, the particles further degradation, visible in large quantities Nano hydroxyapatite crystal. At 6th week all bony matrix had become mature. Proliferation and maturation of fibrous tissue can be found. More cells in pores showed more degradation. At 10th week more bony matrix, more cells in pores, and further degradation can be found. There was only a little Nano- hydroxyapatite material left (Fig. 4.13D).

4.3.3.4 Mechanical Strength

For the details refer to Figs. 4.14–4.17. It showed no significant differences between groups ACB, ACB + ACB + Nano-HAC and Nano-HAC + BMP-2,

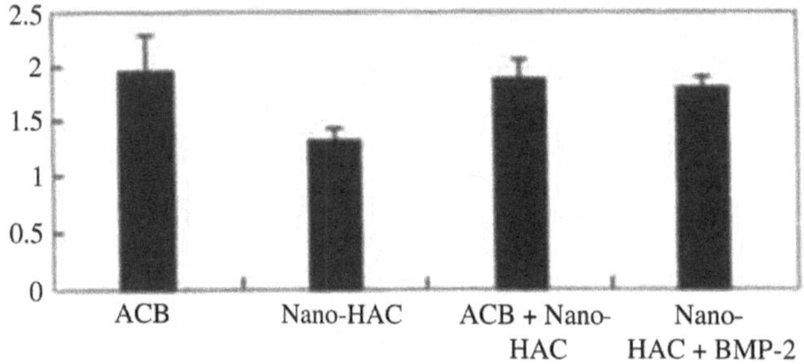

FIGURE 4.14 Max strength for each group at 6 weeks.

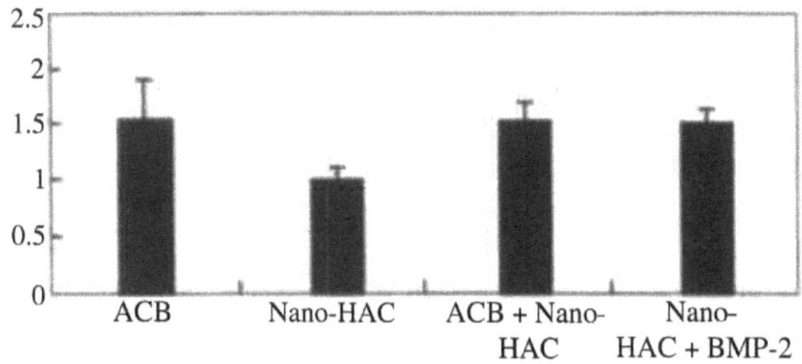

FIGURE 4.15 Stiffness for each group at 6 weeks.

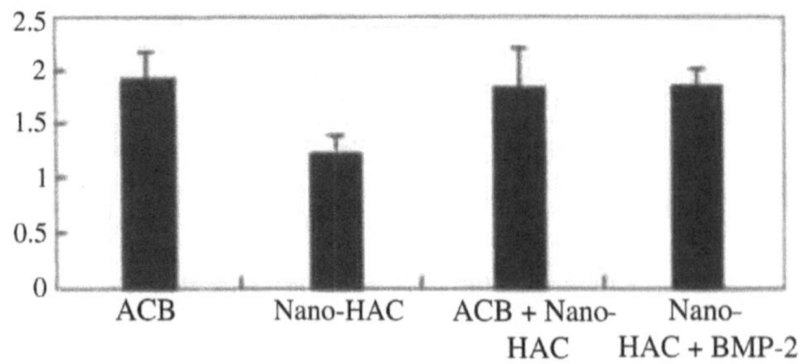

FIGURE 4.16 Max strength for each group at 10 weeks.

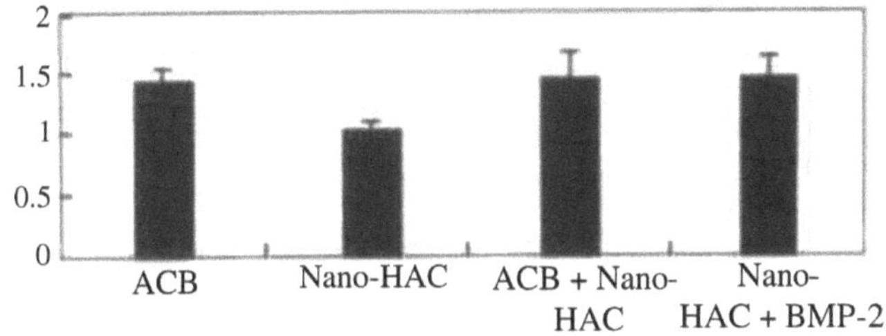

FIGURE 4.17 Stiffness for each group at 6 and 10 weeks.

with significant level set at 5%. The strength and the stiffness of group Nano-HAC were lower than the other four groups.

4.3.4 Discussion

The bone grafting materials can only serve as scaffold materials due to lack of osteoinductive and osteoconductive components. Two weeks after implantation of MC based materials, cells including polykaryocytes, osteoblasts, and fibroblasts were growing into the pores. They degraded the material and hydroxyapatite crystals were deposited. New bony matrix was formed. At 4th, 6th, and 10th weeks more cells have grown and more fibroblasts were found in the pores of materials and degraded the material further. More hydroxyapatite crystals can be found with more new bony matrix. The experiment has indicated that MC based materials have fast biodegradability, fine bone-bending ability, high performance osteoconductivity, and are easy to use for new bone formation.

4.3.5 Conclusion

The nanohydroxyapatite/collagen composite is a promising bone replacement substitute that has quickly biodegradability, fine bone-bending ability, high performance osteoconductivity, and is easy to use for new bone formation.

4.4 POSTEROLATERAL SPINAL FUSION IN RABBIT MODEL

4.4.1 Objective

The purpose of the study is to investigate the safety, effectiveness, biocompatibility, and veterinary clinical use of MC based materials using the New Zealand white rabbit spine fusion model; and to evaluate the potential events in human clinical use, minimize the risk in clinical trial, and develop the clinical trial protocol.

TABLE 4.5 Study Design

Group	Lumbar Level	Time-Point (weeks)			Rabbits
Empty (negative control)	L4/5 (or L5/6)	4	8	12	15
Autograft (positive control)		4	8	12	15
BG alone		4	8	12	15
BG + BMA		4	12	12	15
BG + AGB		4	12	12	15

4.4.2 Study Design

4.4.2.1 Design

A total of 75 New Zealand white rabbits were utilized for the study of MC based materials' safety, effective, biocompatibility. The animals were divided into five groups and four groups were treated with MC based materials alone and in combination with autograft and bone marrow aspirate compared with autograft alone, and outperformed decortication alone with no graft material. The study design is outlined in Table 4.5. Animals were euthanized at 4, 8, and 12 weeks after surgery for analysis and gross evaluation at preliminary stage, (i.e., radiological method consisted of X-ray analysis and micro-CT scanning) was conducted to measure bone formation around implants. Afterwards, histologic and biochemical evaluations were performed to study the fusion at the end of the 4th, 8th, and 12th weeks.

4.4.2.2 Materials

MC based materials.

4.4.2.3 Methods

Twenty four hours before surgery the animals were prohibited of feeding. The animals were anesthetized for surgery. A midline 6 cm incision was made in the skin, and the intermuscular plane between the multifidus and longissimus muscles was bluntly incised to expose the L5 and L6 transverse processes. An electric burr was used to decorticate the transverse processes and expose cancellous bone, make a slotting with size 20 mm × 3 mm × 3 mm. The filling materials (autologous, BG alone, or with bone marrow aspirate/autologous) were placed between the transverse processes in the paraspinal bed (1.5 cc per side). In the empty group, no graft materials were placed between the transverse processes. At 4, 8, and 12 weeks after surgery, routine inspection was performed.

4.4.2.4 Observation

1. Clinical gross observations

   Observe the animal, wound healing, hematoma, effusion and infection, and the material status after implant.
2. Histological observation

   X-ray image analysis was performed at 4, 8, and 12 weeks after surgery to assess fusion site integrity.
3. Histological evaluation

   Access the interface between material and host bone; the in-growth of new bone; vascularization, inflammatory and degradation of material.

4.4.3 Results

4.4.3.1 Clinical Gross Observations

All animals completed their designated in-life term respectively in good health and without incident. All of the incisions and tissues were found to be well-healed and there was no evidence of infection or any adverse tissue reaction to the implant materials in any instance.

4.4.3.2 Histological Observation

1. X-ray radiography: no significant differences were found between group AGB, BG + BMA, and BG + AGB, with significance level set at 5%. However, BG group had significant difference from the other three groups. After mixing with AGB or BMA, BG showed a slightly higher fusion rate than BG alone. This has been shown in Fig. 4.18.
2. 3D-CT imaging analysis: 3D-CT images are shown in Fig. 4.2. Four weeks postsurgery in the group BG, BG + BMA and BG + AGB there were still boundaries between new bone and the host bone. The autograft group had demonstrated greater amount of new bone in the fusion site. The empty treatment group has very minimal bone fusion. Twelve weeks postsurgery showed complete bone fusion for the group ABG, BG, BG + BMA, and BG + AGB. Whereas the empty group did not show any fusion (Fig. 4.19).

4.4.3.3 Histological Observation

As shown as Fig 4.3, at 4th weeks postsurgery, while there were predominantly inflammatory tissue and connective tissue formation in the empty group; trabecular bone regeneration within bone matrix and revascularization had already occurred in the autograft implanted fusion site. BG group demonstrated scattered new bone formation while some materials were still

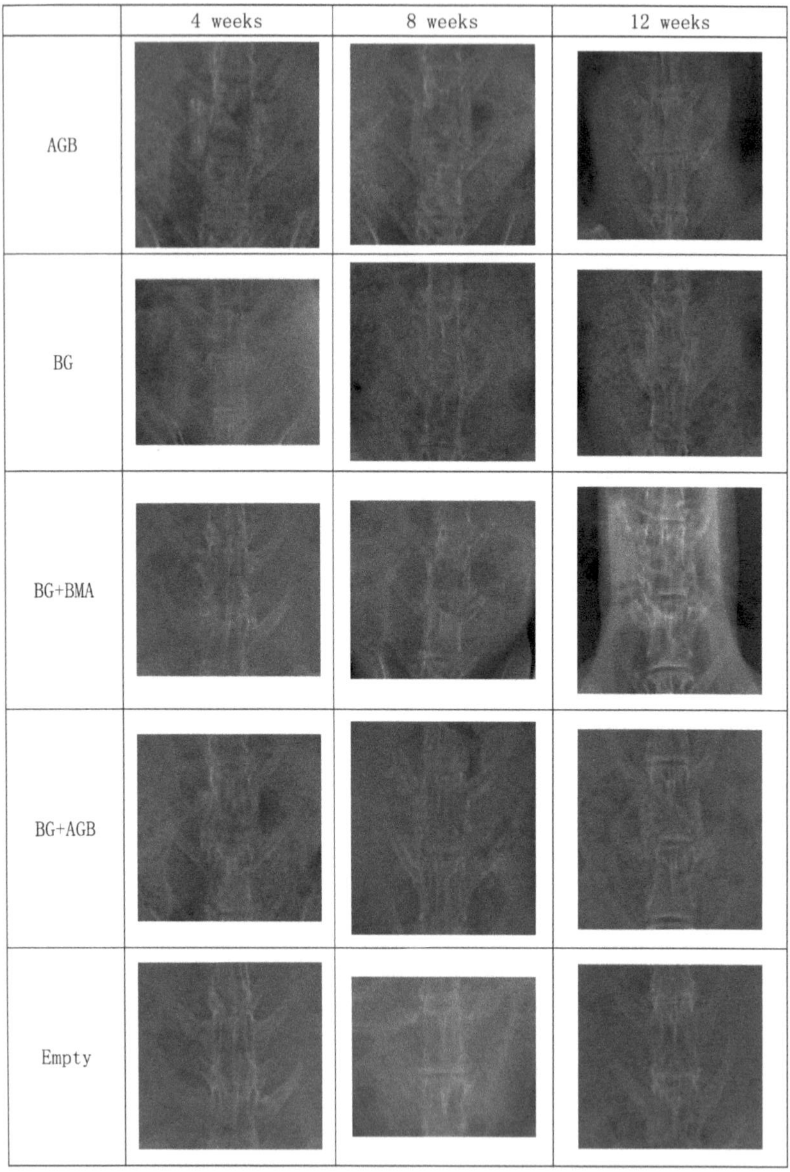

FIGURE 4.18 X-ray radiography.

present. At 8 weeks postsurgery, in the empty group there was presence of osteoblasts and osteoclasts, but no bone marrow revascularization and reperfusion. Whereas other groups demonstrated new bone formation (Fig. 4.20).

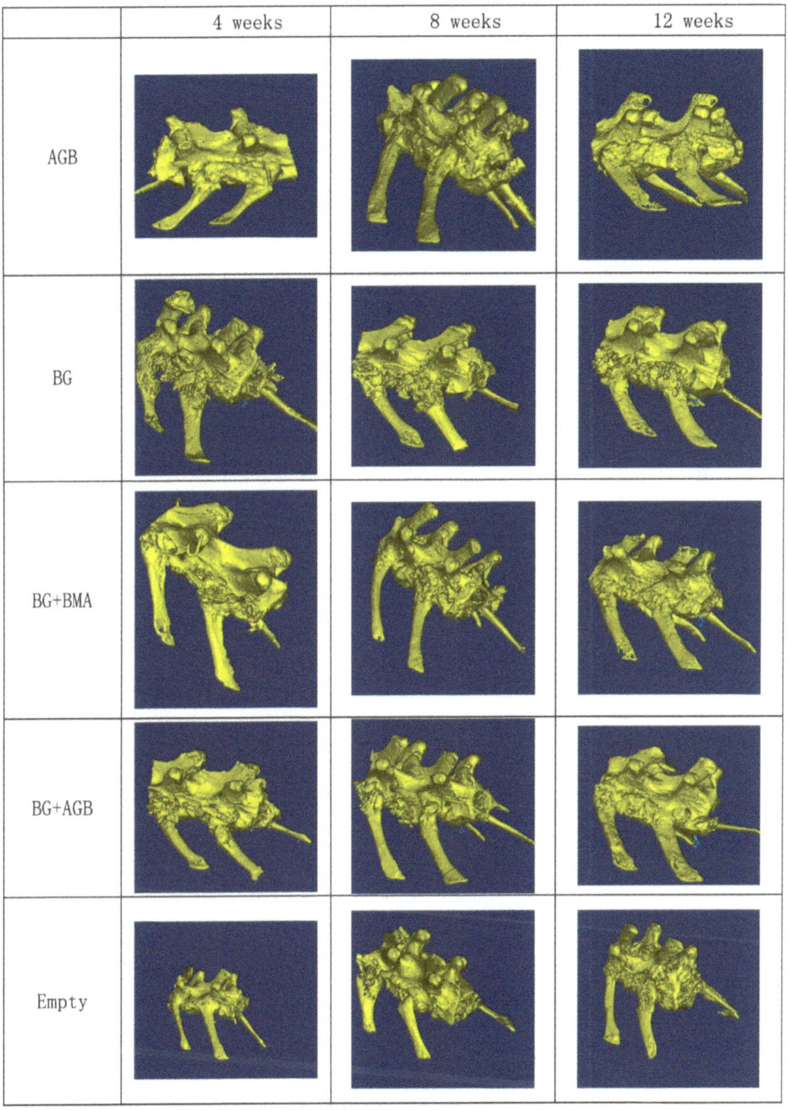

FIGURE 4.19 3D-CT images.

4.4.4 Conclusions

MC based materials can be used for bone defect. Compared with positive control, there is no significant difference.

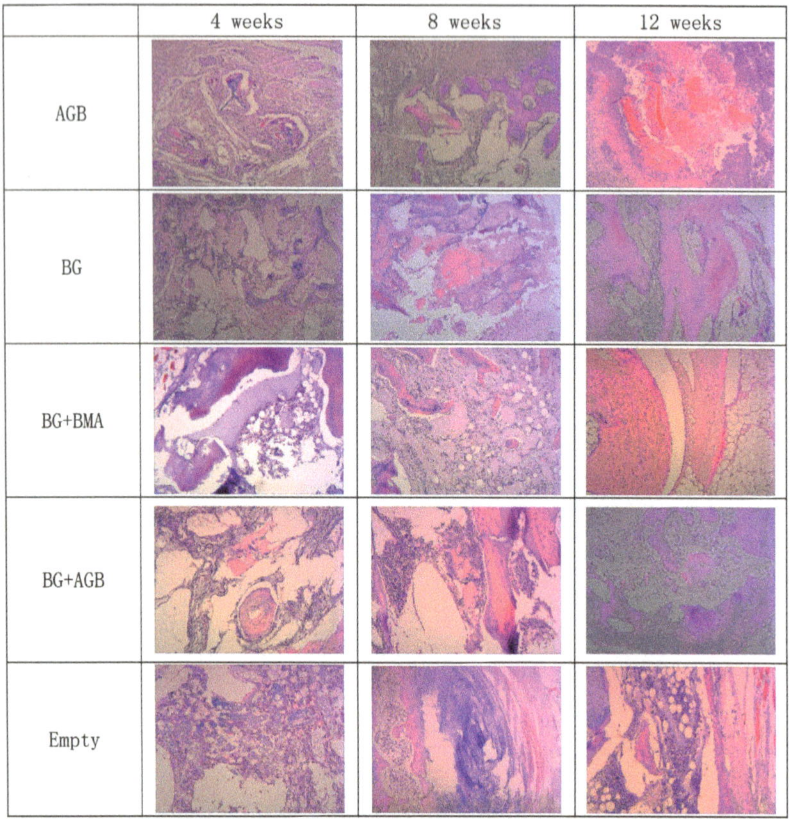

FIGURE 4.20 Images of HE staining.

4.5 THE BONE REPAIRING CAPABILITY OF CALVARIAL DEFECTS IN RATS

4.5.1 Experiment Purpose

To explore the effect of MC on skull repair in rats.

4.5.2 Testing Method

4.5.2.1 Experimental Scheme

The skull defect (5 mm in diameter) was established on the right side of the rat skull, which did not damage the dura mater, and MC was implanted for the repair of cranial bone.

4.5.2.2 Methods the Experiment Groups

The experiment was divided into two groups. The experimental group was implanted with MC, and the blank group was not implanted with any materials.

4.5.2.3 Experimental Materials

Mineralized collagen.

4.5.2.4 Experimental Methods

The skull defect (5 mm in diameter) was established on the right side of the rat skull, which did not damage the dura mater, and MC was implanted for the repair of cranial bone.

4.5.2.5 Experimental Observation

1. Imaging observations

   X-ray and CT scan were performed at 4, 8, and 12 weeks after surgery.
2. Histological observation

   The histological observation of the defect area was performed at 4, 8, and 12 weeks after surgery.

4.5.3 Experimental Results

4.5.3.1 Imaging Analysis

Micro-CT and X-ray films were observed at 4, 8, and 12 weeks after surgery. In the experimental group, the new bone tissue grew along the pore of MC, and the defect site was occupied gradually by the MC. In the blank group, there were no obvious signs of healing, and no obvious changes in the shape of the defect (Fig. 4.21).

4.5.3.2 Histological Observation

Four weeks after the surgery, a large amount of fibrous tissue was inserted into the biomimetic MC material to occupy the pores of the material. Eight weeks after surgery, there was a large amount of new bone tissue in the material. In the 12 weeks after the surgery, there was a large amount of mature new bone tissue in the area of skull repair, and bone healing was achieved in the skull defect. However, only a small amount of fibrous scar tissue was formed in the blank control group, and no obvious signs of osteogenesis were observed (Figs. 4.22 and 4.23).

4.5.4 Discussion

Biomimetic MC has similar composition and microstructure to natural bone, and its biggest advantage is nutrition and metabolic waste exchanging and transfering by bone tissue network channel composed of the newly formed blood vessels and bone tubular structure, which is involved in the metabolism of human body normal process. This study showed that the MC can be used for good repair of rat skull defects.

Imaging observations		Mineralized collagen group	Blank control group
4 weeks after surgery	Computed tomography scan	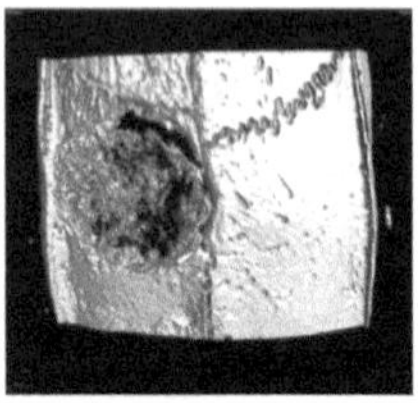	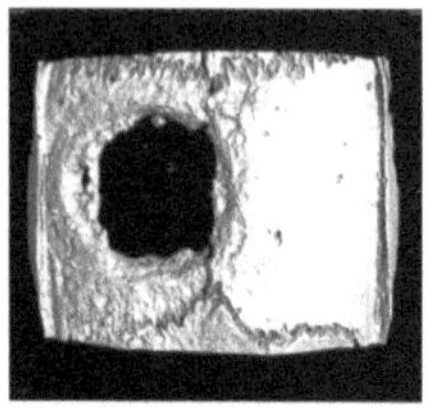
	X ray film	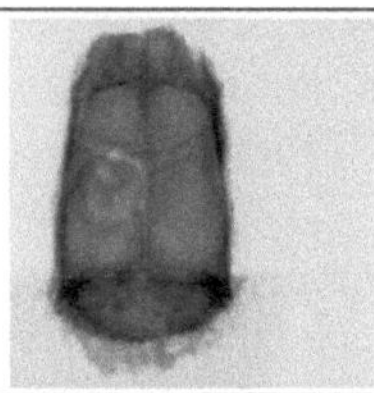	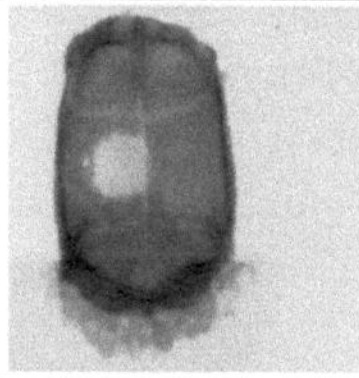
8 weeks after surgery	Computed tomography scan	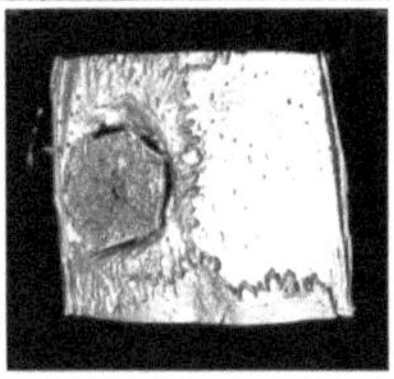	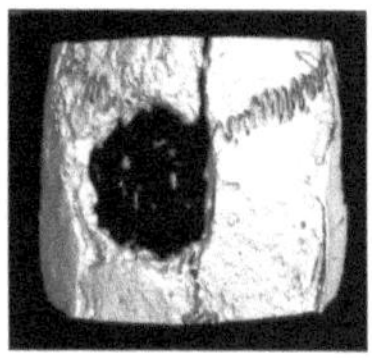
	X ray film	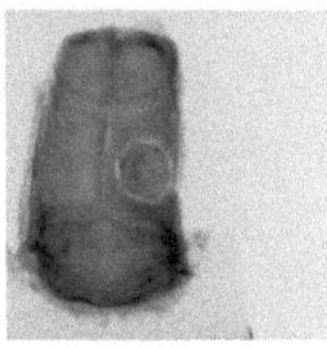	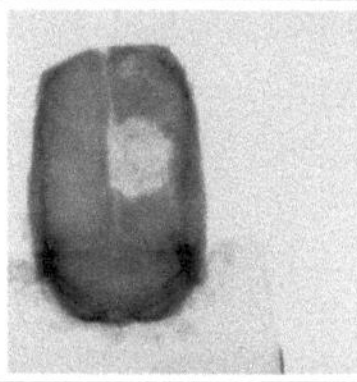
12 weeks after surgery	Computed tomography scan	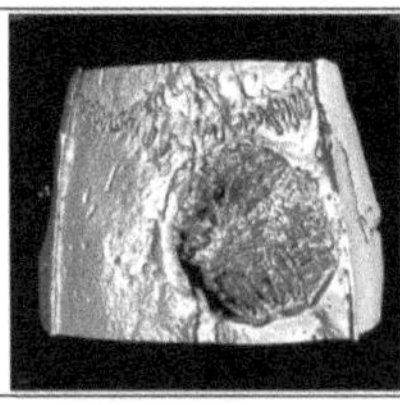	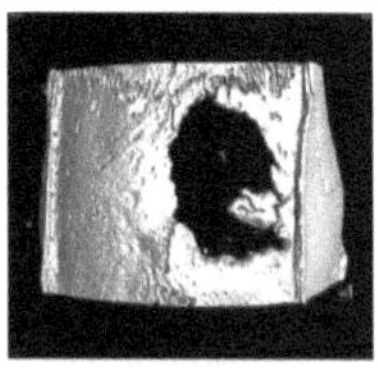
	X ray film	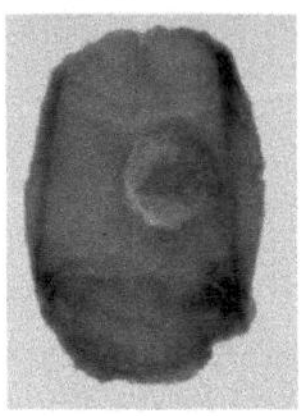	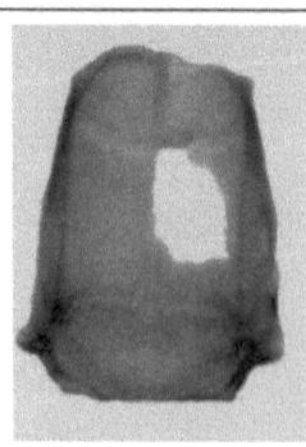

FIGURE 4.21 Imaging observation of 4, 8, and 12 weeks after surgery.

Histological observation	Mineralized collagen group	Blank control group
4 weeks after surgery	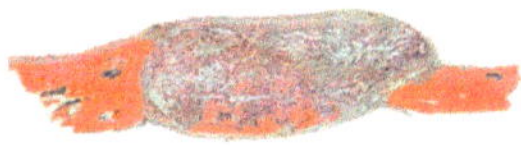	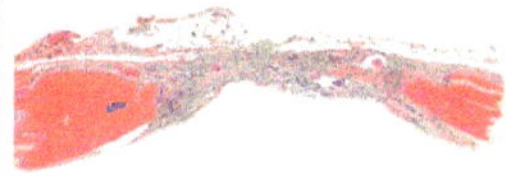
8 weeks after surgery	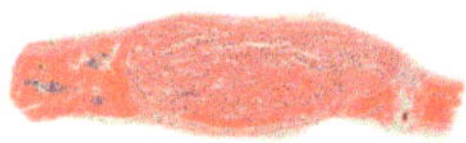	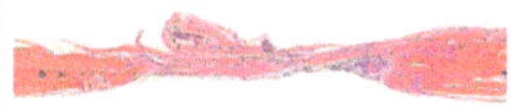
12 weeks after surgery	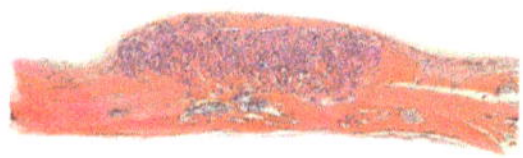	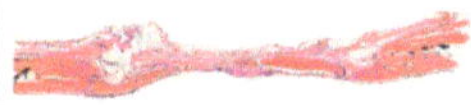

FIGURE 4.22 Histological observation of 4, 8, and 12 weeks after surgery.

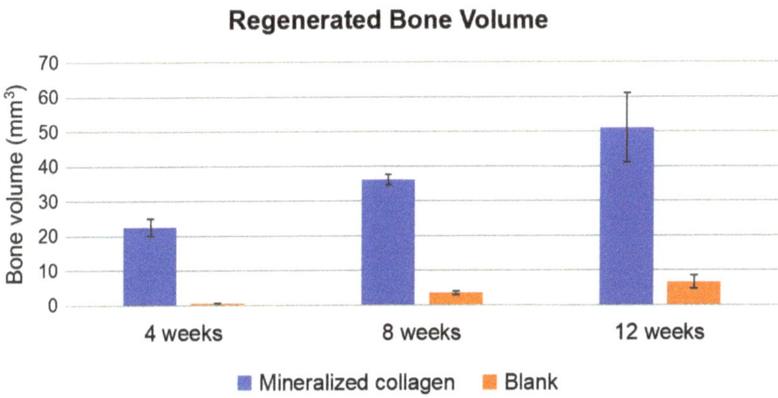

FIGURE 4.23 The newly formed bone mass 4, 8, and 12 weeks after surgery.

4.5.5 Conclusion

The MC material can repair the skull defect well, and the repair effect is good.

4.6 CRANIAL BONE REGENERATION IN DEVELOPING SHEEP [4]

4.6.1 Experiment Purpose

The effect of MC for the repair of large cranial bone defects in a developing animal was investigated by animal experiment.

4.6.2 Testing Method

4.6.2.1 Experimental Scheme

A critical-sized cranial bone defect (3 cm in diameter) model was used to evaluate the bone regeneration under the bone materials repair. Eight healthy one-month-old sheep were used in this study. The sheep were randomly divided into three groups of two animals each: defect without implantation (blank group), MC implantation (MC group), and titanium mesh implantation (Ti-mesh group). The bone regeneration ability was evaluated by visual observation, histological sections, and so on.

4.6.2.2 Methods: The Experiment Groups

The sheep were randomly divided into three groups: Ti-mesh group, MC group, and blank control group.

4.6.2.3 Experimental Materials

MC material, Ti-mesh.

4.6.2.4 Experimental Methods

Under general anesthesia by the injection of 3% sodium pentobarbital (30 mg/kg weight), the sheep were shaved and the incisions were made upon the calvarias with the periosteum partially removed to expose the cranial bones. A 30-mm-diameter round defect in the center of calvaria was then drilled by bone drill as well as rongeur forceps, keeping the dura mater intact. After the implantation of MC, or Ti-mesh, the wound was sutured. The MC and Ti-mesh were fixed on the defects by direct suture, plastic connection pieces, and screws, respectively. After the surgeries, 1,600,000 IU penicillin was injected intramuscularly to the sheep once a day for 5 days (Fig. 4.24).

4.6.2.5 Experimental Observation

1. Gross observation

   The physical and mental status of animals after implantation were observed.

2. Imaging observations

   Computed tomography (CT) scans were taken immediately postsurgery and 3 months after the operation to get 3D reconstructed images through which the status of cranium regeneration could be observed.

3. Histological observation

   Samples of calvarial bone containing both the implants and surrounding original cranial bone were harvested at 3 months after operation for histological evaluation.

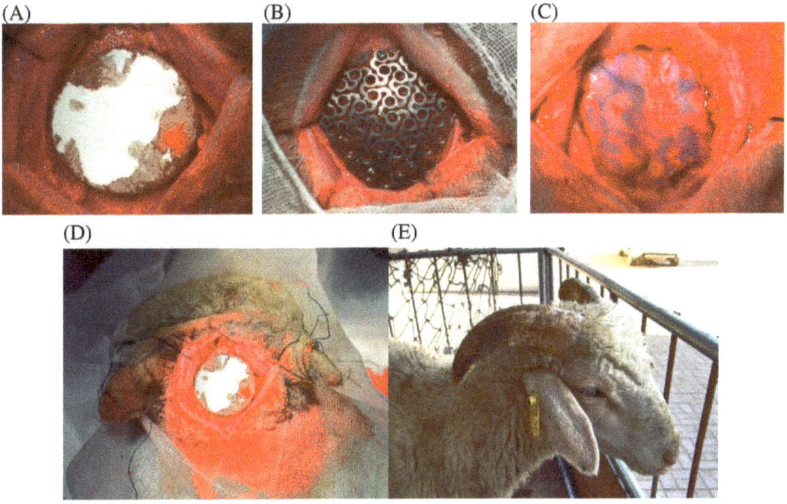

FIGURE 4.24 Implantation process and follow-up of sheep skull. (A) Experimental group. (B) Ti-mesh group. (C) Blank control group. (D) Implantation of the minerlized collagen in the experiment. (E) 3 months after the surgery.

4.6.3 Experimental Results

4.6.3.1 Gross Observation

After the operation, the sheep maintained a good mental state, and the rapid growth is shown in Fig. 4.24.

4.6.3.2 Imaging Observation

At 3 months after surgeries, the CT 3D reconstruction images revealed that the skull perimeters of all the experimental sheep increased dramatically, indicating the rapid growth of the baby sheep. The round defect in the blank group could still be seen only with a little new bone formation along the edge of the defect. a mass of bone regenerated at the defect position and substituted the MC scaffold (Fig. 4.25). Blood was collected around the surgical area 3 months after surgery, and the expression of osteogenic related factors in the blood was compared (Fig. 4.26).

4.6.3.3 Histological Observation

Fig. 4.27 showed the histological assessment of the cranial bone samples from pMC group at 3 months postoperation with Masson's trichrome and H&E staining, respectively. The histology images confirmed the bone restoration of the defect site as observed in the previous CT images. It can be seen that the new bone infiltrated throughout the porous MC scaffold so as to make the scaffold disassembled into pieces accompanying its

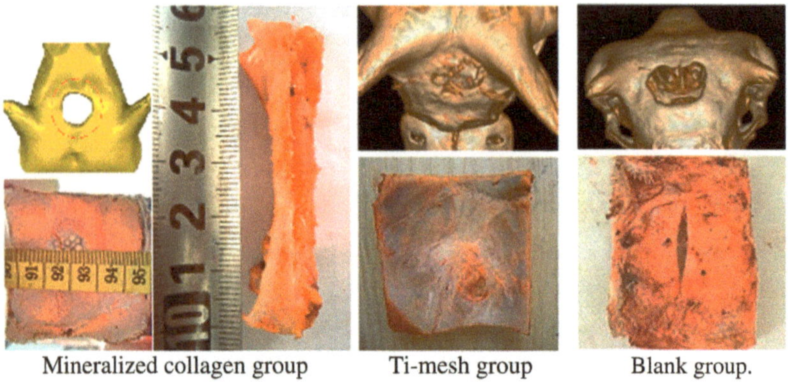

FIGURE 4.25 CT 3D reconstructed images at 3 months postoperation.

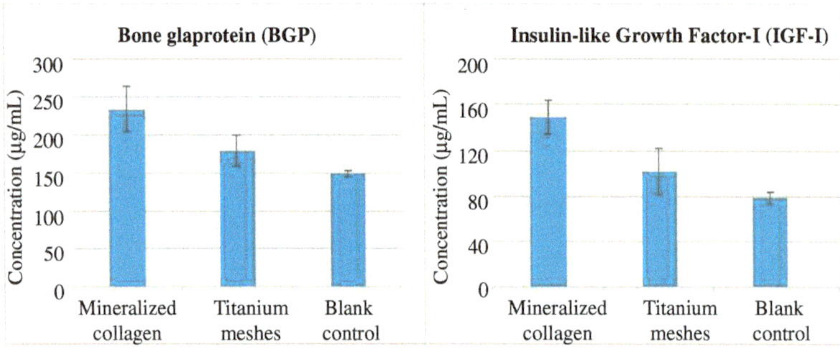

FIGURE 4.26 Bone defect healing contrast.

biodegradation. The tissue stained red indicated MB, whereas the tissue dyed blue represented immature nascent bone (IB).

4.6.4 Discussion

Skull reconstruction remains a great challenge for infants and young children whose skulls are in a period of rapid growth. Because current cranioplasty materials will restrict the growth of the surrounding bone in the growing craniofacial skeleton, thereby leading to the risk of deformation of the skull, there's still a widespread controversy on the timing of surgery for a developing skull. In our study, one-month-old sheep was first applied as a growing skull model. The CT images clearly showed the fast growth of the sheep skull in 6 months. And the Ti-mesh caused the calvarial distortion. In the Ti-mesh group, two obvious protuberances existed on the cranium, because the mechanical properties of the Ti-mesh were much higher than cranial bone. On the other hand, the MC scaffold did not arouse any distortion, although

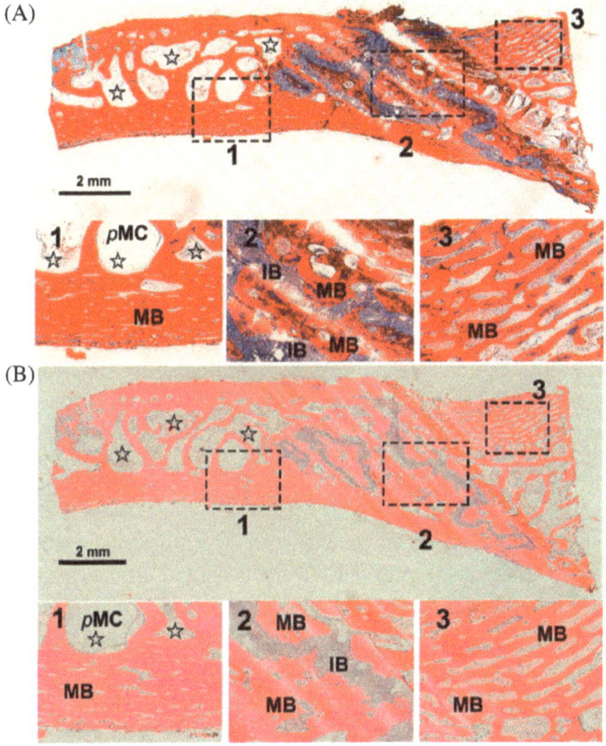

FIGURE 4.27 Histological assessment of the cranial bone samples from MC group at 3 months postoperation with (A) Masson's trichrome and (B) H&E staining. *MB*, Mature bone; *IB*, immature nascent bone.

MC also had little biodegradation in 6 months, which should be attributed to its similar strength and elastic modulus to natural bone.

4.6.5 Conclusion

The MC-based composite bone material was developed successfully in this study.

4.7 REPAIR OF BONE DEFECT BY USING MINERALIZED COLLAGEN DENTAL BONE POWDER AND GUIDING TISSUE REGENERATION MEMBRANE IN MINI PIG MODELS [5]

4.7.1 Experiment Purpose

The aim of this study was to compare the clinical and histologic outcomes of bone regeneration using two different graft materials: deproteinized bovine bone mineral (Bio-Oss) and demineralized collagen bone materials with absorbable collagen membrane, to evaluate the effect of demineralized collagen materials on bone regeneration.

4.7.2 Testing Method

4.7.2.1 Experimental Scheme

The molars of the mini pig were extracted, a 10 mm × 10 mm bone defect was created. Bone defect was filled with Bio-Oss and MC dental bone powder respectively and with absorbable membrane as well. Cone-beam CT was taken 12 weeks after surgery and bone samples were stained with Goldner's Trichrome. The new regenerated area was calculated by the image analysis software Image-Pro plus 6.0 and the percentages of newly formed bone were compared between two groups using SPSS 22.0 software package.

4.7.2.2 Methods the Experiment Groups

The molars on both sides were extracted from two mini pigs, thus there were seven alveolar sockets in all pigs and were assigned into group A1, group A2, group B1 and group B2 respectively. The upper jaw group A1 ($n = 2$, A11, A12) and the lower jaw group A2 ($n = 3$, A21, A22, A23) were implanted with MC dental bone powder. The upper jaw group B1 ($n = 1$) and the lower jaw group B2 ($n = 1$) were implanted with Bio-Oss. There was not any treatment in the blank group ($n = 1$).

4.7.2.3 Experimental Materials

MC bone powder and MC membrane; Bio-Oss, Bio-Gide periosteum,

4.7.2.4 Experimental Methods

Two 13-month old miniature pigs were fasted and deprived of water 12h before surgery and intramuscular injection of ketamine 0.2 mL/kg and a new 0.10 mL/kg. After the success of the general anesthesia, left side, disinfection, spread towels, opening week and mouths open mouth, in the first premolar far nearly cut the gums, and third premolar open trapezoidal disc, gum, collar loose teeth, complete removal of four quadrant of the second premolar. The bone defect of 10 mm × 10 mm × 5 mm was worn on the buccal side of tooth extraction. According to the grouping, the bone powder and collagen membrane were filled respectively, and the mucous membrane was sutured closely. After surgery, penicillin sodium was injected into 3 days, one time a day, 400,000 U.

4.7.2.5 Experimental Observation

1. Gross observation

   Observe soft tissue healing in general.

2. Imaging observations
   The morphological changes and bone density changes of BBB 0 were observed by CT scan with 16-slice CT scan in 12 weeks.
3. Histological observation
   The specimens were collected, embedded, and sected, and the growth of the new bone was observed under the light microscope.
4. Statistical analysis
   The shape and bone density of the defect area were analyzed by the analysis of Cone Beam Computed Tomography (CBCT), and the new bone mass in the defect area was calculated by image analysis software Image-Pro Plus 6.0. The SPSS 22.0 software package was used for comparison between the two groups, and $P < .05$ was significant. Using Image-Pro Plus 6.0 digital microscopic image analysis system, at 1.25 times the microscopic analysis and Goldner trichromatic staining slice of new bone in bone defect area of area percentage, draw new bone percentage, and compare the difference between groups.

4.7.3 Experimental Results

4.7.3.1 Gross Observation

All the defects were covered by mucosal tissue, and the wound healing was good in each group.

4.7.3.2 Imaging Observation

The bone defects in each group were found to be new, the alveolar ridge was highly restored, and the alveolar ridge was seen in the continuous bone cortex (Fig. 4.28). Image-Pro Plus 6.0 was used to calculate the cumulative optical density value of the bone defect area in the bone defect area, and the change of bone density in the defect areas of different groups was determined. A2:20.28 ± 1.31; Bl: 22.02 ± 0.51; B2:20.56 ± 1.08; Blank group: 16.66 plus or minus 1.04. Statistical analysis showed that the MC bone meal and Bio-OSS bone repair maxillary and mandibular defects, with the forming of new bone mineral density (BMD); there no significant differences between groups compared with the blank group ($P < .05$).

4.7.3.3 Histological Observation

Thin sections stained by Goldner's trichromatism were observed under multifunctional microscope, and the boundaries between osteoid, newly mineralized and mature bone were obvious osteoid amaranth, new precision bone to blue-green or light blue (Fig. 4.29). The new mineralized bone and the endogenous Haversian system are not obvious. The cavity in the bone defect area is an unabsorbed bone material. All of the groups were in the proximal portion of the membrane, and the missing bone particles were visible in the

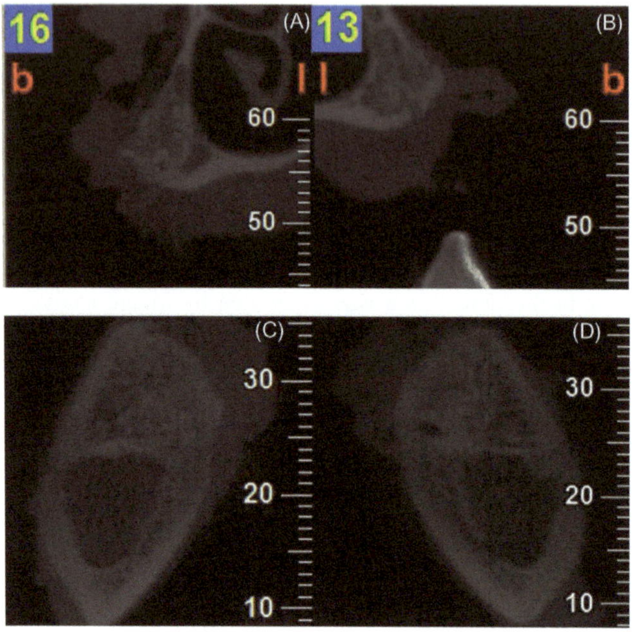

FIGURE 4.28 CBCT finding 12 weeks after operation. (A–D) refer to the four experimental groups A1, B1, B2, and A2, respectively. New bone was observed in all collected samples. Continuous alveolar ridge of group A was not satisfied; some material dropped out of the bone defect. The line between new regenerated bone and maxilla was clear. In (C) and (D), it was difficult to determine the exact point at which the residual particle ended and newly formed bone began.

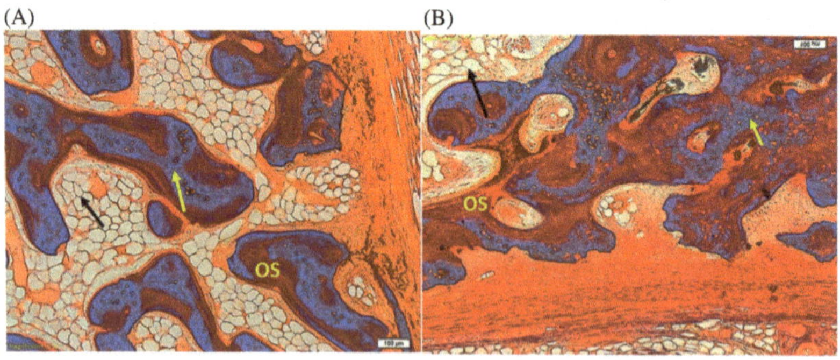

FIGURE 4.29 Goldner's trichrome stain (×10). (A) Group A1; (B) Group B1. OS: red area referred to osteoid; yellow arrow: blue area, referred to newly formed bone; black arrow: residual materials. The regions of residual graft particles had a similar appearance regardless of graft type, and so did the process of new bone formation. Along with the Bio-Oss and degradation, the osteoblast secreted bone matrix, which mineralized into osteoid and the mineralized collagen bone powder, and then woven bone.

inner region of the defect. There was no significant difference in bone mass between group A and group B. As a whole, the upper jaw of the mandible is better than the maxillary bone (Fig. 4.30).

4.7.3.4 Statistics

Image-Pro Plus 6.0 was used to compare the bone area of each group of bone defects (Table 4.6). From Table 4.6, it can be seen that the addition of bone powder group has a large amount of bone mass, and the osteogenesis area of the mandible is significantly increased than that of the maxillary bone, and group B is larger than that of group A, but the difference is not significant.

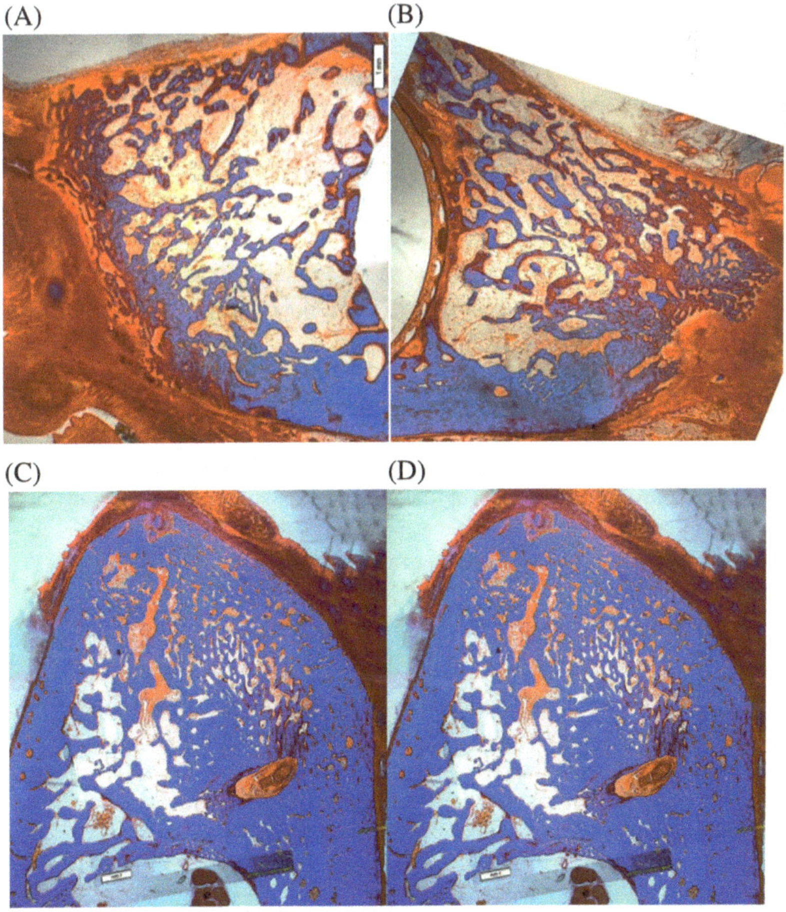

FIGURE 4.30 Goldner's trichrome staining 12 weeks after operation (×1.25). (A–D) refers to A1, B1, B2, and A2 groups, respectively. More regenerated bone can be seen in the mandibular defect than the maxillary defect. There was no significant difference in the newly formed bone area between group A and B.

TABLE 4.6 Percentage of New Regenerated Bone Area Among Different Groups

Group	New Bone Area (mm^2)	Defect Area (mm^2)	New Bone Area Ratio (%)
A1 group	24.85724	43.18075	0.575655587
B1 group	25.02539	42.98743	0.582155993
A2 group	41.96084	54.62592	0.76712034
B2 group	47.57076	57.83858	0.822474549
Blank group	7.497984	27.21009	0.275558956

4.7.4 Discussion

The results of this experiment can be seen 12 weeks after surgery. The new bone mass of maxillary defect is less than that of mandible. It may be that gravity causes the upper maxillary region to be filled with bone loss more than the mandible. Then the new bone mass is decreased. It can be observed from CBCT that the white defect area of some materials is shed. From macroscopic observation and imaging, the bone defect areas of two kinds of materials were filled with new bone tissue, with no obvious difference. Postoperative CT showed that the bone density of each group was basically the same. In histological sections. In the bone defect area repaired by the two materials, some of the materials were replaced and reconstructed by new bone, and the amount of bone formation in the defect area was basically the same. The wounds in the bone defect area were well healed without infection, indicating that they were the same as bio-oss bone powder. It is expected to be one of the engineering materials of bone tissue.

4.7.5 Conclusion

In the past few decades, bone tissue material has been developed rapidly from the original single bone component to mimicking the natural bone ultrastructure and composition of the complex. The results of this experiment showed that the application of MC bone powder and MC membrane to repair the bone defect of tooth extraction fossa of small pig can obtain better osteogenic effect. Although the bone loss was slightly reduced compared with the application of Bio-Oss bone powder and Bio-Gide membrane to repair tooth extraction area, the difference was not significant. It is indicated that MC bone powder has the same effect as Bio-Oss bone powder, which can induce new bone formation. However, the sample size of this experiment is small, and the next step is to expand the sample size to further evaluate the osteogenic effect of MC bone powder on tooth extraction fossa bone defect.

4.8 TEST IN CANINE EXTRACTION SITE PRESERVATIONS BY USING MINERALIZED COLLAGEN PLUG WITH OR WITHOUT GUIDED BONE REGENERATION MEMBRANE FOR DOG TOOTH [6]

4.8.1 Experiment Purpose

The aim of this study was to discuss the feasibility of MC plug and bilayer MC guided bone regeneration membrane in site preservation in extraction sockets.

4.8.2 Testing Method

4.8.2.1 Experimental Scheme

Beagles were randomly divided into A, B, and C groups, with four beagles in each group. The third mandibular premolars on both sides were extracted. Each alveolar socket of group A was immediately implanted with a porous MC plug and covered with a bilayer MC-guided bone regeneration membrane after tooth extraction. Alveolar sockets of group B were implanted with porous MC plug only, and group C was set as blank control without any implantation. The healing effects of the extraction sockets were evaluated by gross observation, morphological measurements, and X-ray micro-computed tomography after 12 weeks.

4.8.2.2 Methods: The Experiment Groups

Twelve beagles were randomly divided into three groups, A, B, and C, with four beagle in each group. The third mandibular premolars on both sides were extracted. Each group was implanted with different materials. The animals were killed by lethal injection at 12 weeks after experiment.

4.8.2.3 Experimental Materials

1. Experimental animals: this study investigated 12 male beagles (approximately 12 months old and weighing 13–15 kg) offered by the Experimental Animal Center of Dalian Medical University.
2. Materials: porous MC plug and bilayer MC guided bone regeneration membrane.

4.8.2.4 Experimental Methods

All surgical procedures, extractions, and experimental protocol were performed under general and local anesthesia. The general anesthesia is induced with intravenous atropine (0.05 mg/kg) and intramuscularly with Xylazine Sailaqin (0.08–0.1 mL/kg). Routine dental infiltration anesthesia with articaine (0.05 mg/kg) was used at the surgical sites.

The bilateral mandibular third premolars were surgically minimally invasively extracted without any destruction to the bone to any of the 12 beagles. The beagles were randomly divided into A, B, and C groups: group A was immediately implanted with porous MC plug covered with bilayer MC Guided Bone Regeneration (GBR) membrane in alveolar sockets, and group B was implanted with porous MC plug only, while group C was left unfilled as a negative control. All of the experimental sites were sutured with 3–0 sutures.

4.8.2.5 Experimental Observation

1. Gross observation

   Diet, general activity, and the presence of infection were observed after the surgery. Next, the degradation process of the material in the surface of the extraction area and bone formation was observed within 12 weeks.
2. Imaging observations
   1. Traverse-continuous-rotation CT observation: 12 weeks later, specimens line head spiral CT scanning, using double spiral CT (SOMATOM definition Spirit, German SIEMENS company), the scanning layer thickness of 1.0 mm, reconstruction interval is 1.0 mm, 130 kv voltage, electric current 45 ma, in the image of coronary to choose from alveolar ridge top to 5 mm from the root, measure the target area for the radius of 2 mm round of CT values of the area of interest, unit of measure (Hounsfield unit, HU). The maximum, minimum, and two intermediate values of the area were recorded, and the mean value was the bone density of a single tooth extraction nest on the side of the experimental dog. Use the same method to measure another tooth extraction nest on one side and two tooth extraction nests on the opposite side.
   2. X-ray microcomputed tomography images: 12 weeks later, the block sections and the surrounding alveolar bones extracted from the extraction sites were made into a block with the length of 20 mm and the height of 15 mm and preserved in 10% neutral buffered formalin for 10 days. The fixed specimens were scanned using X-ray microcomputed tomography (X-_CT; Xradia Versa XRM-500, ZEISS, Germany) at a resolution of 22.4814_m (80 kV and 80_A). The overall topography of the extraction sites was visualized in a 3D reconstructed image, which allowed many structural parameters to be calculated.
3. Histological observation
   1. Histopathological observation: the animals killed by lethal injection at 12 weeks after experiment, and liver and kidney tissues were taken

out and fixed in 10% formaldehyde solution for HE staining and histological observation.

2. Histomorphometric observation: the vertical distance (H) between buccal and lingual bone crests measures the vertical distance between the highest point of the buccal and lingual crest. Firstly, L–L was parallel to the long axis and also the central axis of the socket. LBC and BBC are the lingual and buccal alveolar crest, respectively. Subsequently, horizontal lines perpendicular to L–L connecting with the buccal and lingual bone crest to L–L were drawn. The difference of vertical distance between the buccal and lingual intersections with L–L was measured.

4. Statistical analysis

Data analysis was performed by using SPSS 17.0, then Student's t-test and ANOVA were used; p value less than 0.05 was considered to be statistically significant. All the results showed as the mean_standard deviation.

4.8.3 Experimental Results

4.8.3.1 Gross Observation

Most experimental dogs were in poor diet or in unfavorable condition within 3 days after surgery due to pain stimulus, while the diet went back to normal in 1 week after operation. The overlying mucosa showed slightly hyperemia 1–3 days after surgery, which was back to normal 5 days later and the surface of extractions was completely covered by mucosal epithelium. After 2 weeks, all of the experimental sites healed uneventfully. There were no signs of extensive wound dehiscence and infection during the entire observation period. Twelve weeks later, the sockets were covered with a tough and rubbery mucosa as normal (Fig. 4.31). In group A, a newly formed alveolar ridge with a full profile was observed, whose texture was as solid as that of

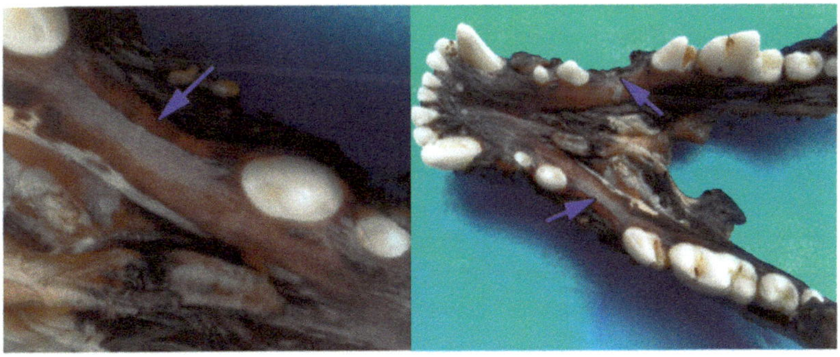

FIGURE 4.31 Twelve weeks later, the sockets were covered with a tough and rubbery mucosa as normal.

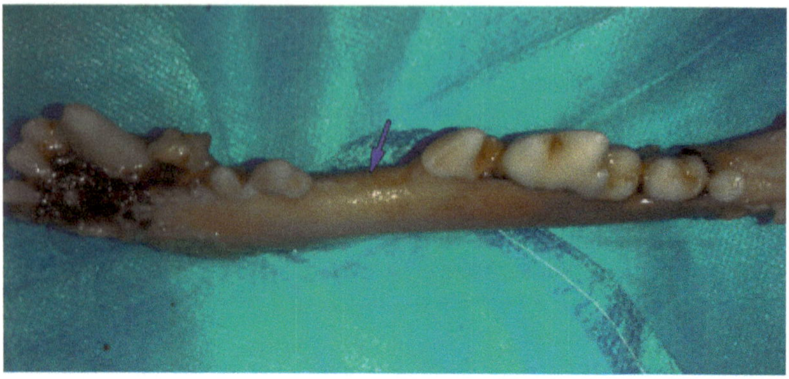

FIGURE 4.32 Newly formed alveolar ridge with a full profile was observed.

the adjacent teeth, with no residue on the surface (Fig. 4.32). In terms of fullness and texture of the alveolar ridge, group B was slightly inferior to group A. A little residue could be seen on the surface. Furthermore, the alveolar ridge resorption was clearly observed in the direction of buccal bone plate in group C, with an obvious reduction in height and width.

4.8.3.2 Imaging Observation

1. Traverse-continuous-rotation CT observation: 12 weeks later, group A's alveolar socket had completely disappeared, alveolar socket inside the scattered gradually transformed into with the jaw bone structure organization with no difference; its density is significantly higher than the surrounding alveolar bone imaging in cancellous bone [7]. The alveolar socket of group B disappeared, and the internal bone tissue was reconstructed, and the structure was basically the same as that of the surrounding jaw bone. Group C's alveolar socket largely disappeared, but The bone density in the alveolar fossa was lower than that in the area of interest of the surrounding jaw tissue, and the relative gray value of the CT of the jaw was different among the groups (Table 8.1), CT value maximum experimental group A areas of interest.
2. X-ray microscopic CT: At 12 weeks, X-ray microCT showed that all the mineralized collagen materials and the new composite mineralized collagen membrane materials were absorbed and degraded, and the surface of the new bone tissue was loose and porous, with obvious boundaries with the surrounding buccal-lingual bone plate (Fig. 4.33). A group of new bone tissue is filled with the tooth socket, orderly arranged closely (Fig. 4.34A). Ultrastructure showed a large amount of new trabecular bone tightly arranged into a 3D network structure, most of which has been converted to form MB (Fig. 4.34B), and some new bone trabecular is undergoing renovation. In group B relative arrangement of new bone

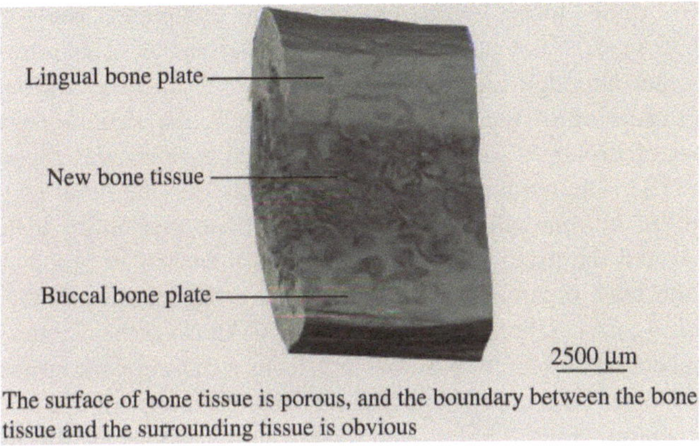

FIGURE 4.33 The new bone tissue and surrounding tissue are distinct.

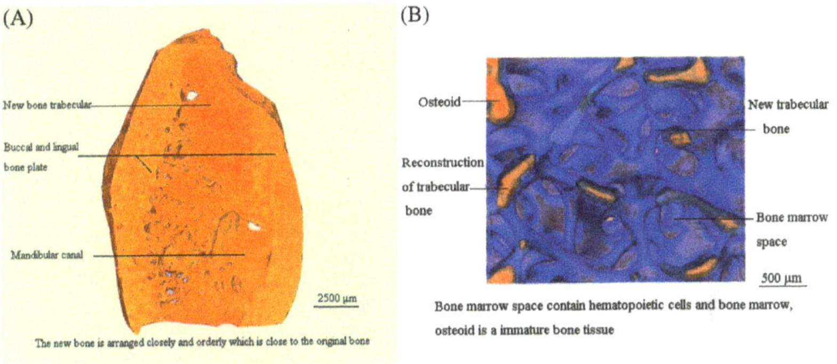

FIGURE 4.34 (A) The new bone trabecula in the experimental group A was filled with alveolar socket and basically completed the reconstruction. (B) The microanatomical structure of the newly formed bone trabecula was observed and the structure of the mature bone trabecula was basically reconstructed.

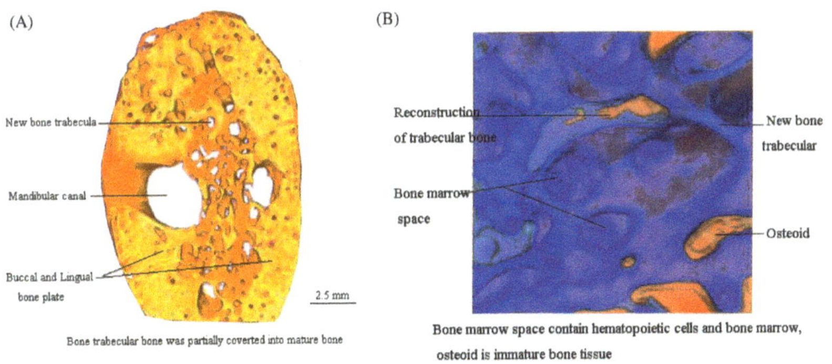

FIGURE 4.35 (A) The new bone trabecula in group B was reconstructed and matured. (B) The microanatomical structure of the new bone trabeculae in group B has been reconstructed and transformed into mature.

tissue is quite loose, with no order, a compared with group A (Fig. 4.35A), and the amount is less than group A. The ultrastructure showed that although the reticular structure was formed in group B, the compact-ordering of the three-dimensional reticular structure was worse than that of group A, and only part of the new bone was reconstructed (Fig. 4.35B). The number of mature bone was less than that of group A, the number of mineralized heterogeneous bone was more than that of group A, and the osteogenic effect was less than that of group A. Group C was the least organized, with the loosest arrangement and most disorder (Fig. 4.36A). Ultrastructure of group C showed the amount of new bone trabecular is scarce and does not form a 3D network structure, and there is almost no reconstruction of the MB, a number of classes of bone mineralization (Fig. 4.36B), and osteogenesis effect is the worst. In groups A, B, and C three sets of new bone tissue areas were selected at constant volume of 6.25 mm^3 rectangle for areas of interest (ROI) for areas of interest (Figs. 4.37 and 4.38), and the ROI areas respectively analyzed per unit volume of BMD, bone volume fraction (BV/TV), bone trabecular thickness (Tb. Th), bone trabecular number (Tb. N), and bone trabecular separation degree (Th. Sp) of the mean and standard deviation,

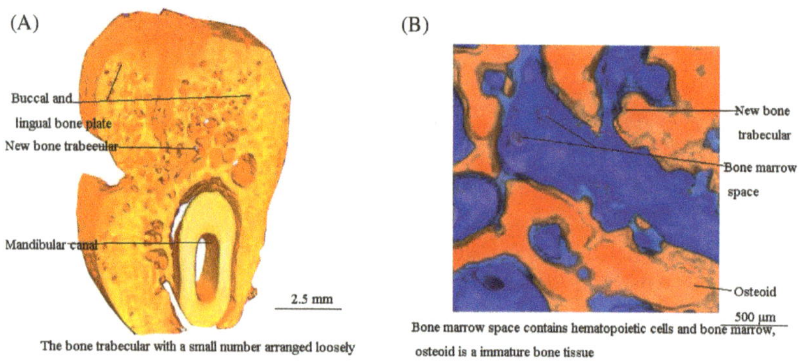

FIGURE 4.36 (A) In group C, the new bone trabecula was loosely arranged, and the number was small, and the reconstruction was hardly completed. (B) The microanatomical structure of the newly formed bone trabeculae in group C was observed.

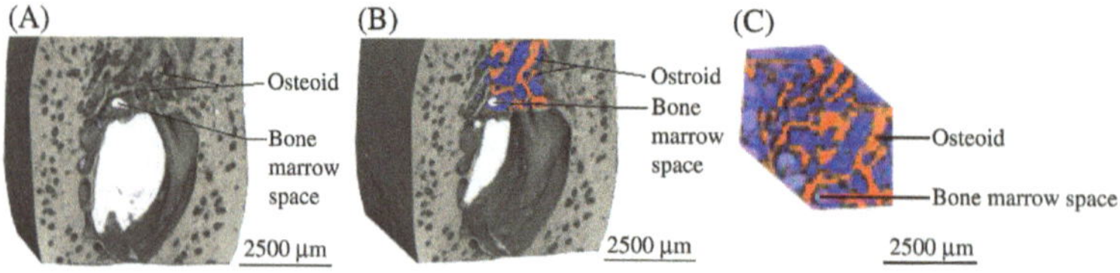

FIGURE 4.37 (A, B) Select a rectangular area as the base (the colored area in B) and then extend the inner side to form a cuboid (C).

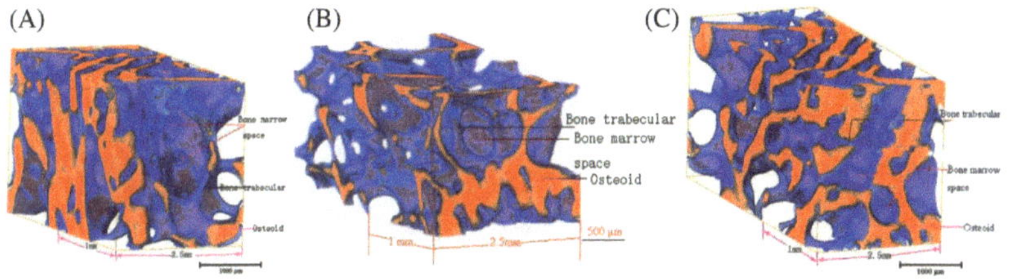

FIGURE 4.38 (A–C) Respectively for the experiment groups A, B, and C selected cuboid region ROI; ROI area of 2.5 mm × 2.5 mm × 1 mm cuboid.

TABLE 4.7 The CT Values in Region of Extraction Interest After Operation at 12 Weeks

Group	Case Number	Minimum Value	Maximum	$\bar{x} \pm S$
Group A	8	142	560	506.8 ± 106.9[a,b]
Group B	16	140	483	445.5 ± 104.1[a]
Group C	16	121	365	265.8 ± 81.4

[a]*Compared with group C, P < 0.05.*
[b]*Compared with group B, P < 0.05.*

as shown in Table 4.7. The differences between the two groups were statistically significant. The larger BMD, TMD, BV/TV, Tb.Th, Th.N, the more stable and mature the bone structure was; On the contrary, the larger Th.Sp is, the greater the distance between bone trabeculae is, the less compact and orderly the three-dimensional mesh structure is, and the worse the bone structure is. Group A BMD, BV/TV, Tb.Th, Th. N are all greater than the B, C group, Th.Sp minimum. It is suggested that the experimental group A is ideal (Table 4.7).

4.8.3.3 Histological Observation

1. Histopathological observation: liver tissue HE staining (Fig. 4.39): there was no significant abnormality in liver tissue structure of group A. The structure of hepatic lobules is complete and clear, and the hepatocytes are arranged radially in the central vein. The liver cells are polygonal and the nuclei are large and round, located in the middle of the hepatocytes. No obvious tissue edema, inflammatory cells, and tissue damage were observed. Pathological section of renal tissue (Fig. 4.40): there was no obvious abnormality of renal tissue structure in group A. Normal glomerulus distribution, assumes the circular or elliptic, peripheral neat, small renal capsule cavity and irregular, usually formed by simple cubic or

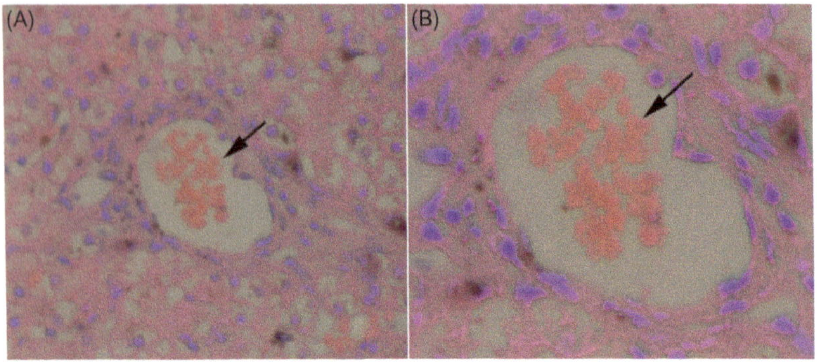

FIGURE 4.39 Liver biopsy was performed 12 weeks after surgery. (A) HE, 100 ×; (B) HE, 200 ×; the black arrow is the central vein.

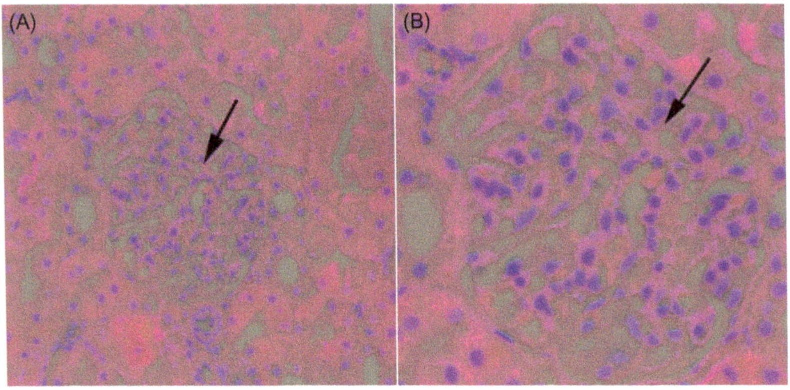

FIGURE 4.40 Pathological section of renal tissue 12 weeks after operation. (A) HE, 100 ×; (B) HE, 200 ×; the black arrow is shown as the renal capsule cell.

Pyramidal epithelial cells, free surface with brush border cells, nuclear circle located near base, a strong eosinophilic cytoplasm dyed dark red. The renal tubular lumen is compact and small. No inflammatory cells were found and tissue structures were not damaged.

2. Morphological observation of the tissue: 12 weeks of measurement of buccal alveolar alveolar height difference in each group (Table 4.8).

4.8.4 Discussion

New composite MC membrane and collagen mineralization materials jointly applied in canine tooth extraction sites preservation can create synergies, reduce alveolar bone absorption, promote the new bone formation, and improve the quality of healing. After 12 weeks group A had alveolar ridge height and width decrease significantly less than groups B and C, and The

TABLE 4.8 **The Vertical Height Loss of the Buccal Bone Plate $\bar{x} \pm S$ (mm)**

Group	Case Number	Minimum Value	Maximum	$\bar{x} \pm S$
Group A	8	1.8	2.4	2.1 ± 0.2[a,b]
Group B	16	2.5	3.2	2.8 ± 0.4[a]
Group C	16	2.9	4.8	3.7 ± 0.5

[a]*Compared with group C, P < .05.*
[b]*Compared with group B, P < .05.*

quality and density of bone formation were better than those of the other two groups. The spatial structure of bone trabeculae was more hierarchical, and the tight and orderly arrangement was closest to the autologous bone, and the bone composition effect was the most ideal. The reasons for this are as follows. (1) The main components of the MC materials are type I collagen and hydroxyapatite, new composite MC membrane composition is also composed of type I collagen and hydroxyapatite, the biocompatibility of the two materials can achieve the best, at the same time new composite mineralization rate slower than the MC collagen membrane materials, in the process of repairing the membrane has been maintaining a space barrier and the role of inducing osteogenesis, new bone formation rate, and degradation rate of two kinds of materials can achieve the ideal effect of matching, to accelerate the early tissue healing process, shorten the time to repair. (2) The MC material with three dimensional network structure has a distributed mutually supportive structure for various nutrients and growth factors to surrounding cells and promotes bone growth providing a good space. The MC of the new composite MC membrane can provide growth support for bone marrow cells, induce bone regeneration, and form new adhesion and new bone tissue. The two materials form a double scaffold and play a synergistic effect to slow the absorption of alveolar bone, promote the formation of new bone and improve the healing quality. (3) The new type of composite mineralized collagen has a certain mechanical strength, and it can bond with the mineralized collagen material after blood infiltration in the alveolar fossa to play a physiological bonding role, improve the strength of mineralized collagen, and play an important role in the early repair process of healing. (4) To cover the membrane material contact with the top tooth extraction at the soft tissue, strict isolation of contact with the outside world, because of the mineralization rate of the degradation of collagen in the body faster than new compound MC material, as time prolonged, the gradual degradation of bone repair materials lost space support role, but the new composite MC membrane are still around for cell migration, value-added, continue to provide differentiated support role, relative to extend the time effects of cytokines, make its role in alveolar socket healing extended, thus, compared with other two groups had better bone healing effect. It is believed that the new composite MC membrane and MC material will be used together with good preservation effect of alveolar ridge, which will provide a new idea for the future development of absorbable collagen membrane and its clinical application. The experiment scale is small, the number of experimental subjects is small, and there is insufficient data, so we need to increase the sample size for further discussion.

4.8.5 Conclusion

The results suggest that the new composite MC membrane and collagen mineralization joint bone repair materials applied in canine tooth extraction sites preservation can create synergies, slow down the alveolar bone absorption, promote new bone formation, and improve the quality of healing.

4.9 SMALL PIG EXPERIMENTAL STUDY OF MINERALIZED COLLAGEN MEMBRANE INDUCED OSTEOGENESIS IN EARLY STAGE [7]

4.9.1 Experimental Objective

To explore the ability of new compound MC membrane as GBR barrier membrane to induce early osteogenesis after implantation in vivo.

4.9.2 Experimental Method

4.9.2.1 Experimental Method

Three 8 mm × 8 mm total defects were prepared by dental drills at mandibular bone of the small Bama pig, respectively, and covered with the MC membrane Bio-Gide covering and without covering the defect area. The animals were executed after the first month after surgery, in the first 1 or 2 weeks before the death of the intramuscular injection of tetracycline solution and 2 cresol orange solution. After fixing the samples, the hard tissue slices were prepared. Under fluorescence microscope and optical microscope (toluidine blue and methylene blue one acid magenta), the degradation degree of the film and the new bone formation ability under the membrane were observed, and the bone morphogenetic and bone maturation were evaluated.

4.9.2.2 Experimental Groups

The experiment was divided into three groups. Three experimental animals were implanted with MC membrane, Bio-Gide, and the blank control group had no material implanted.

4.9.2.3 Materials

MC membrane, MC bone repair material, Bio-Gide collagen membrane.

4.9.2.4 Experimental Method

The lateral mandible of small Bama pig was located along the anterior edge of the masseter muscle, the lower mandibular margin was 5 mm, and the parallel mandibular lower margin was used to cut the skin, 5–6 mm long, and the blunt separation muscle and periosteum to the bone surface, the periosteum was removed and the operation field was fully exposed. 0.9% three parallel 8 mm × 8 mm whole-layer bone defect models were prepared with split drill under saline cooling, and the peripheral blood vessels, nerves, and muscles were protected. The BFM was mixed with blood and implanted into the bone defect area. The first two bone defects were treated with MC membrane and Bio-Gide; these defects were covered with titanium membrane nail, and the last bone defect area was not covered. Layered suture closed the incision.

4.9.2.5 Experimental Observation

1. General observation
2. Histological observation: fluorescence analysis, toluidine blue staining, methylene blue–acid magenta staining

4.9.3 Result

4.9.3.1 General Observation

After 4 weeks of operation, there was no infection, no degradation of the MC membrane and the Bio-Gide group, and there was no local inflammatory reaction.

4.9.3.2 Histological Observation

1. Fluorometric analysis

   Fig. 4.41 is a fluorescent image of hard tissue slices at 4 weeks after GBR operation. The orange stripe is formed by excitation of 2 cresol orange, indicating the position of bone at 2 weeks before the animal is killed, and the green stripe is formed by the activation of tetracycline, indicating the bone position at 1 week before the animal is killed, The area between the two bands represents the new bone formed between 2 weeks and 1 week before the execution. The results showed that there was obvious bone formation in the MC membrane and Bio-Gide group, but the new bone tissue was disorganized, the trabecular structure was messy, and the fibrous connective tissue was obvious. The fluorescence of the experimental group was stronger than that of the control group and the film-free covering group, the orange fluorescence of the film-free covering group was weak, and was almost invisible at 100 ×, which showed that the bone-forming capacity was very weak at 2 weeks before the death. In addition, although the fluorescence intensity of the control group in Bio-Gide group was weaker than that of MC membrane group, the new bone formation thickness was obviously larger than that of the experimental group, and the trabecular meshwork structure was obvious.

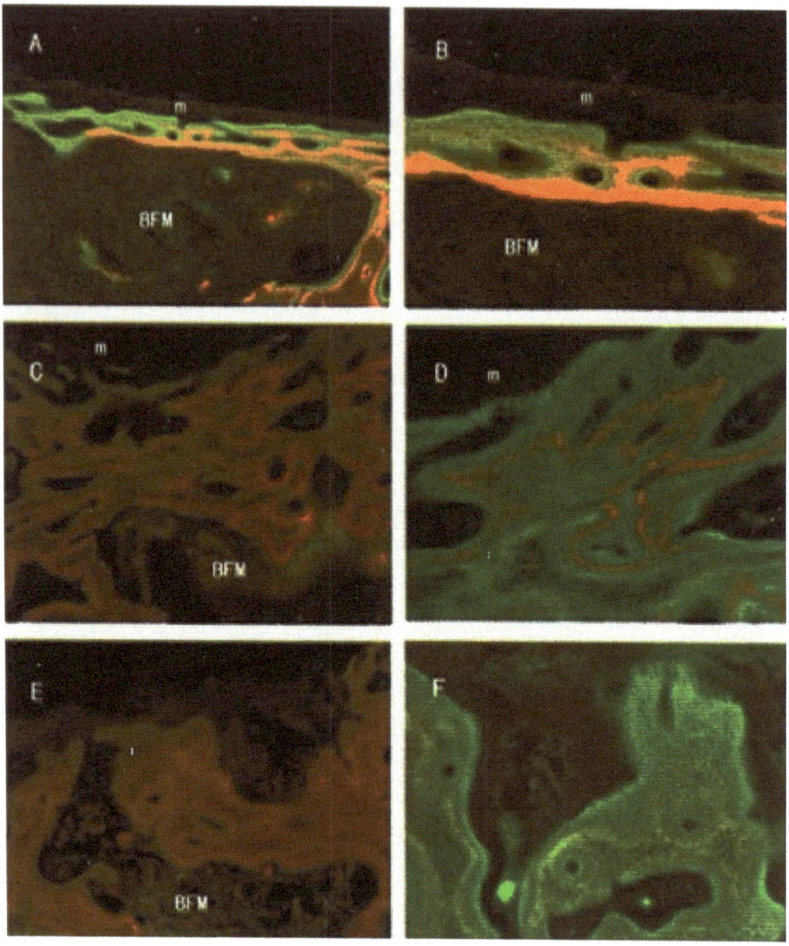

FIGURE 4.41 Fluorescence microscope image. (A, B) Mineralized collagen membrane. (C, D) Bio-Gide. (E, F) Film-free covering group. (A, C, E) ×40; (B, D, F) ×100. *m*, Barrier film; *BFM*, bone filling material.

2. Toluidine blue staining

Toluidine blue staining is very suitable for the observation of bone tissue staining; especially in the observation of the degree of bone mineralization, the distinction between new bone and old bone is very obvious. Fig. 4.42 is a toluidine blue staining image of hard tissue slices at 4 weeks after GBR operation. In both the experimental group and the control group, there was obvious barrier membrane osteogenesis. The old bone (the host bone, gray) and the newly formed bone (dark blue) are clearly visible in A and C. The newly formed bone grows from the edge of the barrier membrane to the bone defect area, the BFM is filled in the

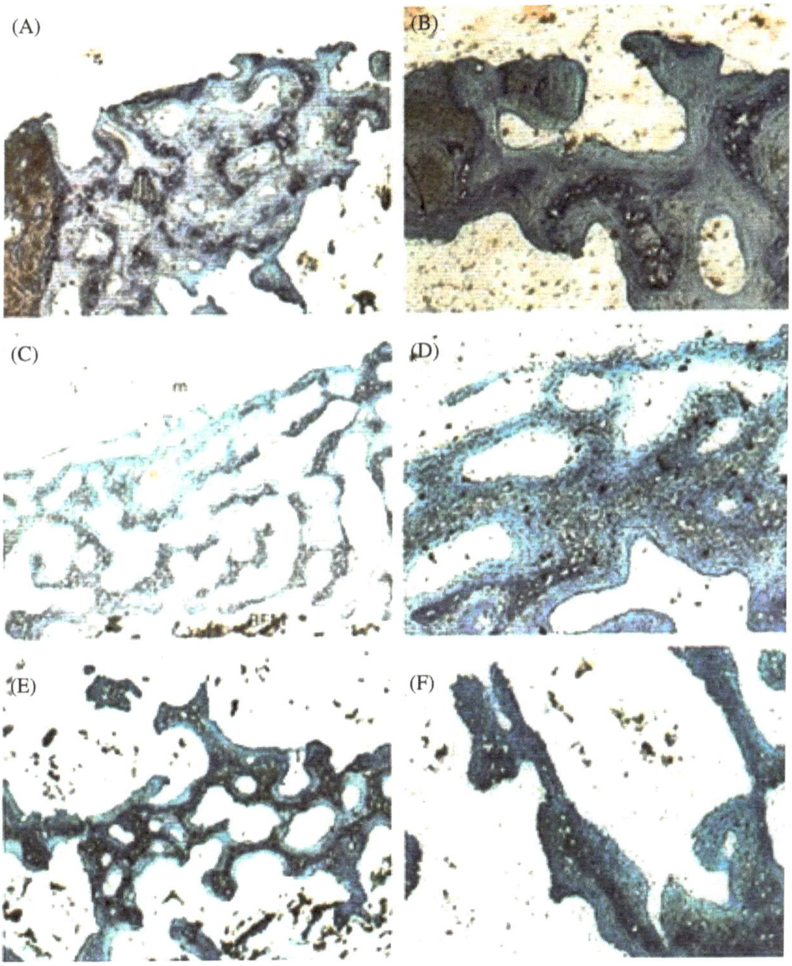

FIGURE 4.42 Photo of toluidine blue staining. (A, B) Mineralized collagen membrane; (C, D) Bio-Gide. (E, F) Film-free covering group. (A, C, E) ×40; (B, D, F) ×100. *m*, Barrier film; *BFM*, bone filling material.

defect area, the new bone is not fully filled with the bone defect area, and the volume and thickness of the new bone in the control group are significantly higher than that of the experimental group. But the mineralization degree of the two groups of newly formed bone was close. B and D showed clear trabecular bone structure, visible osteoblast and original blood vessel structure, and BFM not fully absorbed in trabecular bone. In the membrane-free covering group, the new bone tissue was disorganized, the trabecular structure was disorganized, and the fibrous connective tissue length was obvious (Fig. 4.42E and F), and no experimental group and control group were formed. The mineralization of the

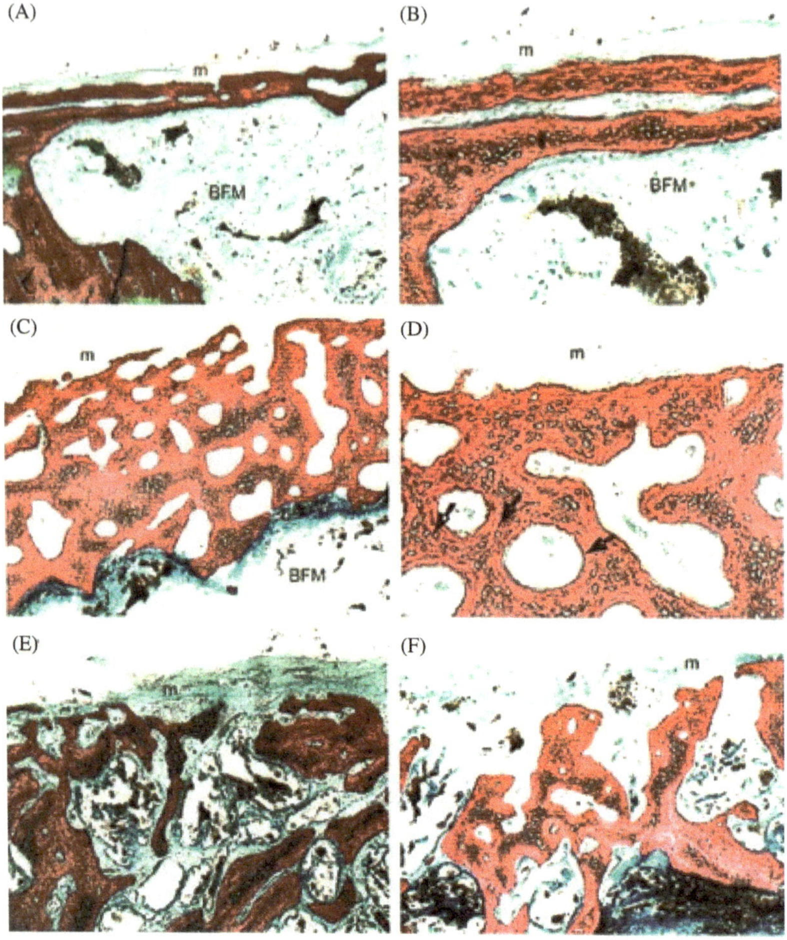

FIGURE 4.43 Dyeing of methylene blue–acid magenta. (A, B) Mineralized collagen membrane; (C, D) Bio-Gide. (E, F) Film-free covering group. (A, C, E) ×40; (B, D, F) ×100. *m*, Barrier film; *BFM*, bone filling material.

newly formed bone was good, but there was no similar vascular structure in the newly formed bone.

3. Methylene blue–acid magenta staining

The results showed that the osteoblasts and nucleus and bones of the methylene blue–acid magenta were clear: the osteoblast was dark blue, the bone was blue-green, the bones were purple, the collagen and muscle were blue, and the different mineralization stages of bone tissue were not obvious. Fig. 4.43 is the methylene blue–acid magenta stain of the hard tissue section 4 weeks after GBR operation. The results showed that there was obvious barrier membrane osteogenesis in both the experimental group and the control group. The old bone (host bone, dark purple) and newly formed bone (purple) are visible in A and C, and the newly formed bone is under the barrier membrane. From the edge of the defect area to the bone defect area, the BFM was filled in the defect area, the new bone incompletely filled the bone defect area, and the volume and thickness of the new bone in the control group were significantly higher than that of the experimental group. A clear bone trabecular structure is visible in Fig. 4.43D, and the deep blue osteoblasts are arranged along the Trabecular bone rows of the bone and the original vascular structure (shown in the arrows), and the BFM s that have not yet been fully absorbed are visible in the small beam of bone. The fibrous connective tissue long bone defect cavity was clearly visible in the membrane-free covering group, the new osseous tissue was separated, the new bone was disorganized, the trabecular structure was disordered (Fig. 4.43E and F), and no experimental group and control group were formed. There was no similar vascular structure in the newly formed bone.

4.9.4 Discussion

The MC membrane used in this experiment consists of type I collagen and mineralized type I collagen (type I collagen:mineralized type I collagen = 9:1). The collagen type I was obtained by dissolution of the extracted collagen and the mineralized type I collagen was composed of hydroxyapatite and type I collagen, which was consistent with autogenous bone composition. By controlling the mineralization process, hydroxyapatite can arrange the type I collagen protein to prepare the MC granular material. The effective combination of type I collagen and hydroxyapatite preserves the excellent biocompatibility of collagen membrane, the good osteogenic induction ability of hydroxyapatite can be obtained, and the mechanical strength of the membrane [wet state (saline wetting) is ≥ 10 N], the ability of keeping the void space is good, and the degradation rate of the film can be decreased. Through technical adjustment, the structure of porous-shaped cancellous bone for the bone defect site was prepared, and the pore size of the new bone was prepared by controlling the porosity of the membrane. The experiment used Bio-Gide as a control group, the collagen membrane was implanted into the animal body, the titanium nail was used for solid retention, and the ability of the membrane osteogenesis was evaluated by gross observation, fluorescence detection, and staining.

The results of toluidine blue staining and methylene blue–acid magenta staining showed that there was obvious barrier membrane osteogenesis in the MC membrane group and Bio-Gide group, that the new bone incompletely filled the bone defect area, and the new bone mass of MC membrane was less than that of the Bio-Gide group. In the absence of membrane covering group, the new bone tissue was disorganized, the trabecular structure was messy, and the fibrous connective tissue was obvious.

4.9.5 Conclusion

The results showed that the MC membrane was not degraded during 4 weeks of implantation, with good biocompatibility, good bone conduction, and the ability of osteogenesis, but the bone induction of new bone is inferior to the Bio-Gide control group. For better clinical results, it is necessary to further improve the production process of collagen membrane to enhance bone induction.

4.10 EXPERIMENTAL STUDY ON THE APPLICATION OF MINERALIZED COLLAGEN IN THE REPAIR OF JAW DEFECT [8]

4.10.1 Purpose

Objective: to study the ability of rabbit bone marrow stromal cells (BMSCs) as seed cells, MC nano-hydroxyapatite bone cement (nHAC) as scaffold material, and rabbit autologous platelet-rich plasma (PRP) as growth factor to repair mandibular defects in rabbits.

4.10.2 Experimental Method

4.10.2.1 Experimental Scheme

Rabbit mandibular 15 mm × 15 mm full layer bone defect was taken as follows: Group A, tissue engineering materials; Group B, autogenous iliac bone; Group C, pure mineral glue raw materials; Group D, control group repair. Radionuclide bone examination, BMD measurement, and histological observation were observed in 1, 3, and 6 months after operation.

4.10.2.2 Group of Experiments

4 groups of Japanese big-eared white rabbit, 10 per group, were randomly divided from a total number of 40. For the first group, one side underwent tissue engineering bone repair, and the other side did not undergo repair of the indwelling defect, for negative control. The second group had one side receive the tissue engineered bone repair, and the other side received autogenous iliac bone repair. The third group received on one side tissue-engineered bone repair, and the other side pure mineralized gum raw materials repair. For the fourth group, one side underwent repair of the defect with the raw material of pure mineralized glue, and the other side did not undergo defect repair. The tissue engineered bone repair sample total was 30 (Group A), autogenous iliac bone repair sample total 10 (group B), pure mineralized

gum raw material repair sample total 20 (group C), negative control group sample total 10 (group D), and normal control group sample total 10.

4.10.2.3 Material

In vitro construction of tissue engineered bone: the rabbit BMSCs and MC were cultured in 10 platelet-rich plasma (PRP) each 3 days for 1 time, continuous culture 14 days.

4.10.2.4 Method

After weighing the animals, 20% urapidil 1000 mg/kg was injected into the ear and the whole body was anesthetized. The rabbit was fixed in supine position on the operating table, the skin of the lower jaw was prepared, followed by routine disinfection and placing of the towel. In the mandible cut form mm × 15 mm full-layer periosteum bone defect; do not destroy the continuity of the mandible. They were implanted with tissue engineered bone, fresh autogenous ilium, raw material of pure mineralized gum, or indwelling blank defect and suture. 40,000 units Gentamicin was given after operation for 3 consecutive days. One second day after the operation, a group of subjects was injected with PRP, 1 time every day, 0.5 mL each time, for a total of 10 injections.

4.10.2.5 Observation

1. 99mTc—MDP radionuclide bone imaging examination:

   In 1, 3, and 6 months after operation, the rabbit was prone to the test bed under general anesthesia, and the "projectile" injection imaging agent 99mTc-MDP. The ROI of the normal control group was evaluated by the image method, and the ratio of the radiation count was obtained.
2. Bone density measurement:

   1, 3, and 6 months after the operation, using Prodigy dual-energy X-ray bone density tester, the new bone tissue in the operation area was taken from cheek to tongue side, and small animal software was used to analyze it.
3. Histological observation:

   In 1, 3, and 6 months after the operation, the normal tissues of the mandibular defect were collected and the implanted material bone block, 10% neutral formalin fixed, 50% formic acid was treated at room temperature, and the time of decalcification lasted for about 2 weeks. The specimens were washed overnight, followed by gradient alcohol dehydration, xylene transparent, conventional paraffin embedding, slicing, HE staining, and light microscopic observation.

TABLE 4.9 The Ratio of Radioactivity Counts in Different Periods of ROI in Each Group

Groups	1 Month	3 Months	6 Months
A	1.89 ± 0.21*1*2	3.02 ± 0.31*1*2	1.06 ± 0.09
B	1.83 ± 0.17*1*2	3.06 ± 0.20*1*2	1.09 ± 0.13
C	1.26 ± 0.31*1	1.01 ± 0.07	1.02 ± 0.05
D	0.98 ± 0.08	0.92 ± 0.11	0.94 ± 0.03

Compared with group D, *1 $P < .01$; compared with group C, *2 $P < .01$.

4.10.3 Result

4.10.3.1 99mTc—MDP Radionuclide Bone Imaging Examination

One month after operation: there was no significant difference between groups A and B. There were statistically significant differences between group A and groups C/D; between group B and groups C/D; and between groups C and D. Three months after operation: there was no significant difference between group A and B. There were statistically significant differences between group A and groups C/D, and between group B and groups C/D. There was no significant difference between groups C and D. Six months after operation: there was no statistically significant difference between the groups (Table 4.9).

4.10.3.2 Bone Density Measurement

The BMD of groups A, B, and C increased with time; at 1 month after operation, the 4 groups of BMD were equivalent to normal bone density: (15.27 ± 1.41)%, (16.05 ± 1.39)%, (8.60 ± 0.97)%, (1.17 ± 0.06)%. There was no significant difference in BMD between groups A and B. The difference between groups A and C/D was statistically significant. There were statistically significant differences between group B and C/D. There were statistically significant differences between group C and group D. At 3 months after operation, the 4 groups of BMD were equivalent to normal bone density (58.69 ± 4.20)%, (956.05 ± 5.25)%, (933.92 ± 6.08)%, (3.56 ± 0.41)%. There was no significant difference in BMD between the groups A and B. There were statistically significant differences between groups A and C/D. There were statistically significant differences between groups B and C/D. There were statistically significant differences between groups C and D. At 6 months after operation, the 4 groups of BMD were equivalent to normal bone density (98.38 ± 2.63)%, (100.05 ± 0.17)%, (60.75 ± 1.94)%, (9.82 ± 1.03)%. There was no significant difference in BMD between groups A and B. The

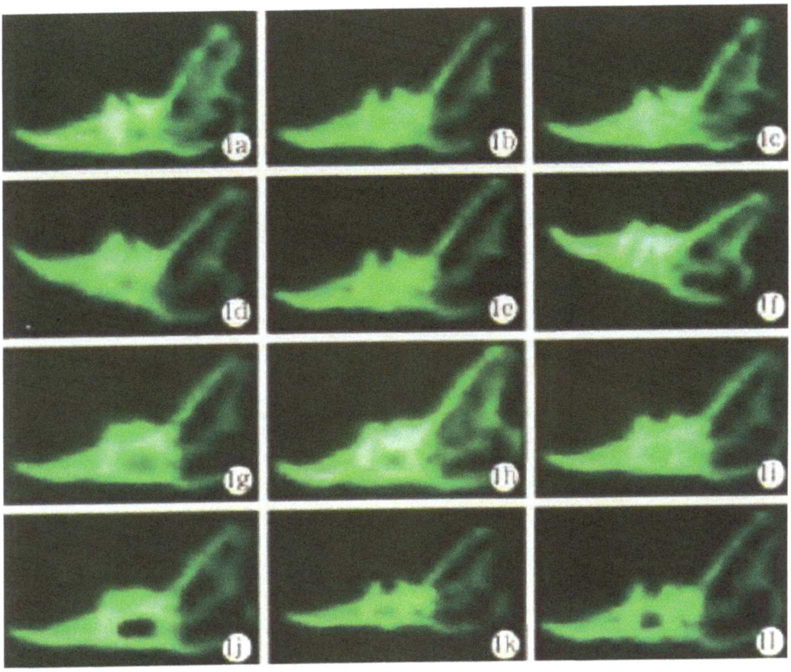

FIGURE 4.44 Results of bone mineral density test. (1a, 1b, 1c: A group after operation 1, 3, 6 月 bone density image; 1d, 1e, 1f: B group 1, 3, 6 months bone density image; 1g, 1h, 1i: C Group after operation 1, 3, 6 months bone density image; 1j, 1k, 1l: D).

TABLE 4.10 Bone Mineral Density Measured at Different Periods in Each Group

Groups	1 Month	3 Months	6 Months
A	0.08 ± 0.01*1*2	0.29 ± 0.01*1*2	0.53 ± 0.02*1*2
B	0.08 ± ± .08*1*22	0.28 ± 0.01*1*2	0.54 ± 0.02*1*2
C	0.04 ± 0.00*1	0.17 ± 0.02*1	0.33 ± 0.01*1
D	0.01 ± 0.00	0.02 ± 0.01	0.05 ± 0.01
Normal bone	0.52 ± 0.01	0.50 ± 0.01	0.54 ± 0.01

Compared with group D, *1 $P<.01$ compared with group C, *2 $P<.01$.

difference between groups A and C/D was statistically significant. There were statistically significant differences between groups B and C/D, and there were statistically significant differences between group C and group D (Fig. 4.44, Table 4.10).

4.10.3.3 Histology Observation

Group A, 1 month after surgery: 2a visible host bone into tissue engineered bone, stent material has been degraded, 2b visible osteoclasts appear near the stent material; 2c visible osteoblasts are present in the stent pores, and 2d can be found in the inside and around the scaffold material. Group A, 3 months after operation: 2e visible more new bone small Liang is in the stent mesh hole, but not connected to the film. Group A, 6 months after the operation: 2f has visibly formed a large mature new bone, and stent material is left. In group C, 1 month after the 2g, the fibrous connective tissue was grown into the scaffold material, and the scaffold material was degraded obviously. In Group C, 3 months after operation, 2h and 2i were found to be more dense in the scaffold material, the trabecular bone was small, and the scaffold material was degraded. In Group C, 6 months after operation, 2j of the stent material was found to increase the trabecular bone, but more fibrous tissue was embedded in it, and the scaffold material was dropped (Fig. 4.45).

4.10.4 Discussion

The results of radionuclide bone detection, BMD, and histological observation at various time points showed that the tissue engineered bone had a strong potential for inducing osteogenesis and revascularization. There was no significant difference in the ratio of radioactivity count and BMD between groups A and B at three different time points. It is proved that the tissue engineered bone and autogenous iliac bone graft have similar osteogenic activity and bone repair process, which can be attributed to the process of constructing tissue engineered bone in vitro. The PRP induces BMSCs to differentiate into osteoblasts and promote its proliferation. The spatial structure provided by MC further promotes the differentiation and proliferation of cells, although some of them are not yet fully differentiated into mature osteoblasts in vitro, but in animals, osteoblasts can secrete some growth factors by means of side secretion, such as bone morphogenetic 2 and so on, to promote this part of the cell into osteoblasts, and then secrete extracellular matrix for the mineralization and formation of bone tissue.

4.10.5 Results

The ability of tissue engineered bone to repair jaw defects was similar to autogenous ilium and stronger than that of mineral collagen alone, and the raw material of mineral glue can be completely degraded in vivo, so the tissue engineered bone constructed by BMSCs and MC and autologous PRP is a good substitute for bone defect.

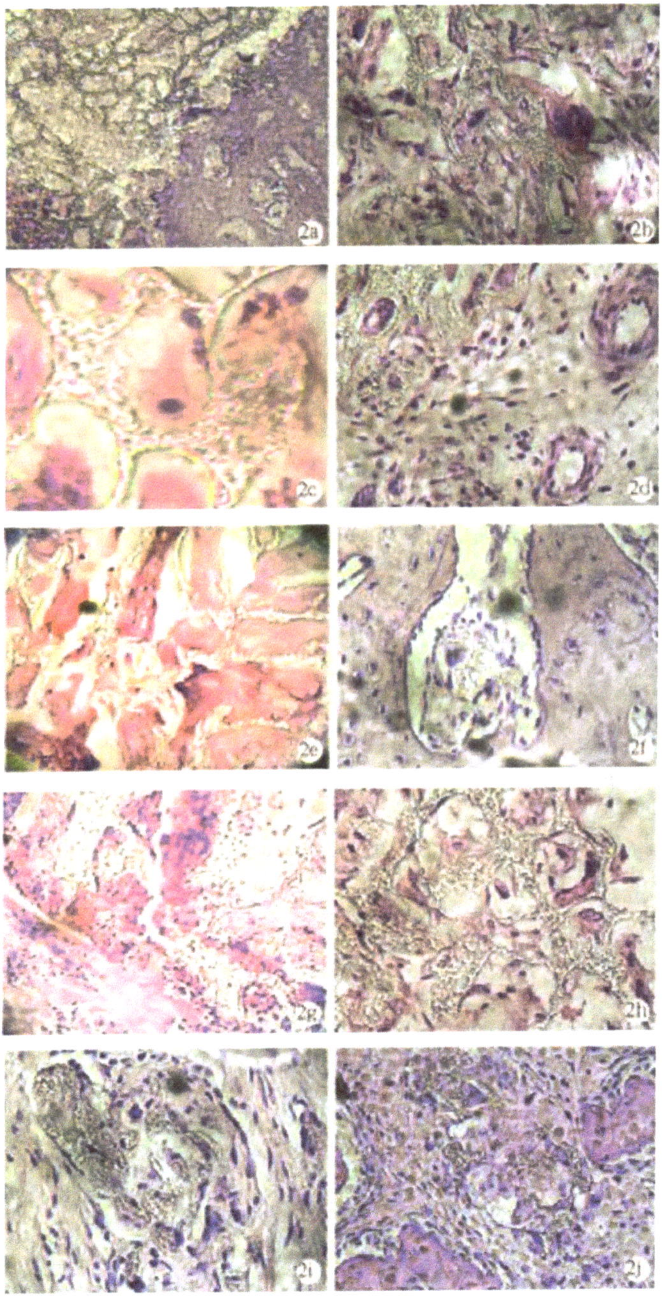

FIGURE 4.45 Results of histological examination. (2a × 100; 2b × 400; 2c × 1000; 2d × 400; 2e × 400; 2f × 400; 2g × 400; 2h × 400; 2i × 400; 2j × 400).

4.11 TISSUE REACTION OF MINERALIZED COLLAGEN IMPLANTED INTO RABBIT FEMUR BONE MARROW CAVITY [9]

4.11.1 Experimental Purpose

To study the tissue reaction of the raw material of mineral glue in the rabbit femur bone marrow cavity.

4.11.2 Experimental Methods

4.11.2.1 Experimental Program

Six New Zealand large-eared rabbits (average weight 3.1 kg) were selected, and intravenous pentobarbital anesthesia (mg/kg weight) was applied to the ear margin. In aseptic conditions, the core of the femoral shaft is drilled (2 mm in diameter), and the MC is pressed into the hole. The conventional feeding conditions were carried out and observations made after 3 months.

4.11.2.2 Experimental Materials

MC cylindrical material: diameter 2 mm, length 4 mm.

4.11.2.3 Experimental Observation

1. Optical microscope observation

   The bone graft was implanted into the backbone of the material, immobilized in 10% neutral formalin followed by graded ethanol dehydration, and poly (methyl methacrylate) was embedded to prepare the calcium-removing slices, followed by toluidine blue staining and light microscopic observation; some of the nonstaining slices were observed under fluorescent microscope. Polarizing microscope was used to differentiate bone tissue and composite materials.
2. Scanning electron microscope (SEM) backscatter electron imaging

   Diamond grinding paste was used to polish the surface of the embedded block after the preparation of the calcium-removing slice, and the carbon was sprayed in the back-scattering electron mode of the SEM (BEI-SEM, KYKY-1000B).
3. SEM two-electron imaging

   Some samples were used in conventional scanning electron microscopy (two-electron mode). Samples with formalin fixation were prepared with 2.5% glutaraldehyde (0.1 M two, pH 7.2). The sample is put into liquid nitrogen to freeze and fracture the shaft to expose the implant material in the medullary cavity. Take the small sample containing the material and the surrounding bone marrow tissue, then fix it by 1%, then the acetone will be dehydrated gradually. The CO_2 critical point is dry and the gold is sprayed under SEM (Hitachi S-450). Component analysis and calculation of ca/p atom ratio in selected area are carried out using spectrometer.

4. Microsclerometry

The embedded block after the preparation of the calcium-cut slice was polished by the diamond grinding paste, which was used for the microhardness determination. Using the $l = 25$ diamond pressure head, load for the GF. The pressure head is wedge-shaped, with two angles of 172.5 (and 130) respectively. In the magnification of x, the length D (m) of the indentation long diagonal is measured with the micrometer. The formula for the calculation of the microhardness was: $hk = 14{,}229$ (L/D2 (kgf/mm^2), measured in the femoral cortex, implanted materials, and the newly formed bone around the implant. As the femur is lengthwise along the backbone axis, the length diagonal of the head can be parallel and perpendicular to the shaft length, and the hardness of the two directions is determined. The hardness of the implanted materials was selected in the middle region of the implant, and the head orientation was the same.

4.11.3 Results

In the calcium-free tissue section, although the implant body has been shed during the production process, most of the interface between the implant and bone marrow tissue is preserved intact. Good contact between the implant and bone marrow was observed under light microscope, and the newly formed bone tissue and cells were found along certain areas of the interface, as shown in Fig. 4.46A. At high magnification, the bone cells and tubules of the trabecular bone are clearly shown, and the composite particles combined with the trabecular bone are clearly visible (Fig. 4.46B). Note that the long axis of the bone cells are parallel to the implant surface, while most bone tubules are perpendicular to the interface; this orientation implies that the trabecular bone has a lamellar structure, and each layer of bone plate is parallel to the implant surface. The bony plates of the newly formed lamellar bone can also be tilted to the interface between the implant and the bone marrow, which can be seen from the light and dark stripes of the bone trabecula under the plane polarization (Fig. 4.47). There is a large amount of tetracycline in the composite at the interface of the fluorescence microscope, indicating that the surface layer of the implant is in active mineralization (Fig. 4.48). The additional growth of the newly formed lamellar bone on the trabecular bone can be seen from two mineralized markers (Fig. 4.48B), from which the formation of the bone can be inferred to grow from the implant surface to the medullary cavity. The growth rate of bone was approximately 0.4–0.5 μm/days by the time interval of double marker line is 10 days.

The technique of electron imaging by SEM can distinguish the implant material, bone and soft tissue, and related interface clearly. As can be seen from Fig. 4.49, after implantation for three months, the central part of the

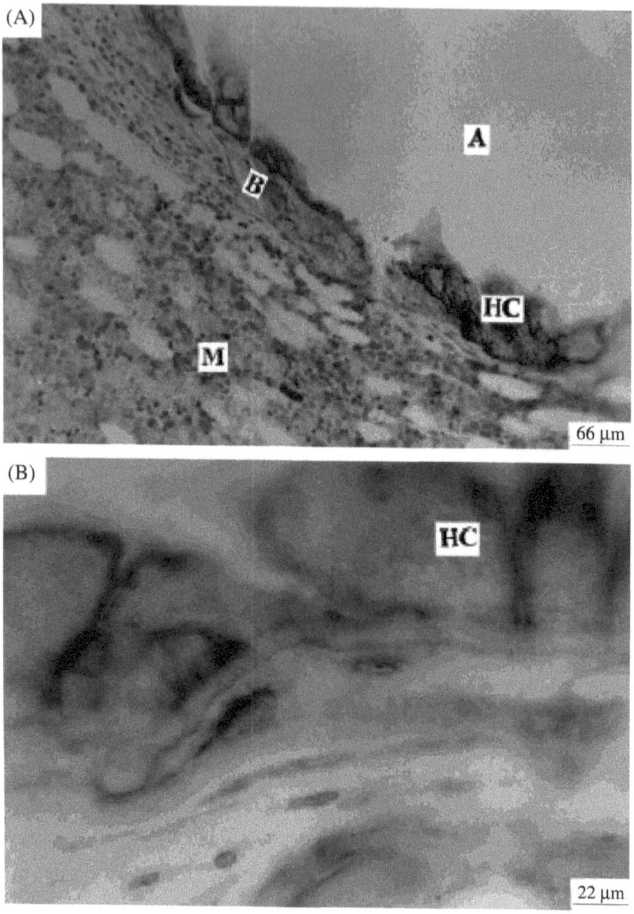

FIGURE 4.46 (A) Non-decalcified tissue sections show good contact between the implant and the bone marrow tissue, and new bone tissue and cells can be found in some areas;150X;(B) Bone cells and bone tubules in the trabecular bone are shown at high magnification. 450 x;

implant is still very dense and unaffected, while the surrounding area of the implant undergoes a greater degree of degradation and is accompanied by the formation of new bone. Fig. 4.49A is a macroscopic picture, showing that the outer contour of the implant is very irregular, and the active absorption of the material has caused many depressions and pipes in the implant, and even formed a cavity inside the implant body. The shallow dish-shaped sag is about a few microns deep, up to dozens of microns long, and resembles a Howship trap formed by osteoclast-absorbing bone tissue. Part of the sag has been filled with newly formed bone trabecular (Fig. 4.49B). Deep implant piping also accompanies the deposition of bones. These pipelines can even penetrate implants (Fig. 4.49C, D), while the cavities formed within

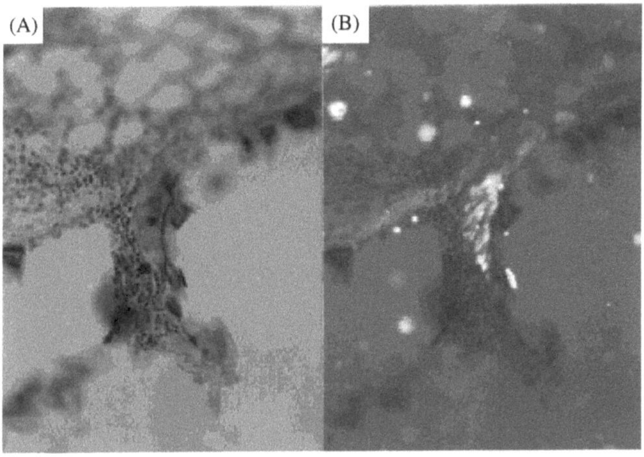

FIGURE 4.47 Common light (A) and polarized polarization (B) showing new lamellar bone.

the dense implant and the growth of new bone on the wall mean that bone marrow tissue and various types of cells invade the implant, and these pipes and cavities are the same as the so-called cutting and filling cone; the latter is a typical feature of the bone remodeling process in the dense bone. A number of cracks can be seen in Fig. 4.49 and may have been formed during the preparation of tissue slices. It is noteworthy that all cracks are produced in the implant, not in the implant–bone interface. The high magnification shown in Fig. 4.50 shows the close contact between bone and implant. Osteogenesis and degradation of the implant were also observed in the samples. Fig. 4.51 shows the bone deposition on the surface of the implant. An osteocyte was closely contacted with the implant in the lacunae. Fig. 4.52 shows the interface between the implant and bone marrow. The composite was globular. Gradient distribution of Ca/P ratio was existed in the entire interface. Such phenomena might be caused by a dissolution–precipitation process. Fig. 4.53 shows another site of the implant–marrow interface with many giant cells aggregated.

4.11.4 Discussion

The study in this chapter shows that dense cylindrical implants that have been implanted into the medullary cavity for three months are degraded to form numerous traps, pipelines, and even cavities within the implant. It is concluded that humoral-mediated dissolution and cell-mediated absorption are two major approaches to material degradation. It is proved that the active mineralization process occurs in the layer of the implant surface; at the same time, the gradient of ca/p ratio can be detected in the interface between the implant and the bone marrow, which indicates the dissolution of minerals,

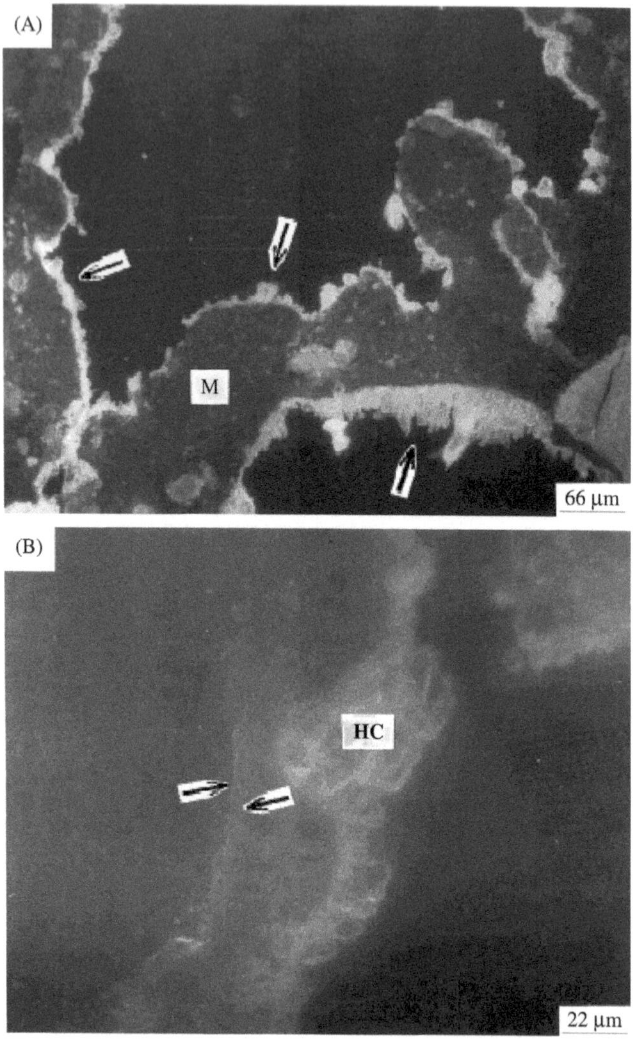

FIGURE 4.48 (A) There is a large number of tetracycline in the composite material at the interface of fluorescence microscope, x. (B) Two mineralized marker lines show the additional growth of newly formed lamellar bone on trabecular bone, 450 ×.

and these phenomena show that the interface layer of the implant is in the dynamic process of dissolution–redeposition. This rapid updating behavior makes the interfacial layer have a certain similarity with braiding bone; the latter is formed in the early stage of bone defect repair, and has the characteristics of rapid growth, disorder of collagen fiber arrangement, and the process of continuous renewal and maturation. The dissolution properties of the synthesized and natural apatite were studied by Daculsi [10], and the

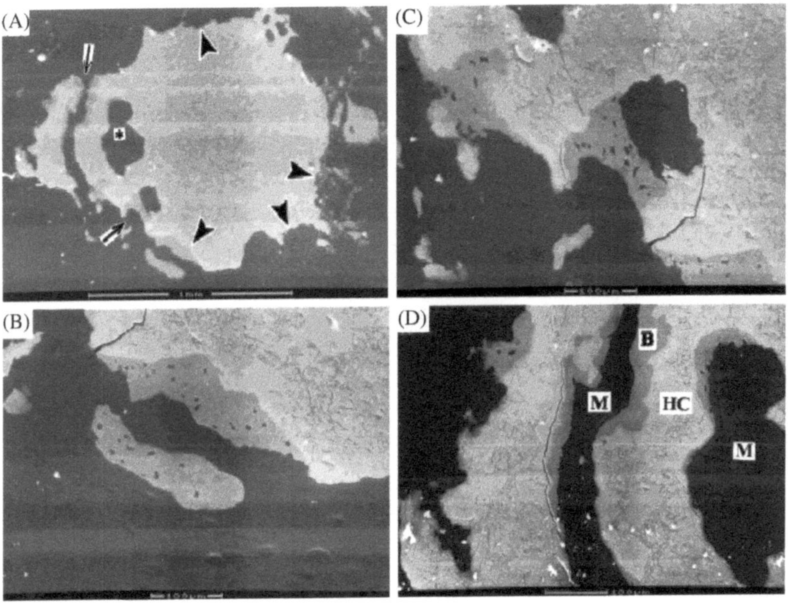

FIGURE 4.49 Scanning electron microscope backscatter electron image shows the degradation of the implant surface and the interior and the subsequent new bone deposition. (A) Macroscopic panorama. (B–D) Local amplification. *M*, Bone marrow; *HC*, implant; *B*, bone.

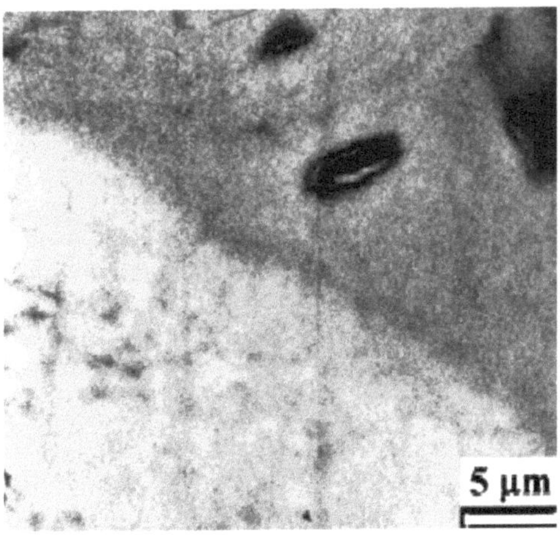

FIGURE 4.50 Scanning electron microscope backscatter electron image; high magnification shows the close contact between bone and implant.

surface and lattice defects of the crystals were proved to be the starting point of dissolution. Therefore, the low crystallinity of mineral phase in MC, the presence of carbonate impurity ions, and the nanometer size of crystals are the key factors that lead to rapid regeneration of the surface layer.

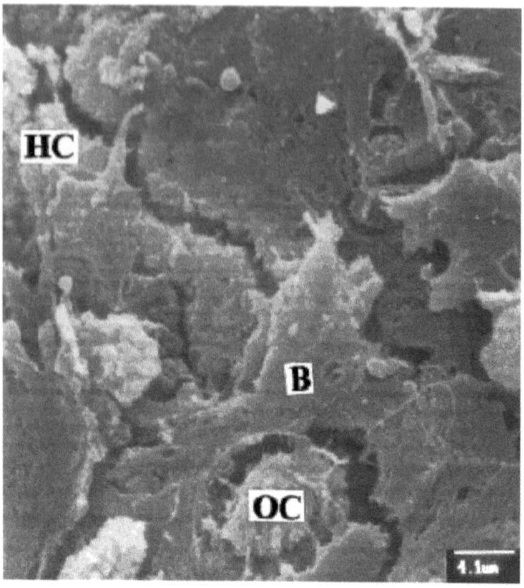

FIGURE 4.51 The scanning electron microscope morphology of frozen fracture specimens showed bone (B) and bone cells (OC) in the surface of implant (HC).

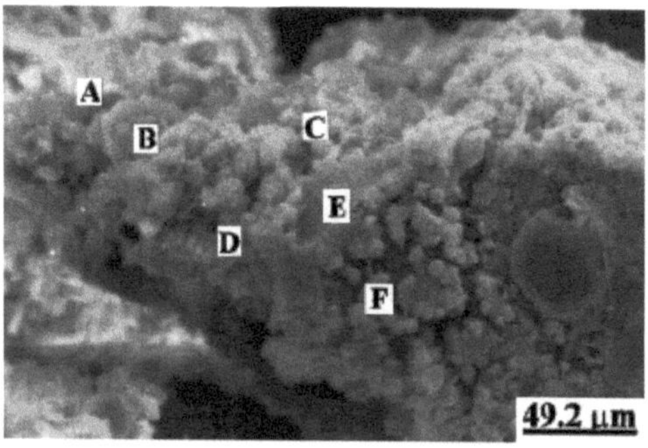

FIGURE 4.52 There is a ca/p gradient in the interface between the implant and the bone marrow tissue, namely (A) 0.614, (B) 0.451, (C) 0.58, (D) 0.044, (E) 0.044, (F) calcium can be neglected.

Cell-mediated absorption is mainly done through giant cells, and the results of morphological observation and ca/p ratio determine that phagocytosis and extracellular degradation are the main ways of interaction between giant cells and N-HAC.

4.11.5 Conclusion

After implantation of MC into the bone marrow cavity, the dynamic rapid renewal process of dissolution–redeposition can occur in the interfacial

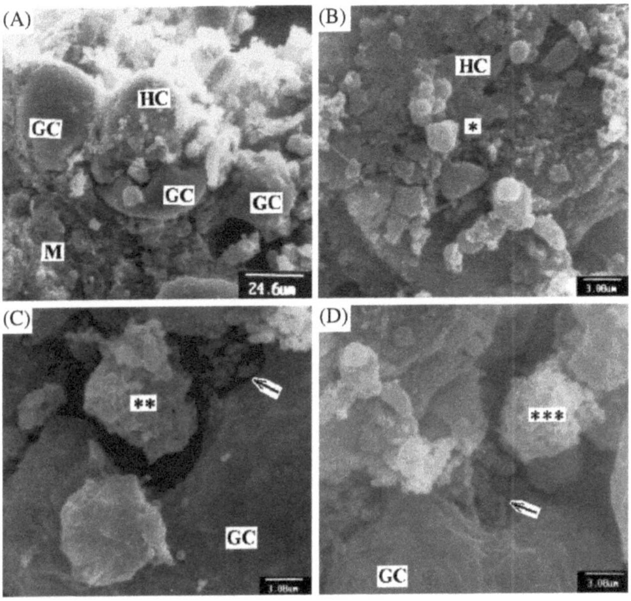

FIGURE 4.53 SEM backscattered electron image. (A) Resorption and bone formation occurred at the peripheral region of the implant. The excavating into the implant led to the formation of large pits (arrowheads), tunnels (arrows), and chambers (asterisk). (B) The resorption pit filled with new bone trabeculae. (C) The tunneling into the implant and new bone deposition. (D) The tunnel through the implant and the chamber inside the bulk of the implant.

layer, and the giant cells can absorb the implant by phagocytosis and extracellular degradation, and after the implant surface and the internal absorption, it is accompanied by the deposition of new bone. This phenomenon is similar to the remodeling process of bone tissue. The results showed that the MC implant could be integrated into the metabolism of living bone and eventually replaced by bone tissue. The raw materials of the mineralized gum are bioactive materials, and the implant and the bone tissue can form the interfacial chemical bonding. The MC composite lacks the complex grading structure of bone tissue, and the mechanical properties are isotropic. However, its microhardness can reach the lower limit of bone cortex microhardness.

REFERENCES

[1] S.S. Liao, The Study on Mineralized Collagen Based Materials for Bone Tissue Engineering, 2003.

[2] Z. Qiu, Y. Zhang, Z. Zhang, et al., Biodegradable mineralized collagen plug for the reconstruction of craniotomy burr-holes: a report of three cases, Trans. Neurosci. Clin. 1 (1) (2015) 3–9.

[3] K. Guan, T.S. Sun, S.S. Shi, et al., The observation of lumbar intertransverse process spinal fusion in rabbits with nano-hydroxyapatite/collagen composite implants, Cervicodynia Lumbodynia 24 (4) (2003) 218–222.

[4] S. Wang, Y. Yang, Z. Zhao, et al., Mineralized collagen-based composite bone materials for cranial bone regeneration in developing sheep, ACS Biomater. Sci. Eng. 3 (6) (2017).

[5] P. Wang, Y. Yao, H. Zhao, et al., Repair of bone defect by using mineralized collagen materials and collagen membrane in minipig models, China J. Oral Maxillofac. Surg. (5) (2017).

[6] Y. Sun, C.Y. Wang, Z.Y. Wang, et al., Test in canine extraction site preservations by using mineralized collagen plug with or without membrane, J. Biomater. Appl. 30 (9) (2016) 1285.

[7] B. Bai, J.T. Zhu, L.W. Wang, Osteoinductive potential in mandibular defects using a novel collagen membrane, Stomatology 35 (3) (2015) 170–174.

[8] C.Y. Wang, Y.S. Yao, S.F. Wang, et al., Experimental study of tissue engineering bone repairing defects of rabbit mandibular bone, Oral Sci. Res. 28 (3) (2012) 213–217.

[9] C. Du, F.Z. Cui, Q.L. Feng, et al., Tissue response to nano-hydroxyapatite/collagen composite implants in marrow cavity, J. Biomed. Mater. Res. B. Appl. Biomater. 42 (4) (2015) 540–548.

[10] G. Daculsi, R.Z. LeGeros, D. Mitre, et al., Crystal dissolution of biological and ceramic apatites, Calcif, Tissue Int. 45 (1989) 95–103.

Chapter 5

Clinical Applications of the Mineralized Collagen

Tian-Xi Song, Yan-Li Hu, Zhi-Min He, Yun Cui,
Qi Ding and Zhi-Ye Qiu
Beijing Allgens Medical Science and Technology Co., Ltd., Beijing, P.R. China

Bone defect is a common symptom where the integrality of the bone is damaged. The main reasons leading to bone defect include trauma, bone tumor, degenerative disease, infection, osteomyelitis, and some congenital diseases. According to the statistics, there are 20 million orthopedic surgeries every year all over the world, and 70% of them need bone graft substitutes to fill and repair bone defects. The global market capacity of bone implants has reached US$30 billion and has been growing rapidly with a compound annual growth rate (CAGR) of 8.2% [1].

In China, annual there were about 6 million orthopedic surgeries in 2016, and 50% of them needed bone graft substitutes. CAGR of bone grafts in China is 15%–20%, which is much higher than that of the world average level. There is also a considerable market of bone graft substitutes in the field of stomatology. In this field in China, dental implants exceeded 600,000, and periodontal surgeries with bone defect repair exceeded 500,000 in 2016. Besides, many other departments, such as craniotomy and skull base reconstruction of neurosurgery, thoracotomy of chest surgery, as well as plastic surgery, E.N.T., ophthalmology, etc. have their own clinical requirements for bone graft substitutes. These various clinical requirements make up a huge market of the biomaterials for bone graft substitutes. According to calculations, the annual market of the bone graft substitutes in China has exceeded 2 billion RenMinBi (RMB), and is growing rapidly with a CAGR as high as 20%. Moreover, with the continuous improvement of the living standards and increased aging of the population in China, the need for bone graft substitutes for various diseases will continuously increase.

As a biomimetic artificial bone repair material that is most similar to human natural bone in terms of composition and microstructure, mineralized collagen (MC) demonstrated good bone regeneration effects in repairing bone defects at different parts of the body. Especially when mixed with

Mineralized Collagen Bone Graft Substitutes. DOI: https://doi.org/10.1016/B978-0-08-102717-2.00005-9

autologous bone marrow, clinical outcomes of the MC were close to autologous bone [2,3]. This chapter will describe clinical applications of the MC for bone defect repair in the fields of orthopedics, stomatology, and neurosurgery, with analyses of clinical cases.

5.1 CLINICAL APPLICATIONS OF THE MINERALIZED COLLAGEN IN INTERVERTEBRAL FUSION

Spinal fusion is a basic skill in the treatment of spinal diseases. Spinal fusion usually implants bone graft substitutes between facet joints, intertransverse, or interbody, or implants fusion cage interbody with bone grafting through various operative approaches, to form osteointegration between joints of adjacent bodies to establish and maintain spinal stability. Such surgical method has good treatment effects on spine instability caused by various reasons. Bone graft fusion is indispensable in the surgery. The purposes of the bone grafting include maintaining anatomic relationship of the spine, restoring stability of axial load on the vertebral bodies, avoiding lumbar foraminal stenosis induced by collapse of intervertebral space, so as to effectively maintain curative effects of decompression procedures, and prevent long-term complications such as progressive kyphosis or spondylolisthesis [3].

5.1.1 Typical Case 1: Cervical Intervertebral Fusion

Beijing Dongzhimen Hospital performed a clinical study and follow-up of MC artificial bone for anterior cervical bone graft fusion. The study demonstrated clinical outcomes of the MC artificial bone were closed to those with autografting. And the use of the MC artificial bone avoided complications caused by autografting, and reduced surgical time. Therefore, MC is an ideal bone graft substitute for anterior cervical bone graft fusion. A typical case is as follows.

A 42-year-old female patient was admitted to hospital for cervical spondylosis for 4 years and progressive numbness and weakness of the limbs for 3 months. Radiographs revealed persistently enlarged prevertebral soft-tissue shadow and decreased disc height at C5-6 and C6-7 (Fig. 5.1A). magnetic resonance imaging (MRI) revealed features of cervical disc disease at C5-6 and C6-7 (Fig. 5.1B). Corpectomy was performed at C6, internal fixation was performed at C5-7, and cervical bone graft fusion was performed at C6-7. A metal fusion cage was used and 1.5 cm^3 MC bone graft was implanted in each intervertebral space. Lateral X-ray shows that at 14 weeks after the surgery C5-6 and C6-7 have achieved solid spinal fusion. (From: Beijing Dongzhimen Hospital).

5.1.2 Typical Case 2: Atlanto-Axial Intertransverse Fusion

A 59-year-old male patient was admitted to hospital for limitation of motion caused by cervical trauma. He was diagnosed as burst fracture at C1.

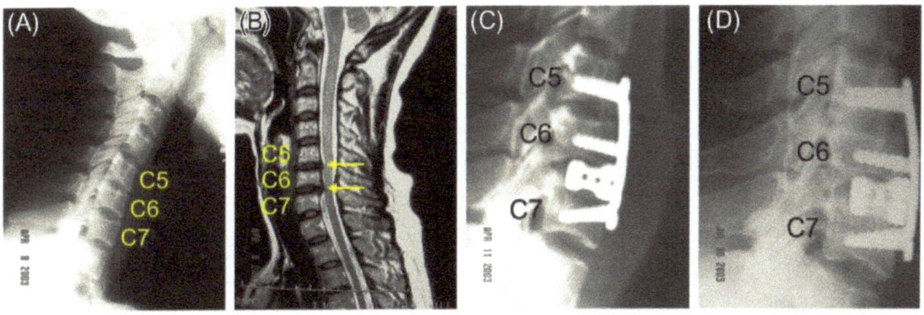

FIGURE 5.1 Preoperative and postoperative imaging observations. (A, B) Preoperative X-ray and MRI image shows spinal cord was compressed by C5-6 disc and C6-7. (C) Postoperative immediate lateral image. (D) Lateral X-ray at 14 weeks after the surgery.

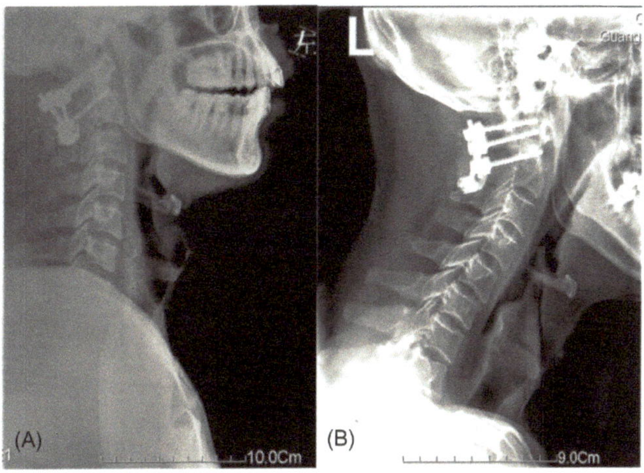

FIGURE 5.2 Postoperative plain radiographs at follow-ups. (A) 2 weeks postoperation. (B) 3 months postoperation.

Decompression was performed at C1-2 with internal fixation by pedicle screw and intertransverse bone graft fusion. 2 cm^3 biomimetic MC artificial bone particle was implanted into both sides of atlanto-axial intertransverse spaces. After 3 months, the implanted MC particles blurred on the edge and became irregular. The atlanto-axial intertransverse fusion was preliminarily achieved (From: Guangzhou General Hospital of Guangzhou Military Command of PLA) (Fig. 5.2).

5.1.3 Typical Case 3: Lumbar Interbody Fusion

A 28-year-old female patient was admitted to hospital for low back pain with radiating pain and numbness at left lower extremity for 2 years, and aggravated for 1 week. She was diagnosed as lumbar spinal stenosis and lumbar disc herniation at L5-S1. Fenestration decompression of the vertebral plate, removal of nucleus pulposus, and interbody bone graft fusion were

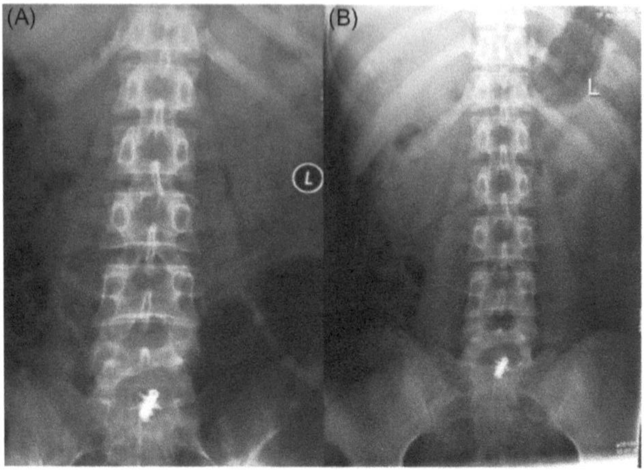

FIGURE 5.3 Postoperative plain radiographs at follow-ups. (A) 2 weeks postoperation, (B) 3 months postoperation.

performed at L5-S1. A lumbar interbody fusion cage filled with 1.5 cm^3 autologous bone particle mixed with biomimetic MC artificial bone particle was implanted. At 3 months postoperation, the width of each intervertebral space was fine with symmetry at both sides. The implanted bone graft particles blurred with obvious ossification and without obvious gap. The interbody fusion was preliminarily achieved. (From: Beijing Dongzhimen Hospital) (Fig. 5.3).

5.1.4 Typical Case 4: Lumbar Interbody Fusion

A 48-year-old female patient was admitted to hospital for low back pain with radiating pain and numbness at both lower extremities for 2 years, and aggravated for 1 month. She was diagnosed as lumbar spinal stenosis and lumbar disc herniation at L5-S1. Fenestration decompression of the vertebral plate, removal of nucleus pulposus, and interbody bone graft fusion were performed at L5-S1. A lumbar interbody fusion cage filled with 2.5 cm^3 biomimetic MC artificial bone particle with pressure was implanted. At 3 months postoperation, the width of each intervertebral space was fine with symmetry at both sides. The implanted bone graft particles blurred with obvious ossification and without obvious gap. The interbody fusion was preliminarily achieved. (From: Guangzhou General Hospital of Guangzhou Military Command of PLA) (Fig. 5.4).

5.1.5 Typical Case 5: Lumbar Interbody Fusion

A 56-year-old male patient was admitted to hospital for low back pain with radiating pain and numbness at both lower extremities for more than 1 year, and aggravated for 2 months. He was diagnosed as lumbar spinal stenosis

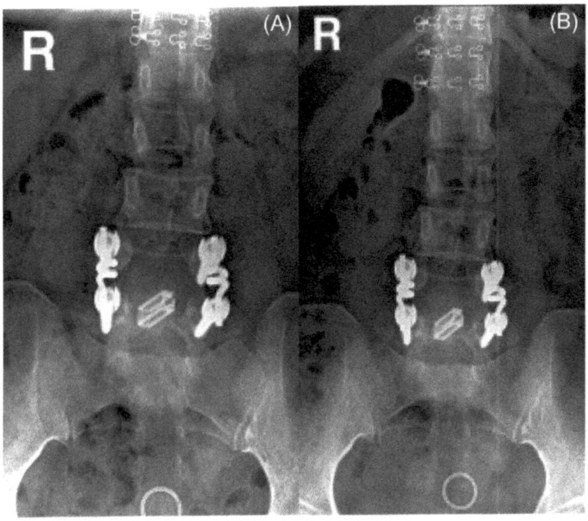

FIGURE 5.4 Postoperative plain radiographs at follow-ups (A) 1 postoperation. (B) 3 months postoperation.

and lumbar disc herniation at L5-S1. Fenestration decompression of the vertebral plate, removal of nucleus pulposus, and interbody bone graft fusion were performed at L5-S1. A lumbar interbody fusion cage filled with 1.5 cm^3 MC artificial bone particle with pressure was implanted into intervertebral space, and 4 cm^3 autologous bone particle mixed with MC artificial bone particles was implanted into intertransverse space. At 3 months postoperation, the width of each intervertebral space was fine with symmetry at both sides. The implanted bone graft particles blurred with obvious ossification and without obvious gap. The interbody fusion was preliminarily achieved. (From: Guangzhou General Hospital of Guangzhou Military Command of PLA) (Fig. 5.5).

5.1.6 Typical Case 6: Lumbar Interbody Fusion

A 57-year-old female patient was admitted to hospital for low back pain and discomfort with radiating pain at both lower extremity for more than 2 years, and aggravated for 2 weeks. She was diagnosed as lumbar spinal stenosis and lumbar disc herniation at L4-S1. Spinal canal decompression with semilaminectomy, removal of nucleus pulposus, and interbody and intertransverse bone graft fusion were performed at L4-S1. Three lumbar interbody fusion cages filled with 1.5 cm^3 autologous bone particle mixed with biomimetic MC artificial bone particle with pressure respectively were implanted into intervertebral space, and 4 cm^3 autologous bone particle mixed with biomimetic MC artificial bone particles was implanted intertransverse space. At 3 months postoperation, the width of each intervertebral space was fine with symmetry at both sides. The implanted bone graft particles blurred with

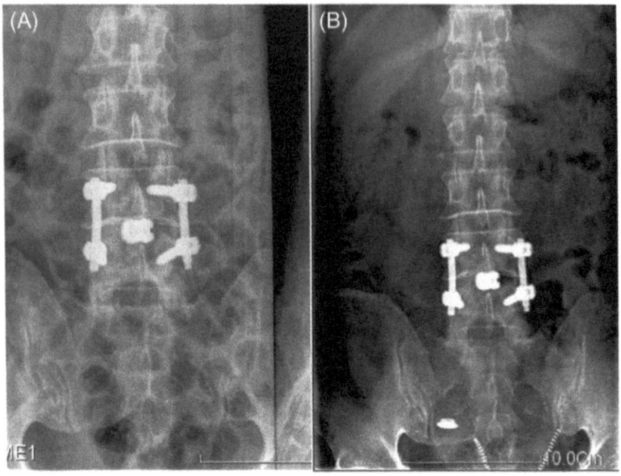

FIGURE 5.5 Postoperative plain radiographs at follow-ups. (A) 2 weeks postoperation (B) 3 months postoperation.

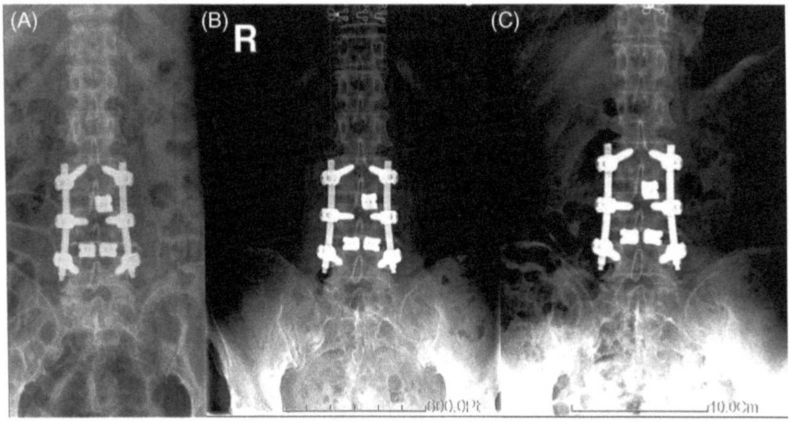

FIGURE 5.6 Postoperative plain radiographs at follow-ups (A) 2 weeks postoperation. (B) 3 months postoperation. (C) 6 months postoperation.

obvious ossification and without obvious gap. The interbody fusion was preliminarily achieved. At 6 months postoperation, the width of each intervertebral space was fine with symmetry at both sides. The implanted bone graft particles could not be identified and the edge disappeared. The interbody fusion was achieved. (From: Guangzhou General Hospital of Guangzhou Military Command of PLA) (Fig. 5.6).

5.1.7 Typical Case 7: Lumbar Interbody Fusion

A 15-year-old male patient was admitted to hospital for low back pain with radiating pain at both lower extremities for 3 months, and aggravated for

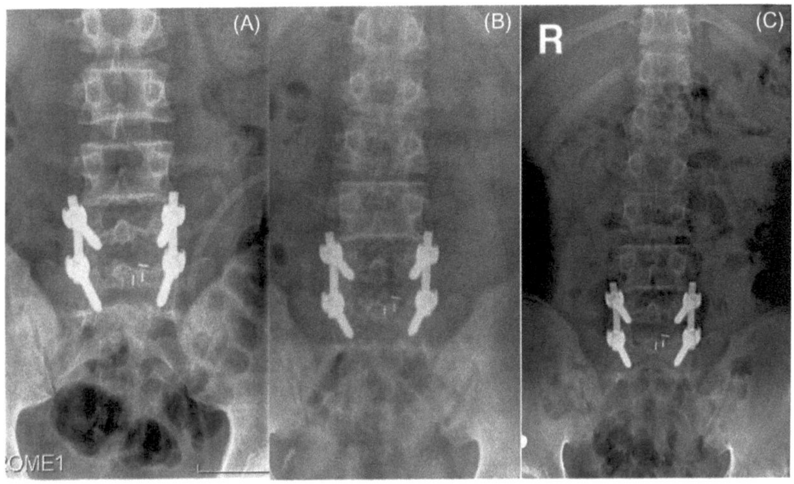

FIGURE 5.7 Postoperative plain radiographs at follow-ups (A) 2 weeks postoperation. (B) 3 months postoperation. (C) 6 months postoperation.

2 weeks. He was diagnosed as lumbar spinal stenosis and lumbar disc herniation at L5-S1. Fenestration decompression of the vertebral plate, removal of nucleus pulposus, and interbody bone graft fusion were performed at L5-S1. A lumbar interbody fusion cage made of polyetheretherketone (PEEK) filled with 1.5 cm^3 autologous bone particle mixed with biomimetic MC artificial bone particle with pressure was implanted. At 3 months postoperation, the width of each intervertebral space was fine with symmetry at both sides. The implanted bone graft particles blurred with obvious ossification and without obvious gap. The interbody fusion was preliminarily achieved. At 6 months postoperation, the width of each intervertebral space was fine with symmetry at both sides. The implanted bone graft particles could not be identified and the edge disappeared. The interbody fusion achieved. (From: Guangzhou General Hospital of Guangzhou Military Command of PLA) (Fig. 5.7).

As a conclusion of the above typical cases, biomimetic MC achieved good clinical outcomes in interbody bone graft fusion surgeries through both anterior and posterior approaches. According to the follow-ups, the bone graft results were close to those using autologous iliac bone. There was no rejection reaction. Complications caused by autografting were avoided. Time of each surgery was reduced. Therefore, biomimetic MC is an idea bone graft substitute for interbody fusion [4].

5.2 CLINICAL APPLICATIONS OF THE MINERALIZED COLLAGEN IN INTERTRANSVERSE FUSION

Intertransverse bone graft fusion is one of the surgical methods for spinal fusion. Such fusion is performed between transverse processes with removal of cortical bone, so as to partially reconstruct stability of the spine after laminectomy. Intertransverse fusion is a commonly used surgical method for the treatment of spinal instability caused by various reasons [5].

5.2.1 Typical Case 1: Lumbar Intertransverse Fusion

A 45-year-old female patient was admitted to hospital for low back pain with radiating pain and numbness at both lower extremities for 3 months, and aggravated for 1 week. She was diagnosed as lumbar spinal stenosis and lumbar disc herniation at L4-S1. Decompression of the vertebral plate, removal of nucleus pulposus, and internal fixation with pedicle screws were performed at L4-S1, and interbody bone graft fusion was performed at L5-S1. Both intertransverse spaces were implanted with 4 cm^3 autologous bone particle and 4 cm^3 biomimetic MC artificial bone particle respectively. At 6 months postoperation, the side implanted with autologous bone fused well, and the other side implanted with the biomimetic MC got close to osseous fusion. The symptoms disappeared and the patient returned to normal life and work. (From: Beijing Dongzhimen Hospital) (Fig. 5.8).

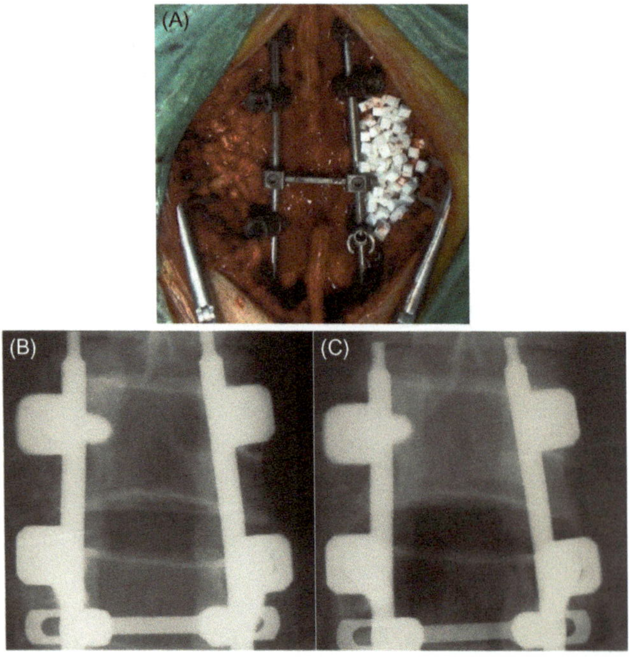

FIGURE 5.8 (A) Implantation of autologous bone and biomimetic mineralized collagen into intertransverse spaces at L5-S1. (B) Plain radiograph at 2-month follow-up. (C) Plain radiograph at 6-month follow-up.

5.2.2 Typical Case 2: Thoracic Intertransverse Fusion

A 75-year-old female patient was admitted to hospital for intradural masses in thoracic vertebrae and incomplete paraplegia. The intradural masses were then determined at T8-9. In the surgery, vertebral plates of T8-9 were removed, spinal dura mater was incised, followed by removal of the masses after neurolysis. Intertransverse bone graft fusion using mixture of autologous bone and biomimetic MC was performed with pedicle screws fixation. At 3 months postoperation, the pedicle screws and rods at T8-9 fixed firmly with fine interbody space. The implanted particles blurred with obvious ossification and without obvious gap. The intertransverse fusion was preliminarily achieved. (From: Beijing Dongzhimen Hospital) (Fig. 5.9).

5.2.3 Typical Case 3: Lumbar Intertransverse Fusion

A 70-year-old female patient was admitted to hospital for lumbosacral pain with radiating pain at both lower extremities for 14 years, and aggravated with involuntary tremor of the extremities for 1 month. She was diagnosed as lumbar spinal stenosis and lumbar disc herniation at L4-5. Decompression by removal of the vertebral plates of L4 and L5, removal of nucleus pulposus, internal fixation with pedicle screws and rods, and interbody and intertransverse bone graft fusions were performed. A total of 5 cm^3 mixture of autologous bone particle and biomimetic MC artificial bone particle was implanted into interbody and intertransverse spaces. At 3 months postoperation, the pedicle screws and rods at L4-5 fixed firmly with fine interbody space. The implanted particles were blurred or invisible. The bone grafting sites were ossified visibly and preliminarily fused. (From: Beijing Dongzhimen Hospital) (Fig. 5.10).

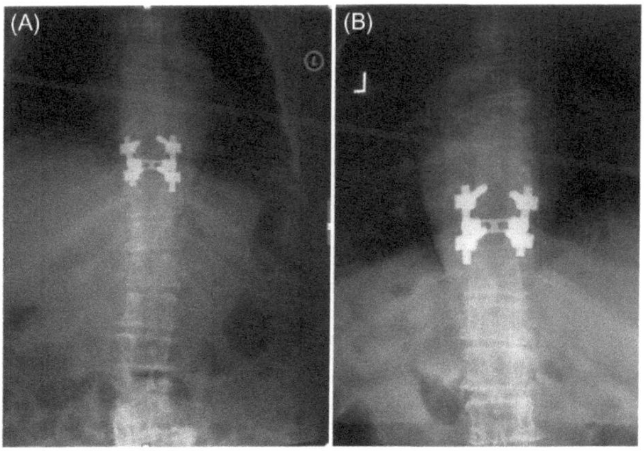

FIGURE 5.9 (A) 2 weeks postoperation. (B) 3 months postoperation.

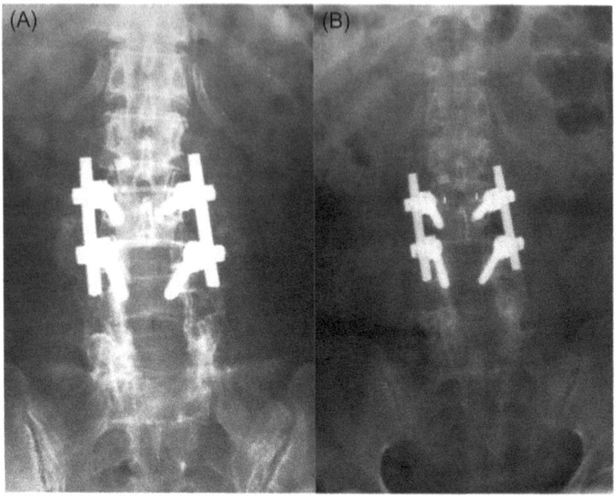

FIGURE 5.10 (A) 2 weeks postoperation. (B) 3 months postoperation.

5.2.4 Typical Case 4: Lumbar Intertransverse Fusion

A 52-year-old male patient was admitted to hospital for low back pain with radiating pain and numbness at both lower extremities for more than half a year, and aggravated for 1 week. He was diagnosed as lumbar disc herniation at L3-4 and L4-5. Decompression by removal of the vertebral plates, removal of nucleus pulposus, internal fixation with pedicle screws, and intertransverse bone graft fusion were performed at L3-5. The intertransverse spaces were implanted with 6 cm^3 mixture of autologous bone particle and biomimetic MC artificial bone particle. At 3 months postoperation, the pedicle screws and rods at L3-5 fixed firmly with fine interbody spaces. The implanted particles blurred with obvious ossification and without obvious gap. The intertransverse fusion was preliminarily achieved. At 6 months postoperation, the pedicle screws and rods at L3-5 were still fixed firmly with fine interbody spaces. Obvious ossification could be observed in intertransverse spaces at right side of L3-4 and both sides of L4-5, without implanted particles. (From: Beijing Dongzhimen Hospital) (Fig. 5.11).

5.2.5 Typical Case 5: Lumbar Intertransverse Fusion

A 74-year-old female patient was admitted to hospital for lumbosacral pain with radiating pain and numbness at both lower extremities, as well as intermittent claudication for 7 months, and aggravated for 2 weeks. She was diagnosed as lumbar spinal stenosis and lumbar disc herniation at L4-S1. Decompression by removal of the vertebral plates, removal of nucleus

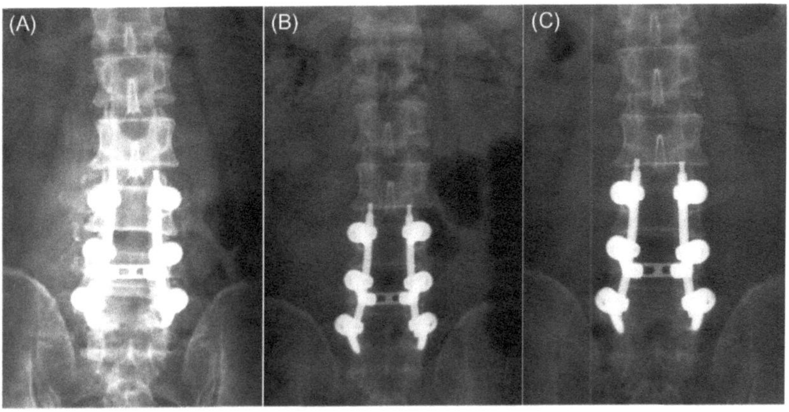

FIGURE 5.11 (A) 2 weeks postoperation. (B) 3 months postoperation. (C) 6 months postoperation.

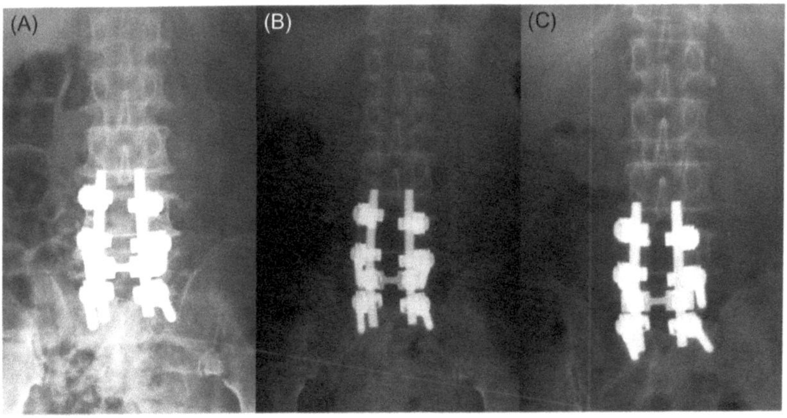

FIGURE 5.12 (A) 2 weeks postoperation. (B) 3 months postoperation. (C) 6 months postoperation.

pulposus, internal fixation with pedicle screws, and intertransverse bone graft fusion were performed at L4-S1. The bilateral intertransverse spaces were implanted with 4.5 cm^3 mixture of autologous bone particle and biomimetic MC artificial bone particle. At 3 months postoperation, the pedicle screws and rods at L4-S1 fixed firmly with fine interbody spaces. The implanted particles blurred with obvious ossification and without obvious gap. The intertransverse fusion was preliminarily achieved. At 6 months postoperation, the pedicle screws and rods at L4-S1 were still fixed firmly with fine interbody spaces. Obvious ossification could be observed in intertransverse spaces at right side of L4-5 and both sides of L5-S1, without implanted particles. (From: Beijing Dongzhimen Hospital) (Fig. 5.12).

5.2.6 Typical Case 6: Lumbar Intertransverse Fusion

A 53-year-old female patient was admitted to hospital for low back pain with radiating pain and numbness at both lower extremities for more than 6 months. She was diagnosed as lumbar spinal stenosis and lumbar disc herniation at L4-S1. Decompression by removal of the vertebral plates, removal of nucleus pulposus, internal fixation with pedicle screws, interspinous fixation, and intertransverse bone graft fusion were performed at L4-S1. The bilateral intertransverse spaces were implanted with 6 cm^3 mixture of autologous bone particle and biomimetic MC artificial bone particle. At 3 months postoperation, the pedicle screws and rods at L4-S1 fixed firmly with fine interbody spaces. The implanted particles blurred with obvious ossification and without obvious gap. The intertransverse fusion was preliminarily achieved. At 6 months postoperation, the pedicle screws and rods at L4-S1 still fixed firmly with fine interbody spaces. Obvious ossification could be observed in intertransverse spaces at right side of L4-5 and both sides of L5-S1, without implanted particles. (From: Beijing Dongzhimen Hospital) (Fig. 5.13).

Beijing Dongzhimen Hospital performed systematic studies and clinical follow-ups for 12 months on interbody and intertransverse bone graft fusions with the biomimetic MC. The clinical outcomes demonstrated that the mixed use of biomimetic MC and autologous bone could achieve similar results to the autologous bone, without obvious rejection reaction. The use of the MC artificial bone ensures sufficient bone graft volume, meanwhile avoids or minimizes complications by harvesting autologous iliac bone. The surgery time could be accordingly reduced. Therefore, the biomimetic MC could be used as substitute or supplement of the autologous bone in interbody and intertransverse bone graft fusions [4,5].

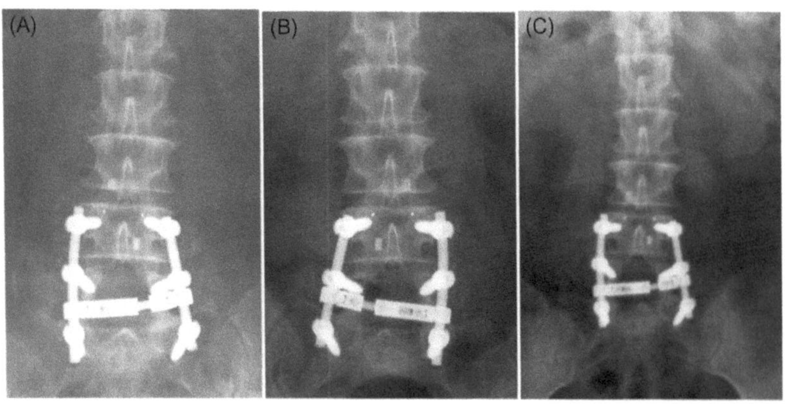

FIGURE 5.13 (A) 2 weeks postoperation. (B) 3 months postoperation. (C) 6 months postoperation.

5.3 CLINICAL APPLICATIONS OF THE MINERALIZED COLLAGEN IN THE TREATMENT OF BONE DEFECT INDUCED BY OSTEOPOROTIC THORACOLUMBAR BURST FRACTURE

Vertebral burst fracture usually occurs due to vertical compression of the vertebral body, and is common in middle and lower lumbar regions. The vertebral body is pressed to burst crush by adjacent bodies, dislodge, or fracture-dislocation. For those thoracolumbar fractures associated with spinal cord injury, surgery should be performed as soon as possible on the basis of definite diagnosis.

The second affiliated hospital of Zhejiang Chinese Medical University (Zhejiang Xinhua Hospital) performed clinical observation studies on the treatment of bone defect induced by osteoporotic thoracolumbar burst fracture with the MC artificial bone graft substitute. During the period from November 2011 to July 2013, 24 patients were selected for the observation. The age of the patients was 55–70 with an average age of 60. Statistical results of these 24 patients showed that the average vertebral height was restored from preoperative $53.2\% \pm 6.2\%$ to $89.1\% \pm 2.8\%$ at the last follow-up, and Cobb's angle was restored from preoperative $23.7^\circ \pm 3.5^\circ$ to $5.0^\circ \pm 1.9^\circ$ at the last follow-up. The results demonstrated that such bone grafting treatment associated with vertebral pedicle screw fixation was safe and effective. This method could reconstruct the spinal stability and retain a portion of motion segment of the spine with less trauma. The MC has good bioresorbability and osteoconductivity, thus promoting growth of osteocytes and minimizing trauma within the injured vertebral body, decreasing "shell-like" change and increasing stability of the injured vertebral body. Sagittal balance can also be restored, and antirotation force of the spine would be increased. Therefore, the biomimetic MC is a good bone graft substitute in the treatment of bone defect caused by thoracolumbar burst fracture [6].

5.3.1 Typical Case 1

A 49-year-old male patient was admitted to hospital for difficulties of daily activities induced by lumbar pain for 1 week. The patient was diagnosed as pathological fracture at L3 vertebrae and tumor-like lesion was determined by biopsy. The L3 vertebral body was almost completely destroyed to form a large cavity, as shown in Fig. 5.14A and B. Fat-suppression sequence MRI (Fig. 5.14C) indicated cystic lesion with liquid inside the L3 vertebral body, and T1 sequence MRI (Fig. 5.14D) indicated space-occupying lesion with an irregular cavity in the L3 vertebral body.

In the surgery, lesion of the fractured L3 was removed via a posterior approach. Then, MC bone graft was implanted into the vertebrae via a transpedicular approach. The MC bone graft was mixed with a small amount autologous bone particles harvested from nearby zygopophysis, vertebral

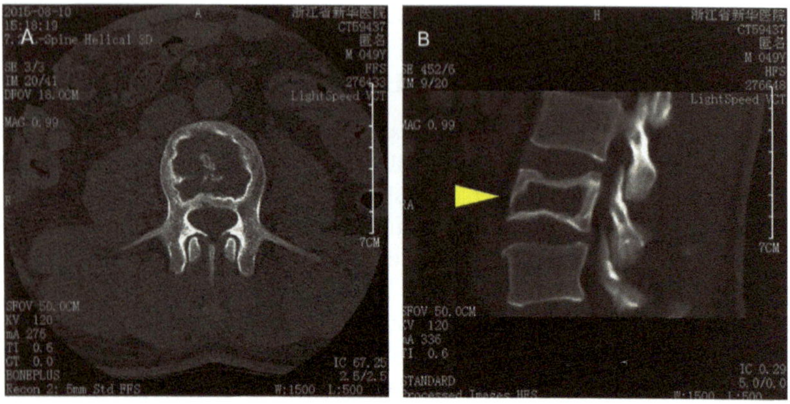

FIGURE 5.14 Preoperative computed tomography (CT) observations of the injured vertebral body. (A) Transverse plane CT. (B) Sagittal plane CT.

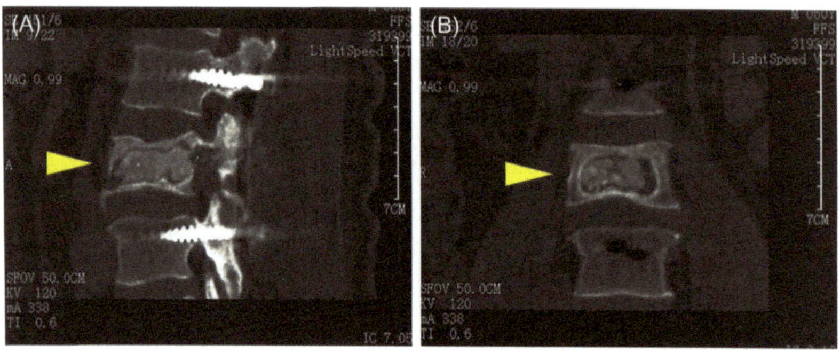

FIGURE 5.15 Postoperative computed tomography (CT) scans and three-dimensional (3D) reconstruction of the injured vertebral body at 3 months after the surgery. (A) Transverse plane CT. (B) Coronal plane CT.

plate, and spinous process surfaces. The amount of the MC bone graft was 20 cm^3, and the intraoperatively harvested autologous bone was about 1 cm^3. Finally, titanium alloy screw-rod system was applied for internal fixation.

Computed tomography (CT) observations were performed in follow-ups at 3 and 18 months postoperation (Figs. 5.15 and 5.16). As shown in Fig. 5.15, bone defect gradually healed at the injured body; the cavity of the injured L3 vertebrae was well filled with bone grafts 3 months after the surgery. However, there was still a gap between the bone graft and the host bone. In the follow year (Fig. 5.16), the gap disappeared with the new bone regeneration and creeping substitution. Bone fusion could be observed at the interface between the grafts and the host bone. three-dimensional (3D) reconstruction of the injured L3 vertebrae indicated that the height restored as a normal vertebral body.

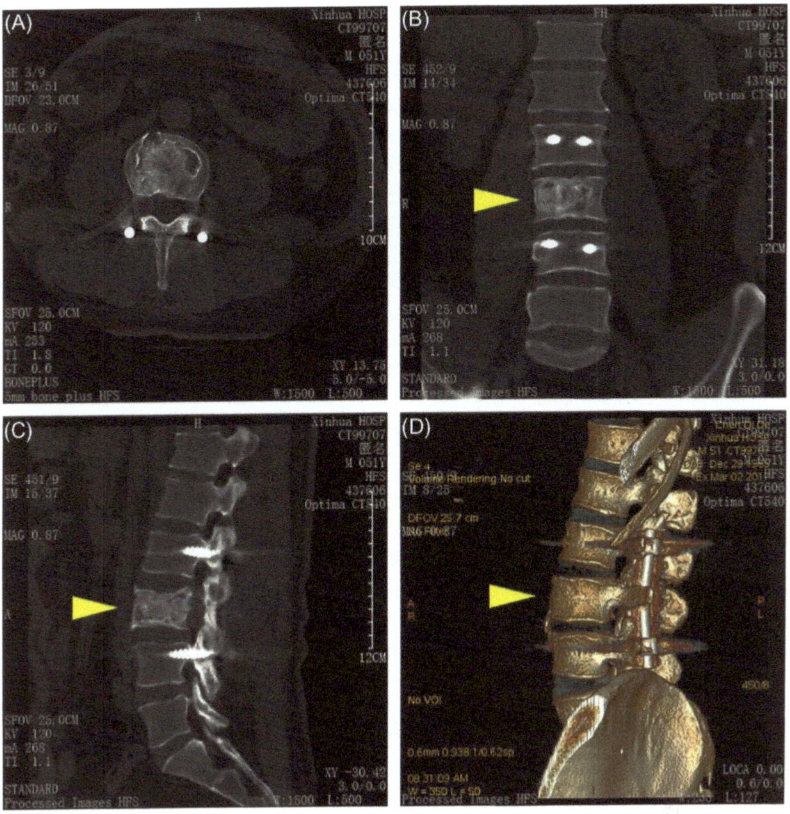

FIGURE 5.16 Postoperative computed tomography (CT) scans and three-dimensional (3D) reconstruction of the injured vertebral body at 18 months after the surgery. (A) Transverse plane CT. (B) Coronal plane CT. (C) Sagittal plane CT. (D) 3D reconstruction of CT scans. Yellow arrow: the healed vertebral body.

5.3.2 Typical Case 2

A 38-year-old female patient was admitted to hospital for limitation of motion induced by lumbar injury and pain for 2 days. She was diagnosed as vertebral burst fracture at L3. Internal fixation at L3, decompression by enlarging interbody space at L2-4, and transpedicular bone grafting at L3 were performed in the surgery. A total of 5 cm^3 mixture of autologous bone particle and biomimetic MC artificial bone particle was implanted into L3, which has been already restored via intraspinal approach. At 6 months post-operation, the pedicle screws and rods fixed firmly, and interbody spaces and intertransverse spaces were normal, without height loss of L3. The implanted bone grafts blurred and invisible with obvious ossification. Osteointegration was preliminarily achieved. At 18 months postoperation, the fracture line at the L3 disappeared, and the vertebral body healed. The heights and spaces of L2-4 were normal without any height loss. (Fig. 5.17).

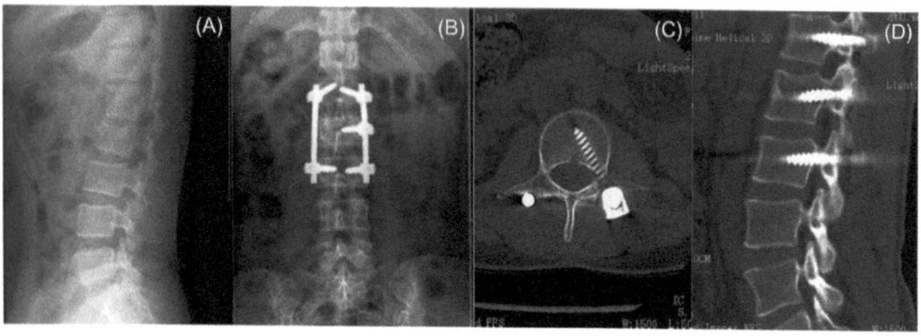

FIGURE 5.17 Imaging observation of the injured vertebral body. (A) Preoperative plain radiograph. (B) Intermediate postoperative plain radiograph. (C) Transverse plane CT at 6 months postoperation. (D) Sagittal plane CT at 18 months postoperation.

5.4 CLINICAL APPLICATIONS OF THE MINERALIZED COLLAGEN IN THE TREATMENT OF BONE DEFECTS INDUCED BY BONE FRACTURE AT THE EXTREMITIES

Bone defects on the extremities induced by trauma, tumor, bone nonunion, and so on are the most common disease in orthopedics [7,8]. This section introduces a variety of typical cases of bone defect repair induced by different reasons with the MC on the extremities.

5.4.1 Typical Case 1: Comminuted Fracture at Right Distal Radius

A 53-year-old male patient was admitted to hospital for posttraumatic pain and swelling of the right forearm, with limitation of motion for 1 day. X-ray showed comminuted fracture at his right distal radius. Open reduction and internal fixation with bone grafting were performed for the treatment of the comminuted fracture. 1.5 cm^3 biomimetic MC particle was implanted for the reconstruction of the bone defect. At 3 months postoperation, the internal fixation of the right distal radius was firm. The fracture was blurred with obvious hypercallosis, and the grafted particle blurred and invisible. The bone fracture was healed. (From: Guangzhou General Hospital of Guangzhou Military Command of PLA) (Fig. 5.18).

5.4.2 Typical Case 2: Comminuted Fracture at Right Olecroanon

A 30-year-old male patient was admitted to hospital for pain and swelling of the right elbow trauma, with limitation of motion for 3 hours. X-ray showed comminuted fracture at his right olecroanon. Open reduction and internal fixation with bone grafting were performed for the treatment of the comminuted fracture. 1.5 cm^3 biomimetic MC particle and putty were implanted for the

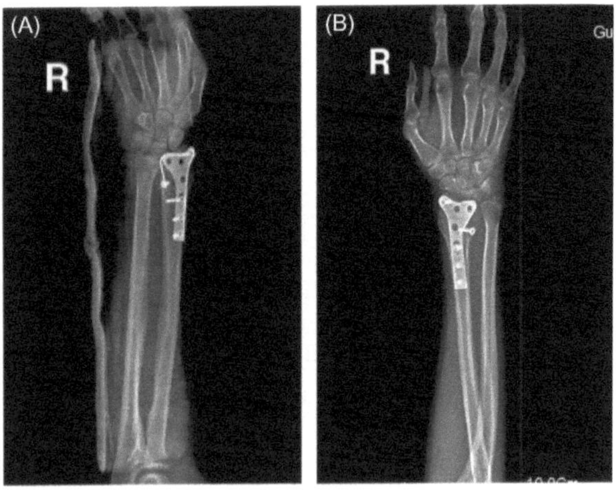

FIGURE 5.18 Plain radiograph of the treated comminuted fracture at the right distal radius. (A) 1 week postoperation. (B) 3 months postoperation.

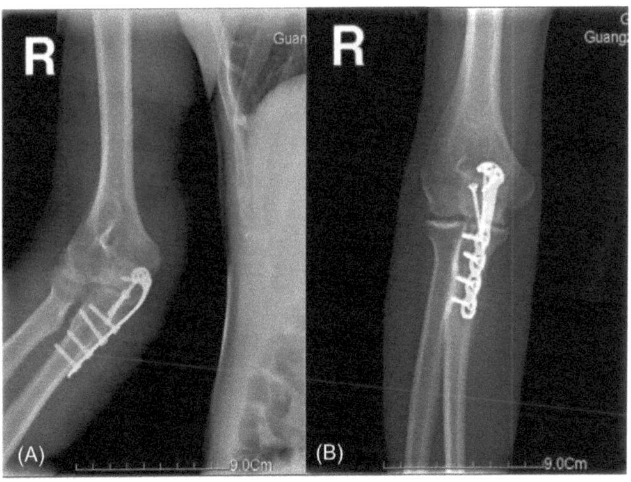

FIGURE 5.19 Plain radiograph of the treated comminuted fracture at the right olecroanon. (A) 1 week postoperation. (B) 3 months postoperation.

reconstruction of the bone defect. At 3 months postoperation, the internal fixation of the right distal olecroanon was firm. The fracture was blurred with obvious hypercallosis, and the grafted particle blurred and invisible. The bone fracture healed. (From: Guangzhou General Hospital of Guangzhou Military Command of PLA) (Fig. 5.19).

5.4.3 Typical Case 3: Osteoporotic Proximal Humeral Fractures

This is a case of 76-year-old female patient who was hospitalized due to the onset of left shoulder pain and swell following an injury and restricted activity for 1 day. Physical examination: old woman, sane, passive position. No obvious abnormalities were observed in cardiopulmonary and spinal examination. Obvious swelling of the left shoulder, visible subcutaneous silting, left shoulder joint tenderness, left shoulder joint axial limited activity, each left radial pulse strong, flexion and right hand point to each function is normal, no feeling, numb, and obstacles. An X-ray film taken before surgery, in which the comminuted fracture of the surgical neck of humerus could be seen and diagnosed as comminuted fractures of the proximal left humerus was treated in the observation group. The authors evaluated X-ray observation of patients before and after treatment with internal fixation and biomimetic MC putty. X-ray film taken before surgery showed comminuted fracture of the surgical neck of humerus (Fig. 5.20A). One day after operation, all fractures showed good contraposition and alignment on the X-ray film (Fig. 5.20B). Bone defect was implanted with biomimetic MC putty, along with satisfactory internal fixation. Three months after operation, the fracture appeared healed with good fixation and union. There was neither osteonecrosis of humeral head nor fracture, proving excellent osteogenesis. The patient was free of pullout or loosening of internal fixation because of increased bone mass and rapid healing of the fracture.

The current study is to observe the effect of the locking system strengthened by biomimetic MC putty for the treatment of senile proximal humeral osteoporotic fractures. From January 2012 to December 2015, 80 cases of senile patients with osteoporotic proximal humeral fractures were randomly divided into an observation group and a control group, each group with a total of 40 cases. For this group study, we used biomimetic MC putty as

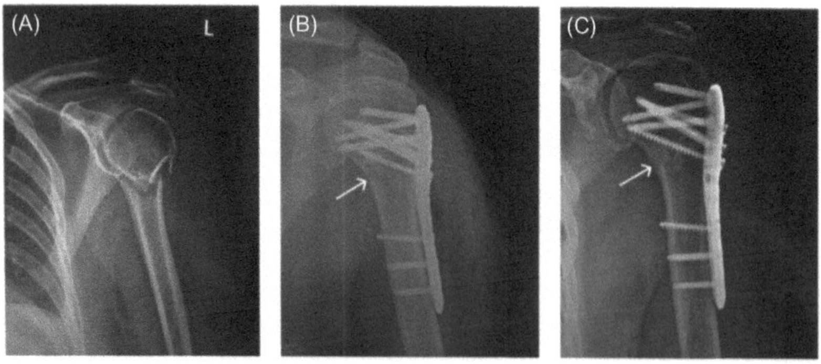

FIGURE 5.20 A case of 76-year-old female patient diagnosed as comminuted fractures of the left proximal humerus. (A) An X-ray film taken before surgery, in which the comminuted fracture of the surgical neck of humerus could be seen. (B) Radiograph was taken 1 day after operation for postoperative reexamination. All fractures showed good contraposition and alignment with satisfactory internal fixation. (C) Radiograph was taken 3 months after operation. Fracture appeared healed with good union. There was neither osteonecrosis nor fracture of humeral head. The internal fixation nails were neither pulled out nor loosened.

bone grafting material, combined with the locking plate in the treatment of senile osteoporotic proximal humeral fracture. Bone defect in 40 cases of senile osteoporotic fracture was packed with biomimetic MC putty. As observed by X-ray and clinical manifestations, fracture healing of the 40 cases of senile osteoporotic fracture were shown to be expedited, with fracture healed and bone graft material absorbed within 12 weeks. Shoulder joint showed better function than the control group while the complication rate is lower than the control group [8]. (From: Jing'an Branch of Shanghai Huashan Hospital).

5.4.4 Typical Case 4: Middle Femoral Shaft Comminuted Fracture

This is a case of 48-year-old female patient who was hospitalized due to left thigh pain and swell following an injury and restricted activity for 4 hours. Physical examination: middle-aged woman, conscious, painful faces, depressed, left lower limbs temporary fixed, passive position. No obvious abnormalities were observed in cardiopulmonary and spinal examination. The left leg is obviously swollen, and the skin shows bruising. The left femoral artery and the left popliteal pulse are clear, the left dorsal artery beats clearly. The left hip joint is restricted and the left ankle is in flexion. No abnormalities were observed in each toe of the left foot. X-ray indicated that middle femoral shaft comminuted fracture. The admitting diagnosis is middle femoral shaft comminuted fracture. After admission to the hospital, "a comminuted fracture of the left femur was cut and the bone marrow internal fixation was performed." Intraoperative implanted BonGold MC artificial bone particles 3 cm^3. Postoperative symptomatic treatment was administered and the patient was discharged 2 weeks later.

The X-ray results following surgery are shown in Fig. 5.21.

Three months after the operation, the right radius of the distal radius was fixed firmly, and the fracture line was blurred. There was obvious callus hyperplasia, the shadow of bone graft was not visible, and the fracture healed. (From: Guangzhou Military Area Guangzhou General Hospital.)

5.4.5 Typical Case 5: Middle Femoral Shaft Comminuted Fracture

This is a case of 24-year-old male patient who was hospitalized due to the right lower extremity pain and swelling following a car accident and restricted activity for 2 hours. Physical examination: young man, conscious, depressed, right lower limb temporary support fixed, passive position. No obvious abnormalities were observed in cardiopulmonary and spinal examination. The right thigh is visibly swollen, and a large area of green silt is seen under the skin. The right popliteal arterial pulse is normal, and the right foot dorsal artery is clear and powerful. The flexion and extension activities

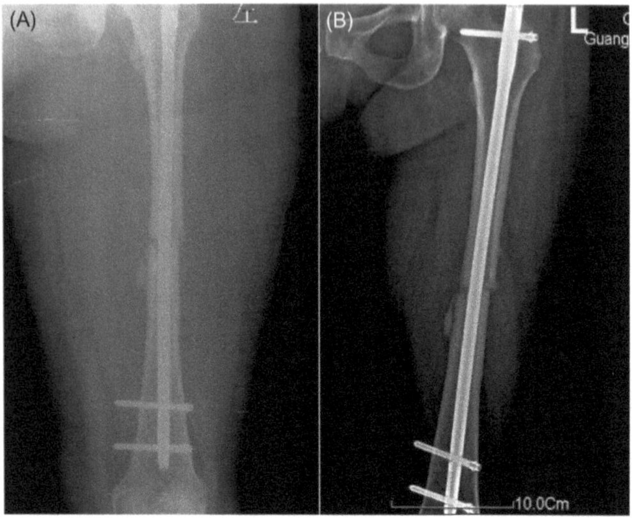

FIGURE 5.21 Results of X-ray examination performed 1 week after surgery (A, left) and 3 months after surgery (B, right).

of right hip knee joint were restricted, and the right ankle and right foot flexion were normal. The X-ray indicated that right femur is comminuted fracture. The admitting diagnosis is midway through the femoral (right). After admission, the "right femoral middle segment comminuted fracture incision and resection of bone marrow internal fixation." Intraoperative implanted BonGold MC artificial bone particles 3 cm^3. Postoperative symptomatic treatment and 3 weeks later discharge.

The X-ray results following surgery are shown in Fig. 5.22.

Three months after the operation, the middle segment of the right femur was fixed firmly, and the fracture line was blurred. There was obvious callus hyperplasia, and the shadow of bone graft was not visible, and the fracture was healed. (From: Guangzhou Military Area Guangzhou General Hospital.)

5.4.6 Typical Case 6: Fracture of Tibial Plateau

A 26-year-old female patient was admitted to hospital for pain and swelling of the right lower extremity, and limitation of motion for 1 day. X-ray showed comminuted fracture of right tibial plateau. Open reduction and internal fixation with bone grafting were performed for the treatment of the comminuted fracture. One cubic centimeter biomimetic MC block was implanted for the reconstruction of the bone defect. At 1 day postoperation, the fractured bone reduced well and the line of force was normal at the right tibial plateau. The internal fixation was firm. The implanted block could be observed with good support effect. At 10 months postoperation, the fracture

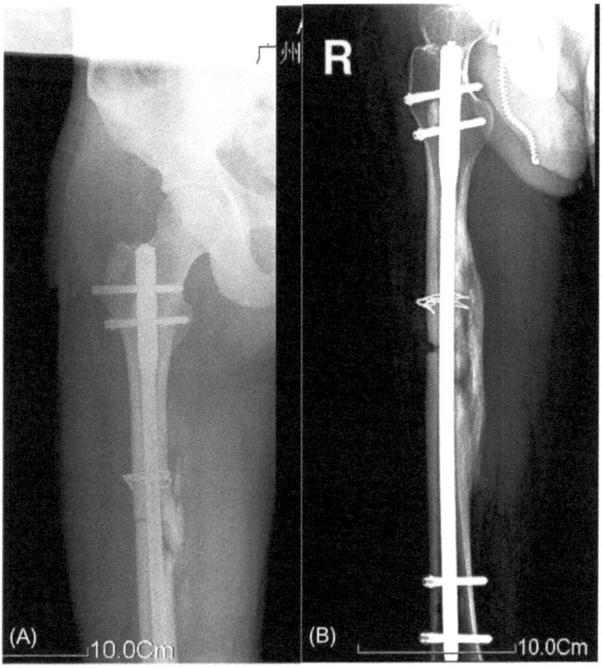

FIGURE 5.22 Results of X-ray examination performed 1 week after surgery (A, left) and 3 months after surgery (B, right).

line of the right tibial plateau blurred. The internal fixation was firm. The implanted block was partially absorbed by creeping substitution, and the edge was a little clear due to bone absorption. (From: Beijing Jishuitan Hospital) (Fig. 5.23).

5.4.7 Typical Case 7: Fracture of Tibial Plateau

A 44-year-old male patient was admitted to hospital for pain and swelling of the left knee, and dared not move for 5 hours. X-ray showed comminuted fracture of left tibial plateau. Open reduction and internal fixation with bone grafting were performed for the treatment of the comminuted fracture. One cubic centimeter biomimetic MC block was implanted for the reconstruction of the bone defect. At 1.5 months postoperation, the fractured bone reduced well and the line of force was normal at the left tibial plateau. Symmetry joint spaces were observed. The internal fixation was firm. The fracture line slightly blurred. The implanted block was partially absorbed and the edge blurred. (From: Beijing Jishuitan Hospital) (Fig. 5.24).

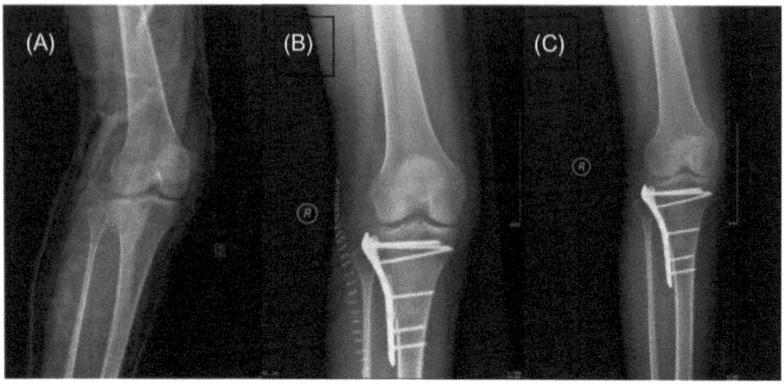

FIGURE 5.23 Plain radiographs of preoperative observation and postoperative follow-ups. (A) Preoperative plain radiograph. (B) 1 day postoperative plain radiograph. (C) 10 months postoperative plain radiograph.

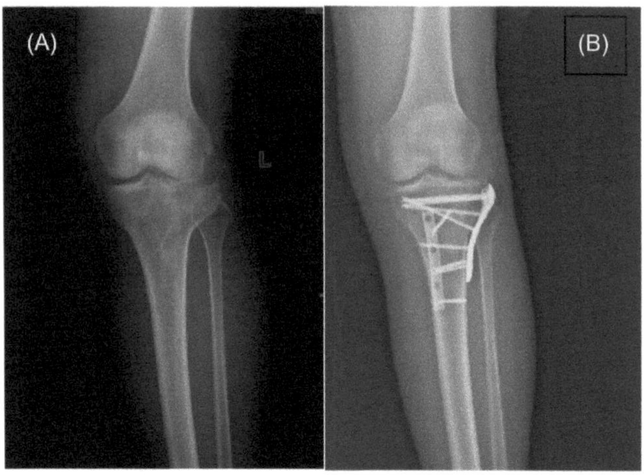

FIGURE 5.24 Plain radiographs pre and postoperaton. (A) Preoperative plain radiograph. (B) 1.5 months postoperative plain radiograph.

5.4.8 Typical Case 8: Fibula Comminuted Fracture

This is a case of 54-year-old male patient who was hospitalized due to right calf pain and posttraumatic swelling and restricted activity for 3 hours. Physical examination: middle-aged man, conscious, his mental health is fine, right lower limb passive position. No obvious abnormalities were observed in cardiopulmonary and spinal examination. The right calf is visibly swollen, a large area of green silt is seen under the skin, with fracture end friction. Right knee joint, right ankle flexion and extension activity are restricted, right foot dorsal artery pulsation is powerful, the right foot flexion and extension function are normal, with no exception. The X-ray indicated right tibia

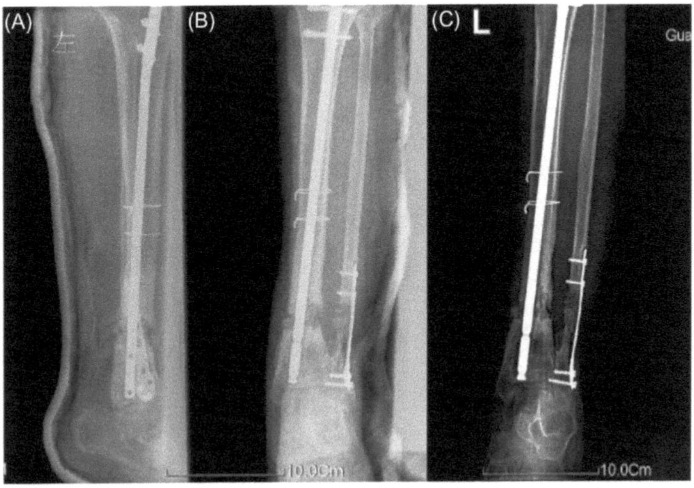

FIGURE 5.25 The X-ray examination results after surgery and follow-up. (A) Preoperation. (B) 1 week after operation. (C) 3 months after operation.

and fibula comminuted fracture. After admission, "the right tibia fibula distal comminuted fracture incision and resection of bone marrow internal fixation. Intraoperative implanted" BonGold MC artificial bone particles 2 cm^3. Postoperative symptomatic treatment and 3 weeks later discharge.

X-ray results after surgery are shown in Fig. 5.25.

Three months after the operation, there was a small amount of callus hyperplasia in the left tibial fibula, the fracture line was blurred, the edge of bone graft was indistinct, and the fracture was initially healed. (From: Guangzhou Military Area Guangzhou General Hospital.)

5.4.9 Typical Case 9: The Disconnection of Limb Bones

This is a case of 32-year-old male patient who was hospitalized due to the fracture of left tibia and fibula in a traffic accident. The tibia was fixed by external fixation, the fibula was fixed in the intramedullary spinal cord, and the fracture was not healed for 15 months after surgery that was performed by another hospital. The admitting diagnosis is the fracture of the left tibial fibular fracture was not healed after operation. After admission to hospital, debride the left tibial fibula and bone transplantation internal fixation. Implanted BonGold MC artificial bone particles 1.5 cm^3 to the nonunion of tibia fracture during operation, and fixation fracture with external fixator. Surgical progress went smoothly.

Postoperative X-ray results are shown in Fig. 5.26.

This patient was followed up for 10 months, and the nonunion of the tibia completely healed and the fracture line disappeared, and the medullary

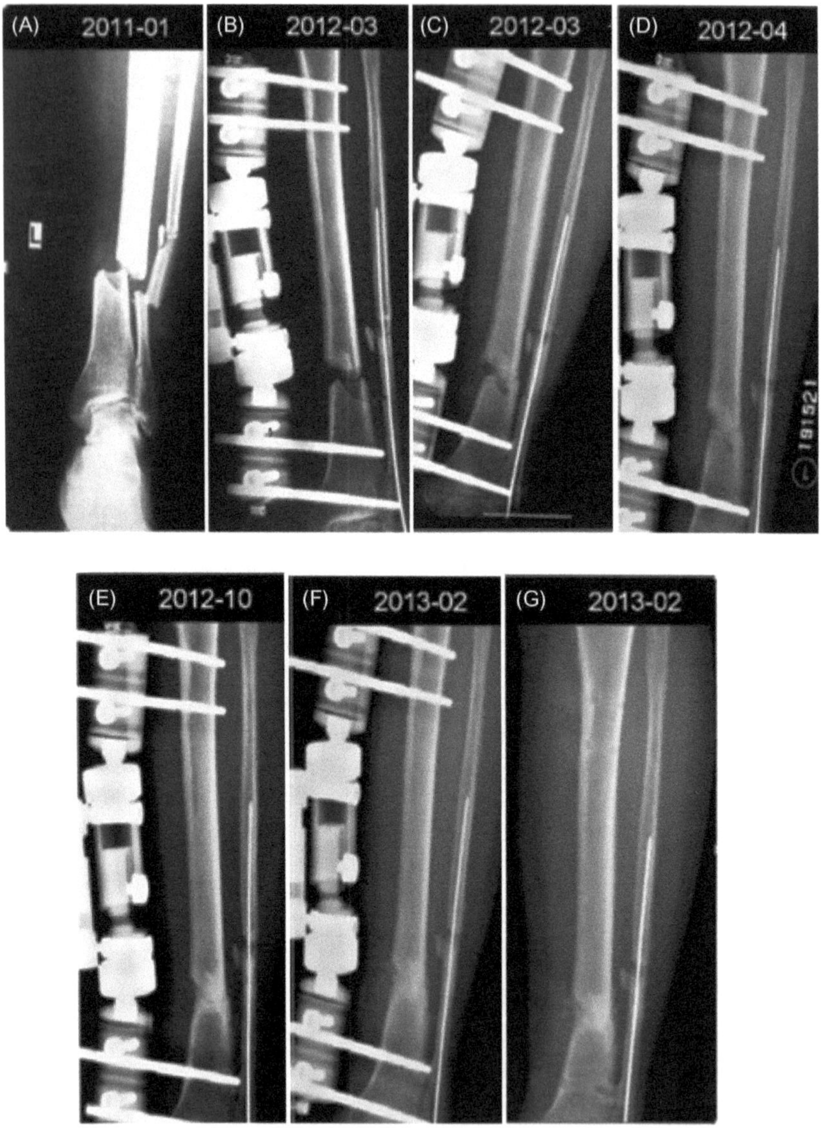

FIGURE 5.26 The X-ray examination results after surgery and follow-up studying. (A) The fracture image after car accident. (B) Bone nonunion 14 months after surgery by one-stage operation. (C) Immediately after the second stage operation. (D) 1 month after the second stage operation. (E) 8 months after the second stage operation. (F) 10 months after the second stage operation. (G) Removal of the internal fixation at 10 months after the second stage operation.

cavity has been partially penetrated. Thus it is indicated that the implant can guide the bone healing. (Data source: The Second People's Hospital of Lianyungang.)

Department of Orthopedics, The Second People's Hospital of Lianyungang presented an evaluation on the clinical effect of MC artificial bone graft incorporated with autologous bone marrow for the treatment of noninfected nonunion [9]. In this clinical case report, 23 patients suffering from noninfected nonunion were treated with MC bone graft combined with autologous bone marrow and proper operational processes. The patients were followed up and clinical and radiologic evaluations were performed to determine healing effects. In summary, the treatment of bone nonunion by using MC bone graft combined with autologous bone marrow obtained satisfactory treatment effects. MC artificial bone graft could serve as an alternative of autologous iliac crest bone graft in the treatment of noninfected nonunion [9].

5.4.10 Typical Case 10: Fracture of Tibia and Fibula

This is a case of 43-year-old male patient who was hospitalized due to the sequelae of poliomyelitis that caused the left tibial fibula to fracture repeatedly, and osteoporosis. The admitting diagnosis is the left tibial fibula fracture, osteoporosis, and sequelae of poliomyelitis. After examinations of admission, the left tibia fibula fracture bone grafting internal fixation. Implanted BonGold MC artificial bone particles 1 cm^3 to the fracture ends of tibia and fibula to increase the bone mass. Surgical progress went smoothly and patient was cured by corresponding treatment and nursing. The patient was discharged after 3 weeks.

The X-ray results of postoperative reexamination as shown in Fig. 5.27.

Six weeks after the surgery, we can see the callus formation visibly and bone healing is good. (From: Guangzhou General Hospital of Guangzhou Military Area Command of Chinese PLA.)

5.4.11 Typical Case 11: Intraarticular Calcaneal Fractures

This is a case of 65-year-old female patient who was hospitalized due to posttraumatic pain and swelling of the right calcaneus, with inability to stand for 1 day. The X-ray results indicated that the right calcaneus is fractured and patient has osteoporosis. All auxiliary examinations were improved after admission. The right calcaneal fracture reduction, bone graft fixation. Implanted BonGold MC artificial bone particles and artificial bone cement particles 3 cm^3 in total to the cavity formed after the percutaneous reduction by leverage and internal fixation. Surgical progress went smoothly and patient was cured by corresponding treatment and nursing. The patient was discharged after 3 weeks.

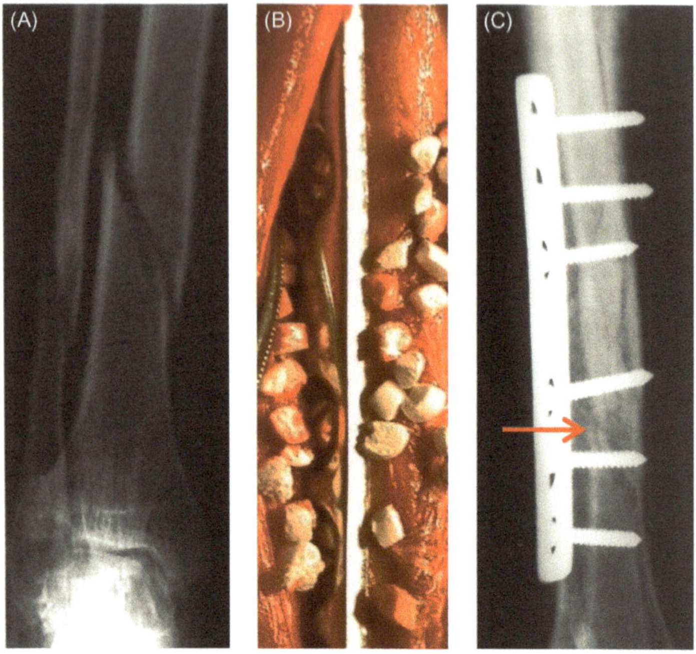

FIGURE 5.27 The X-ray examination results of preoperation and immediately after operation and 6 weeks after operation. (A) The X-ray result of preoperation. (B) Implanted BonGold MC artificial bone particles during operation. (C) 6 weeks after operation.

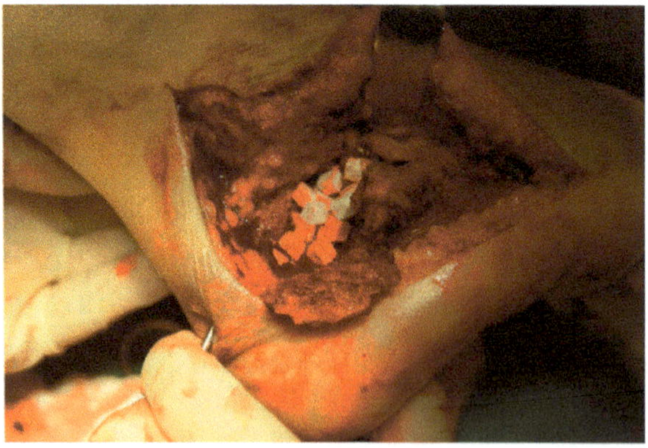

FIGURE 5.28 Implanted mineralized collagen artificial bone particles to the defect site of calcaneal fractures.

A picture taken during the operation is shown in Fig. 5.28.

The results of X-ray postoperative reexamination are shown in Fig. 5.29.

At 6 months postoperatively, CT imaging demonstrated the radiolucent zones between implanted MC and the surrounding bone immediately

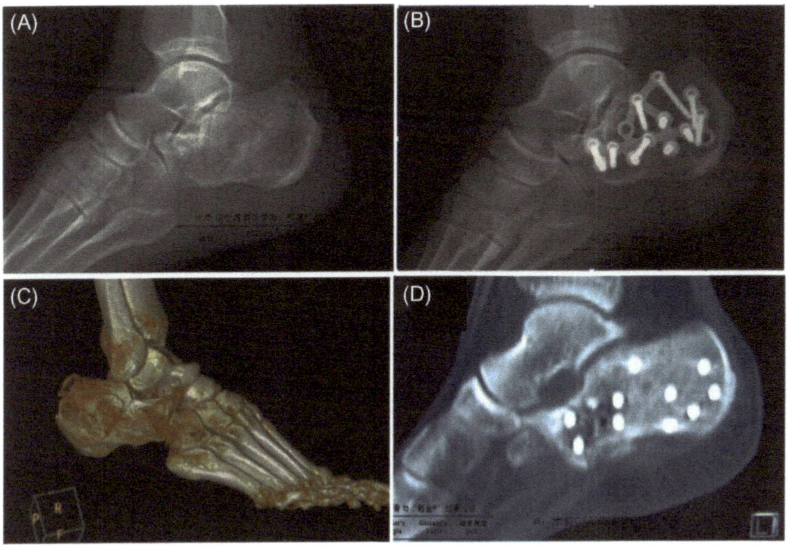

FIGURE 5.29 Images findings of preoperation and 6 months after operation. (A) preoperative three-dimensional CT imaging. (B) 6 month postoperative CT imaging. (C) Preoperative lateral X-ray film. (D) 6 month postoperative lateral X-ray film.)

postoperatively, which gradually disappeared. All areas of implanted MC exhibited intensity that was similar to the surrounding cancellous bone, with evidence of graft incorporation. (From: Hubei Xiangyang Central Hospital and Union Hospital; Tongji Medical College; Huazhong University of Science and Technology.)

Hubei Xiangyang Central Hospital and Union Hospital and Tongji Medical College, Huazhong University of Science and Technology collected 24 pairs of intraarticular calcaneal fractures with trabecular defects were treated with open reduction, internal fixation, and grafting either with MC or autograft. Patient demographics, medical history, and CT fracture classification were matched. Fractures were monitored 6 weeks, 12 weeks, 6 months, and 1 year postoperatively for healing and postoperative complications and results were analyzed. This study demonstrated promising results regarding the efficacy of MC as an extender in displaced intraarticular calcaneal fractures with successful healing rate and clinical scores equivalent to those of autograft graft. MC may be a good autograft alternative in displaced intraarticular calcaneal fractures with trabecular defects [2].

5.4.12 Typical Case 12: Lateral Malleolus Fracture

This is a case of a 62-year-old female patient who was hospitalized due to posttraumatic pain and swelling of the left lateral malleolus with restricted movement for 1 day. Physical examination: middle-aged woman, conscious, her spirit is good, the left calf was fixed by temporary support. No obvious abnormalities were observed in cardiopulmonary and spinal examination. The lower left leg and the ministry of the left external ankle are tender and swollen, with a large area of subcutaneous bruising. There were normal activities of left knee joint function, but the left ankle joint was limited in axial movement, the left foot dorsal artery beats vigorously, the left toe flexion function is normal. No other abnormalities were found. The X-ray indicated distal left fibular comminuted fracture, and distal left tibial avulsion fracture can be seen. The admitting diagnosis is the left ankle fracture (supination–extorsion). After examinations of admission, the patient underwent open reduction of the left lateral malleolus fracture, which was filled with BonGold Bone Sponge and BonGold Bone Putty, and internal fixation. Surgical progress went smoothly and patient was cured by corresponding treatment and nursing. The patient was discharged after 2 weeks.

The results of X-ray reexamination intraoperation and postoperative are shown in Fig. 5.30.

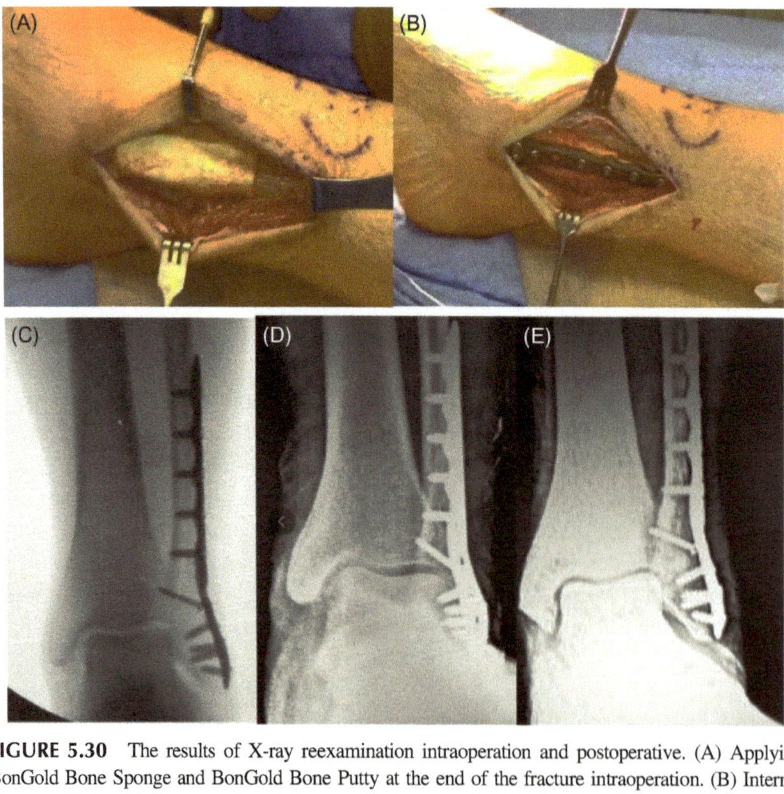

FIGURE 5.30 The results of X-ray reexamination intraoperation and postoperative. (A) Applying BonGold Bone Sponge and BonGold Bone Putty at the end of the fracture intraoperation. (B) Internal fixation. (C) 1 week after operation. (D) 1 month after operation. (E) 3 weeks after operation.

MC materials were applied to the gambrel arthrodesis by being implanted into the collapsed and subluxated metatarsal–cuneiform joint and navicular–cuneiform joint. To evaluate the clinical outcomes, the case was followed up for 13 weeks. The joints fused very well with the MC without inflammatory responses, itching, or exudation at the surgical. (From: Division of Foot and Ankle Surgery, Indiana Regional Medical Center, Indiana.)

5.4.13 Typical Case 13: Hallux Valgus

This is a case of a 59-year-old female patient who was hospitalized due to the ongoing pain located to the right first metatarsophalangeal joint (MTPJ) and medial column, and the pain had been ongoing for 2–3 years and gradually gotten worse. The admitting diagnosis is right first metatarsophalangeal joint arthrophlogosis. After admission examination, treated the right medial column with fusion. The first metatarsal joint of the right foot was fused, and the artificial periosteum was implanted in the fusion part of the joint, and the BonGold Bone Putty was used for filling and internal fixation. Surgical progress went smoothly and patient was cured by corresponding treatment and nursing. Operation of external fixation after 30 days, and patient was discharged after 2 weeks. Follow-up 6 months after discharge.

The intraoperative findings are shown in Fig. 5.31.

The results of X-ray postoperative reexamination are shown in Fig. 5.32.

On this last picture we can see complete consolidation of the medial column with good bone fusion at the medial column. This is 1.5 times faster than expected for this type of surgery. No lucency is seen at the fusion sites [10]. (From: Division of Foot and Ankle Surgery, Indiana Regional Medical Center, Indiana.)

5.4.14 Typical Case 14: Flat Foot

This is a case of a 20-year-old male patient who was hospitalized due to foot pain for 6 years that gradually got worse and restricted movement. The

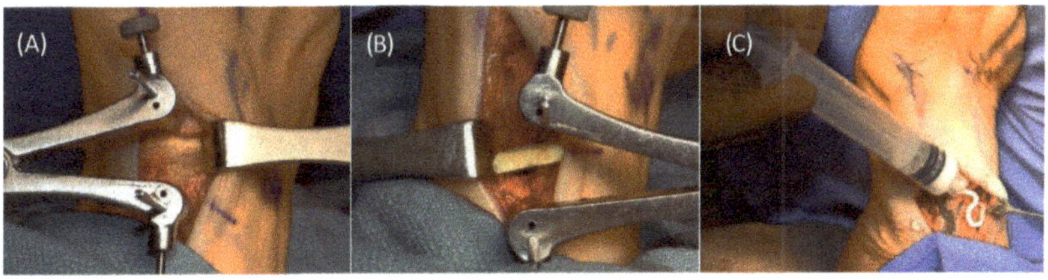

FIGURE 5.31 The progress of implantation intraoperative. (A) Expose the first metatarsal joint. (B) Implantation of BonGold Bone Sponge. (C) Implantation of BonGold Bone Putty.

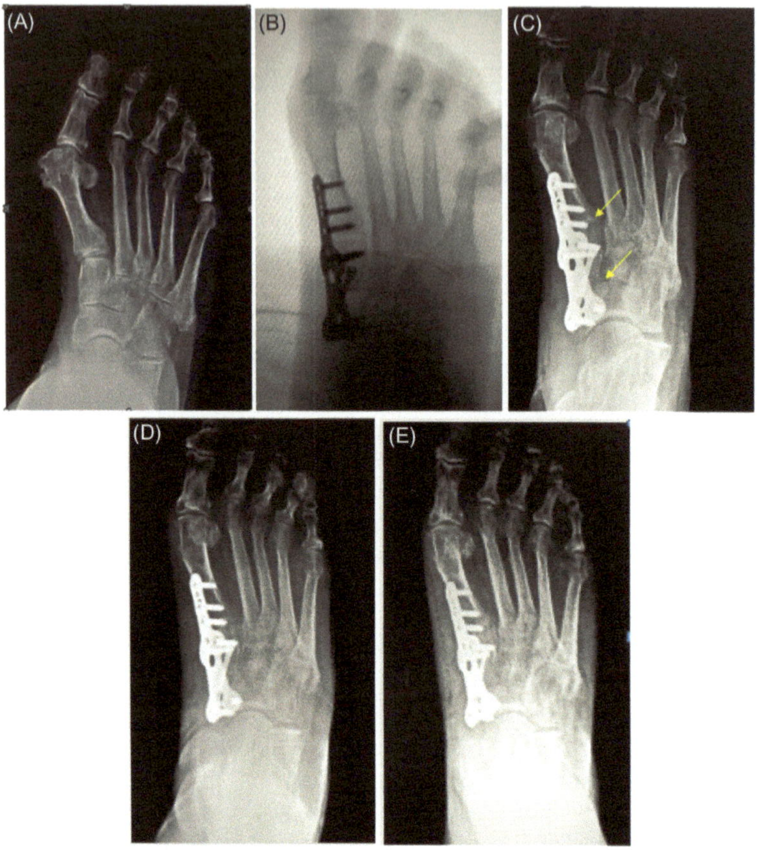

FIGURE 5.32 The results of X-ray postoperative reexamination.A) Preoperative. (B) Immediately postoperative. (C) 4 weeks after operation. (D) 9 weeks after operation. (E) 13 weeks after operation.

admitting diagnosis is flat feet. After examinations of admission, patient was treated as follows: address the equinus by lengthening the gastroc muscle belly then address the abducted right foot by completing a calcaneal osteotomy and placing a wedge to reduce the deformity. The wedge would have BonGold putty placed within it to help facilitate fusion. Once this was complete we fused the medial column again utilizing the putty. Surgical progress went smoothly and patient was cured by corresponding treatment and nursing. The patient was discharged after 2 weeks and followed up 6 months after discharge.

Preoperative, intraoperative, and postoperative X-ray examination results are shown in Fig. 5.33. (From: Indiana Regional Medical Center of America.)

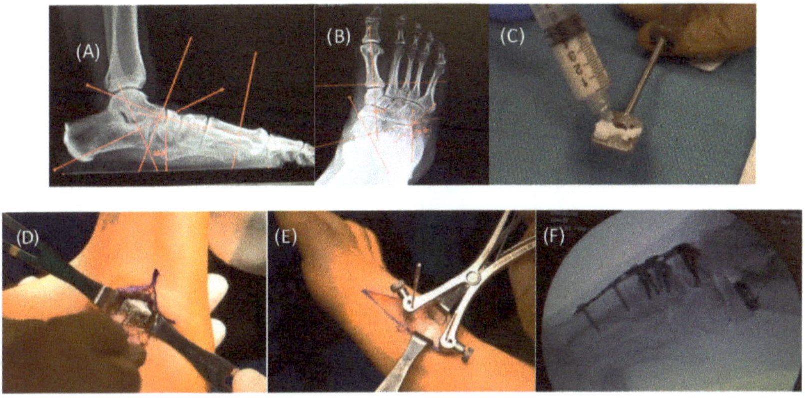

FIGURE 5.33 Preoperative, intraoperative, and postoperative X-ray examination results (A, B) The X-ray examination indicate that double lateral arch flat, arthrostenosis. (C) In the operation, a small joint fusion device was prepared with BonGold Bone Putty. (D) Graft inserted into lateral column. (E) After medial prep and putty in joint space. (F) The X-ray indicated bone formation along the medial column under the plate at the navicular–cuneiform joint after 6 months of discharge). *Division of Foot and Ankle Surgery, Indiana Regional Medical Center, Indiana.*

5.5 THE USE OF MINERALIZED COLLAGEN GRAFT FOR BONE DEFECTS IN REVISION ARTHROPLASTY

Arthroplasty is the replacement of two or more joint prostheses performed on the same joint. Bone implantation materials should be extensively used in the operation of the disease.

Department of Orthopedics, Peking Union Medical College Hospital and Department of Orthopedics, Wendeng Orthopaedic Hospital have made a number of clinical and experimental studies in the use of MC graft for bone defects in revision arthroplasty between February 2010 and June 2013. The study indicated that the MC graft showed no immunogenicity or biodegradation, good conductive osteogenesis, can provide immediate mechanical support, and can be used as an ideal biomaterial for bone tissue engineering. It can be used for joint revision surgery for various clinical reasons [11].

The following are several typical case studies.

5.5.1 Typical Case 1: The Repair of Fractured Acetabular After 4 Years of THA

This is a case of a 58-year-old female patient who was hospitalized due to the prosthetic cup loosening 4 years after total hip arthroplasty (THA). The X-ray indicated that the right bony acetabulum is weak, with the acetabular fracture, and flat fracture can be seen in the pelvic cavity. After examinations of admission, patient was treated with revision of the right hip joint and

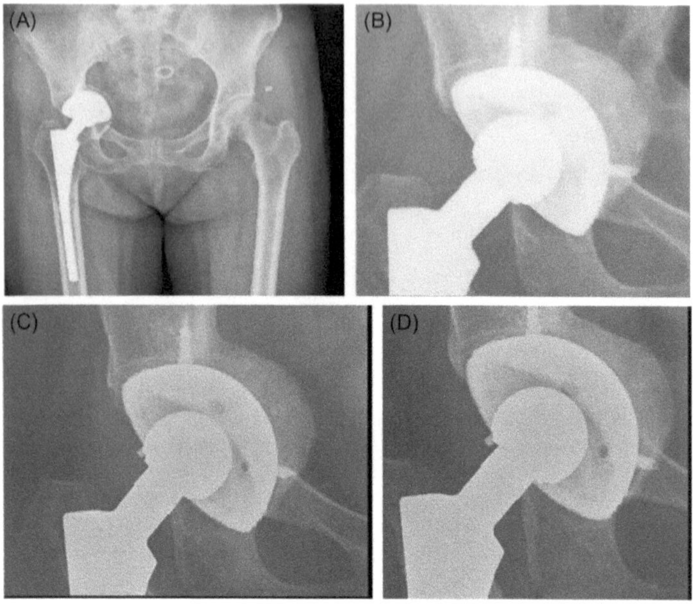

FIGURE 5.34 Postoperative and follow-up X-ray results. (A) Mineralized collagen grafts were used to reconstruct the acetabulum and radiographs taken at third month, (B) sixth month, (C) and final follow-up. (D) Shows the bone grafts were well remodeled. *Department of Orthopaedics, Peking Union Medical College Hospital and Department of Orthopaedics, Wendeng Orthopaedic Hospital.*

acetabular bone grafting. MC grafts were used to reconstruct the acetabulum, the patient recovered smoothly after operation, was discharged after 4 weeks, and followed up 3 years after discharge (Fig. 5.34).

5.5.2 Typical 2: Acetabulum and Femoral Prosthesis Loosen After THA

This is a case of a 65-year-old male patient who was hospitalized due to the prosthesis loosening 4 years after THA. The X-ray indicated lateral osseous defect visible on the left side of the acetabulum prosthesis the left femoral stalk becomes loose and collapses. After admission, he was treated with revision of left hip joint, acetabulum, and femoral bone marrow cavity. MC grafts were used to reconstruct the acetabulum, the patent recovered smoothly after operation, with discharged after 3 weeks. Follow-up was 1 year after discharge.

Preoperative and follow-up X-ray results are shown in Fig. 5.35.

The result indicated that even though reconstruction of the acetabula and femur with massive defects is still a major surgical challenge in revision THA, our findings show that MC graft may be a promising solution for THA

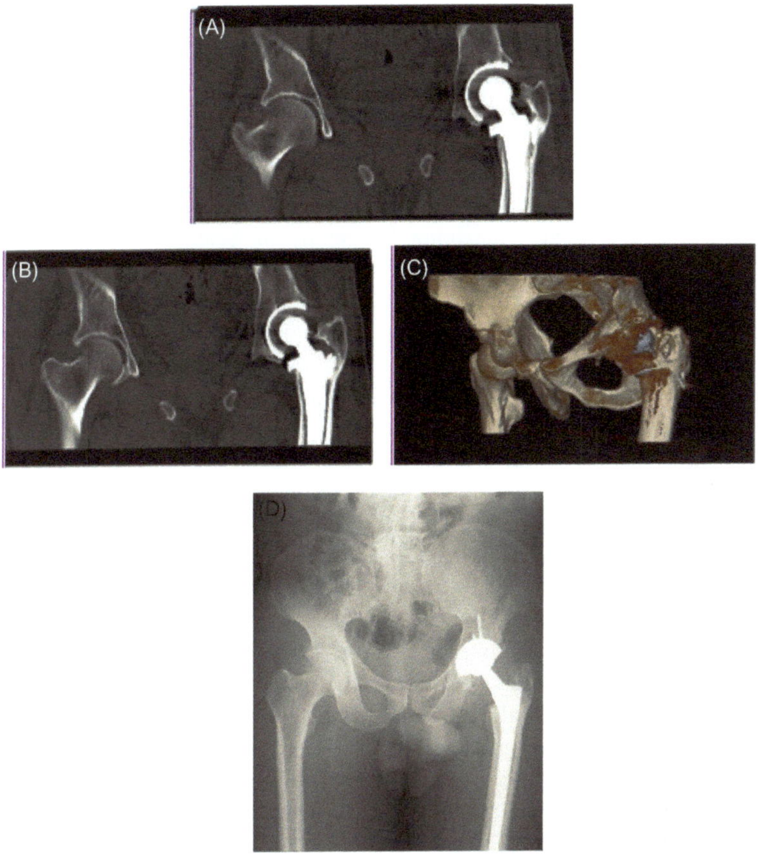

FIGURE 5.35 Preoperative and follow-up X-ray results. Hip computed tomography scan and three-dimensional reconstruction graphs showed bone defects of proximal femur (A–C). Mineralized collagen grafts were used to reconstruct the bone defects and radiographs taken at 3rd month (lost) and 12th month (D) showed that the proximal femur bone grafts were well remodeled. *Department of Orthopaedics, Peking Union Medical College Hospital and Department of Orthopaedics, Wendeng Orthopaedic Hospital).*

revision with massive bone deficiency due to its excellent performance in hip function improvement and few complications. Extended follow-up is necessary to further prove the feasibility of this approach.

5.6 THE MINERALIZED COLLAGEN USED FOR THE TREATMENT OF ADULT EARLY NECROSIS OF FEMORAL HEAD

Femoral head necrosis is a pathological process and occurs at the weight-bearing area of the femoral head initiate. Under stress, the structure of the necrotic bone trabeculae is damaged by microfracture, and then the repair process of the damaged bone tissue follows. The causes of osteonecrosis are not eliminated, the repair is incomplete, and the damage-repair process continues, leading to changes in the structure of the femoral head, the collapse of the femoral head, deformation, joint inflammation, and dysfunction. Femoral head necrosis causes hip joint pain and dysfunction [12].

Clinical data of 104 patients (122 hips) with Steinberg stage Ⅰ–Ⅲ adult necrosis of the femoral head in Department of Orthopedics, Union Hospital, Tongji Medical College, Huazhong University of Science and Technology from March 2012 to November 2014 were retrospectively analyzed. Patients were treated with self-designed nanocrystalline collagen basal allogeneic bone brace combined with allograft. All patients were followed up with osteonecrosis progress and collapse of femoral head. Harris score changes and visual analogue scale/score (VAS scores) before and after operation were compared. Efficacy was evaluated by using the Harris hip scores. The results indicated that using nanocrystalline collagen basal bone brace combined with allograft for the treatment of adult early femoral head necrosis will not destroy the main blood supply of femoral head, and will increase mechanical support in the subchondral bone of femoral head necrosis area, promote rehabilitation of femoral head necrosis and prevent collapse of femoral head, which make it worthy of widespread clinical use.

Sixty patients with osteonecrosis of femoral head in Heibei Hengshui Halison International Peace Hospital were treated with self-designed nanocrystalline collagen basal allogeneic bone brace combined with allograft. All patients were followed up with osteonecrosis progress and collapse of femoral head. Harris score changes and VAS scores before and after operation were compared. Efficacy was evaluated by using the Harris hip scores. The result indicated that the marrow core decompression combined with MC femoral head necrosis reconstruction rods in treatment of femoral head necrosis can obviously improve the function of hip joint and prevent femoral head collapse, and the curative effect is satisfied [13].

5.6.1 Typical Case 1

A 35-year old-male presented to the hospital with left femoral head necrosis (Steinberg stage Ⅱ) and was treated with marrow core decompression combined with MC femoral head necrosis reconstruction of composite allogeneic bone implantation.

Preoperative and postoperative X-ray results are shown in Fig. 5.36.

5.6.2 Typical Case 2

This is a case of 21-year-old male patient who was hospitalized due to the pain of the left hip with restricted movement for 3 years, worsening for 6 months. Physical examination: young man, conscious, passive position.

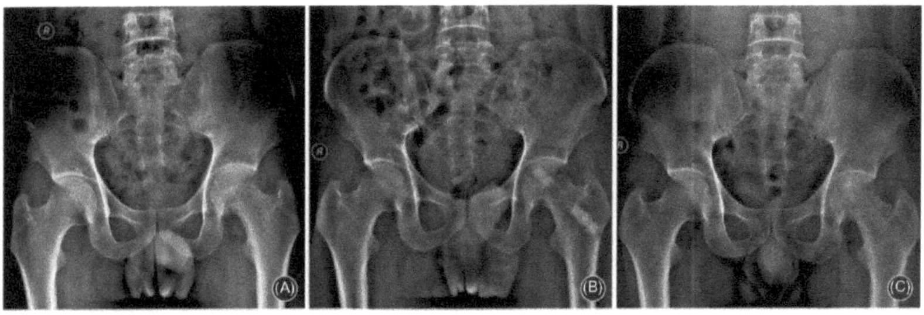

FIGURE 5.36 Preoperative and postoperative X-ray results in the case of a 35-year-old male who suffered with the left femoral head necrosis (Steinberg stage Ⅱ). (A) Preoperative visible femoral head shape, no collapse, no hip osteoarthritis on either side. (B) There was callus formation around the artificial support shelf for 8 months after surgery. (C) 24 months after surgery, the femoral head necrosis area was reossified, and the artificial bone support was obviously absorbed and the shape was blurred.)

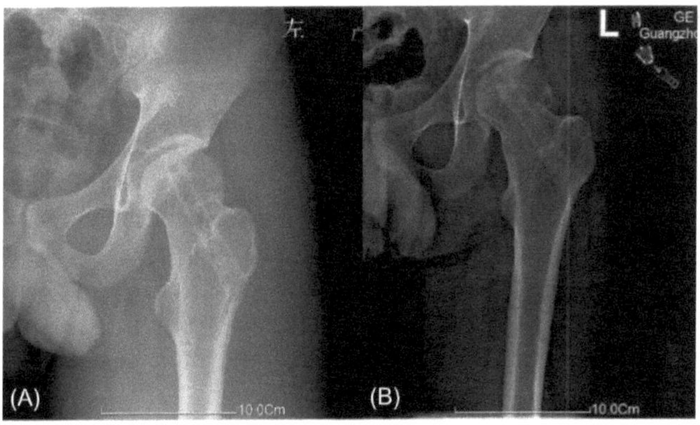

FIGURE 5.37 Preoperative and follow-up X-ray examination results.(A) 1 week after surgery. (B) 3 months after surgery.

vertebral column examination (−), upper limbs (−), and the left hip joint tenderness, no redness. All the abduction activities in the left hip were limited; Patrick sign (+). Left lower limb axial percussion pain(+), left thigh muscles atrophied and skin pigmentation. The dorsal artery beat vigorously. The admission diagnosis was "left femoral head necrosis." After admission, treated with left femoral head necrosis medullary decompression reconstruction stick implantation. Surgical progress went smoothly and patient was cured by corresponding treatment and nursing. The patient was discharged after 2 weeks.

The results of X-ray reexamination are shown in Fig. 5.37.

Three months after operation, the femoral head was normal, with no collapse, no fracture of the femoral neck, and the necrosis of the femoral head was partially degraded, the edges were blurred, and the structure of the bone trabecula was visible in the implant site.

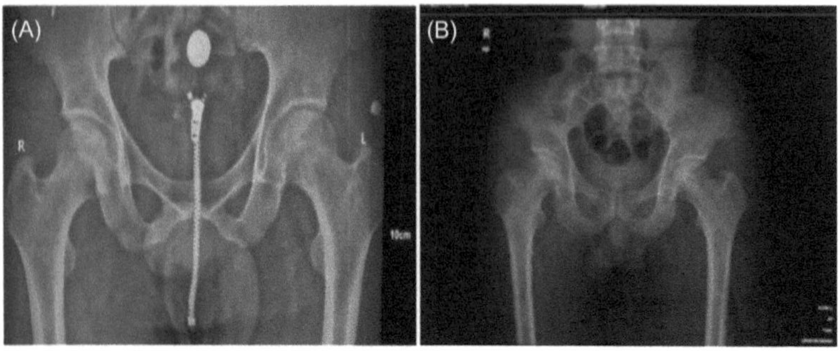

FIGURE 5.38 The results of X-ray reexamination of preoperation and 1 year after operation. (A) Preoperation. (B) 18 months after operation.

5.6.3 Typical Case 3

This is a case of a 48-year-old male patient who was hospitalized due to pain of the left hip and restricted movement for 3 years, worsening for 6 months. Physical examination: middle aged man, conscious, passive position. Cardiopulmonary and spinal examination (−), upper limbs (−). Double hip tenderness and no inflammation. Both hips were restricted in abduction activities. Patrick sign (+), double lower limb axial percussion pain (+). The bipedal arterial pulsation was powerful. No other abnormalities were found. The admission diagnosis was "bilateral femoral head necrosis," and patient was treated with double femoral head necrosis intramedullary decompression and femoral head necrosis reconstruction rod implantation. Surgical progress went smoothly and patient was cured by corresponding treatment and nursing. The patient was discharged after 2 weeks.

The results of X-ray reexamination preoperation and 1 year after operation as shown in Fig. 5.38.

From the X-ray reexamination of 18 months after surgery, we can see that there was no significant collapse in bilateral femoral head, no fracture of the femur neck. The implant was partially degraded and the edges were blurred, the structure of the bone trabecula was visible in the implant site. (From: Wuhan Union Hospital.)

5.6.4 Typical Case 4

This is a case of a 43-year-old male patient who was hospitalized due to the irregular left hip pain and aggravation, with no radiating pain and affected by weather changing. Walking exacerbated the pain with no attenuation after resting. Physical examination: middle aged man, conscious, passive position. Cardiopulmonary and spinal examination (−), upper limbs (−). Left hip tenderness and no inflammation. The left hip was restricted in abduction activities. Patrick sign (+), left lower limb axial percussion pain (−). The bipedal

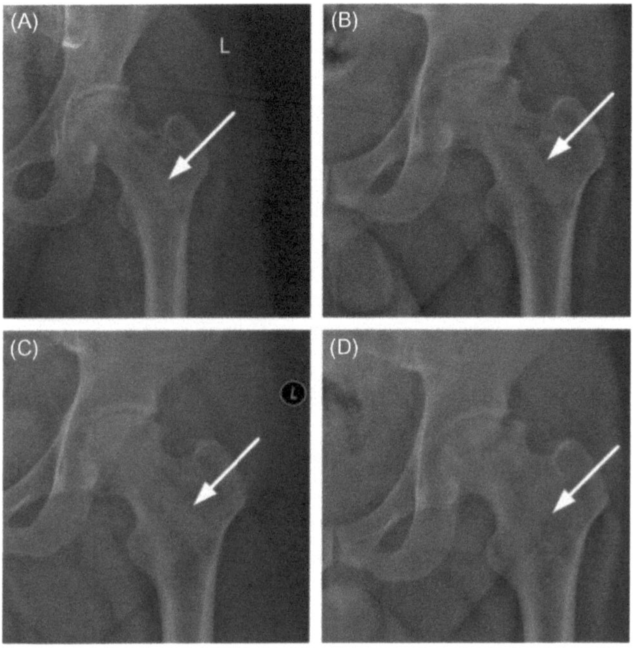

FIGURE 5.39 The results of X-ray examination in the follow-up period. (A) 3 days after operation. (B) 3 months after operation. (C) 5 months after operation. (D) 12 months after operation).

arterial pulsation was powerful. No other abnormalities were found. The admission diagnosis was left femoral head avascular necrosis. According to the femoral head necrosis stage in China, it was II b; According to China-Japan Friendship Hospital (CJFH) classification, it was L2; Harris score was 80 points. After hospital admission, marrow CD and implantation with the MC reconstruction rod were carried out, which attenuated the pain symptoms effectively. Surgical progress went smoothly and patient was cured by corresponding treatment and nursing. The patient was discharged after 2 weeks.

The results of X-ray reexamination are shown in Fig. 5.39.

From the results of X-ray examination 3 months after surgery, we can see there was no significant collapse in bilateral femoral head, and no fracture of the femur neck. The implant was partially degraded and the edges were blurred, the structure of the bone trabecula was fuzzy in the implant site. Five months after operation, there was no obvious enlargement of the collapsed area of the femur, no fracture of the femur neck. The degradation of internal implants was obvious and the edges are further blurred; the structure of bone trabecula was obviously formed in the implant site.

The patient walked a month after surgery, and fell over himself carelessly and caused femoral neck fracture one year after surgery, After hospital admission, the artificial total left hip replacement was carried out 12 months after the primary surgery of marrow CD and MC reconstruction rod implantation. The interception of the femoral head and the part of the femoral neck stump and local slice observation are shown in Fig. 5.40.

Fig. 5.40A indicates that the bone tissue at femoral neck region blended tightly together with MC reconstruction rod. No space was found between host bone and reconstruction rod; it was very difficult to separate the rod from host bone or take it out. The cartilage at the load-bearing region of femoral head was cracked, and a cystic cavity formed due to subcartilage bone necrosis. Host bone and implanted reconstruction rod fused together and formed a curved blurred boundary; at the border region, scattered rich vessel networks were observed. The vessels had a diameter of 20–50 nm (capillary level), surrounded by a thin layer of epithelial cells (darker stained). Osteoclasts and fibrosis were also observed, and debris of degraded implant was phagocytosed by phagocytes (Fig. 5.37B). The partially degraded implant is shown by pink staining and new small vessels could be observed near the border of the host bone (Fig. 5.40A), and the partially degraded implant had mesh structure with irregular size cavities (Fig. 5.40B). Rich lamellae bone-like tissue can be observed at the host bone side of border region with a size >100 nm. A gap region surrounding it can be visualized, which was due to the density difference between the new bone

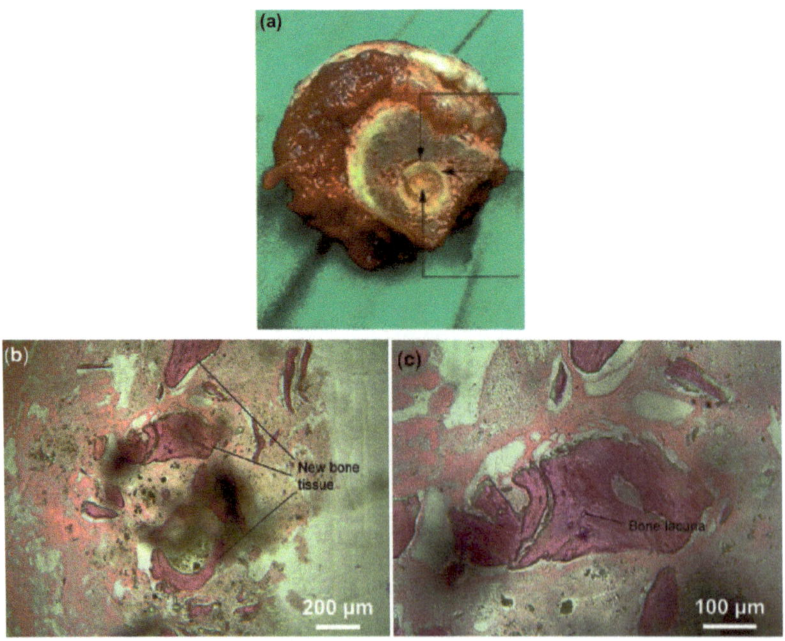

FIGURE 5.40 (A) Transverse section for collum femoris. (B) Pink-stained matrix is degradative implant with irregular shape and scattered cavity and trabecular bone. (C) Osteocytes in lacuna within lamellar trabecular bone.

tissue and material when sectioning, commonly presented in decalcified sample histology [14]. (From: Department of Orthopaedics, 254th Hospital of PLA.)

5.7 APPLICATION OF MINERALIZED COLLAGEN IN THE REMOVAL OF BONE GRAFTING IN BENIGN BONE TUMORS

Benign bone tumor is a benign tumor or other type of tumor that occurs in the whole body bone or its subsidiary tissue. Benign bone tumor is easy to cure and has good prognosis. It is born in the extremities and is prone to bone destruction. Surgery is often required in clinical practice, and it is usually necessary to use bone graft materials to fill the lesion area with internal fixation in parallel with the treatment measures of scraping the lesion, such as to facilitate the regeneration and healing of bone destruction area [7].

5.7.1 Typical Case 1

This is a case of a 13-year-old boy patient who was hospitalized due to the pain of the right lower limb for 1 week. From the X-ray we can see a 4×3 cm low density expansion shadow at the distal end of the right femur, the structural disorders of bone trabeculae, cortical sclerosis was visible at the edge. The admission diagnosis was nonossifying fibroma of the right femur. After admission, nonossifying fibroma of the right femur was removed and bone grafting was performed. Intraoperative implanted BonGold MC artificial bone particles and putty 6.5 cm^3. The X-ray indicated that the tumor cavity has been filled with new bone 9 months after operation. There was no pain or swelling in the patient.

Preoperative X-ray is shown in Fig. 5.41.

X-ray examination results after 1 year of follow-up are shown in Fig. 5.42.

The X-ray immediately after surgery indicated that the defect was completely filled with artificial bone material. Nine months after operation, the defect of bone tumor has been obliterated by new bone and the edge is blurred. (From: Lianyungang Second People's Hospital.)

5.7.2 Case 2: Tibial Plateau Cyst

In a male patient, 28 years old, right knuckle pain caused discomfort for 1 month before entering hospital. The X-ray show that shadow of low density with a size of 3.0*3.5cm in the right tibial plateau and the marginal cortical sclerosis. Diagnosis was right tibial subplateau bone cyst.

The right tibial plateau bone cyst was scraped and bone graft was performed after admission. During operation, the size of the bone defect under the platform was $2 \times 3 \times 3.5$ cm. The MC bone graft material 4 cm^3 and the iliac bone 4 cm^3 were implanted.

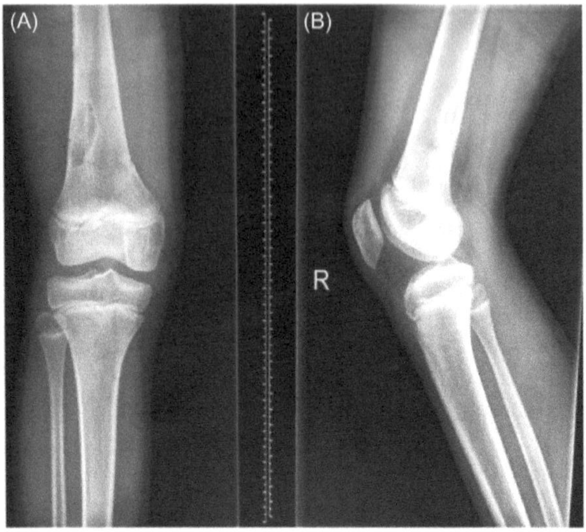

FIGURE 5.41 Preoperative X-ray positive side examination. (A,B) Before surgery, the bone defect was found in the distal proximal joint of the right femur.

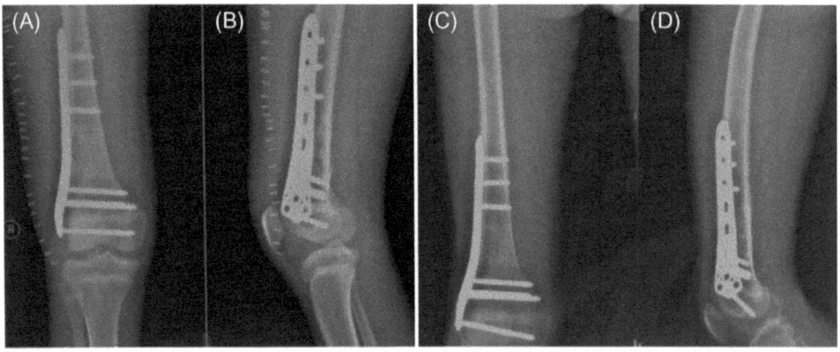

FIGURE 5.42 The results of X-ray examination in the follow-up period. (A, B) Immediately after surgery. (C, D) 9 months after surgery.

Preoperative X-ray film is shown in Fig. 5.43.

The results of X-ray examination during the 1-year follow-up are shown in Fig. 5.44.

The defect site under the platform showed obvious osteogenesis, and the joint had no collapse 3 months after the operation. (From: General Hospital of Guangzhou Military Command of PLA.)

5.7.3 Case 3: Bone Cyst of the Middle Part of the Humerus

A male, 26 years old, was admitted with bone cyst in the middle part of the right humerus. X-ray: a 6 × 4 cm cystic mass is found in the middle part of

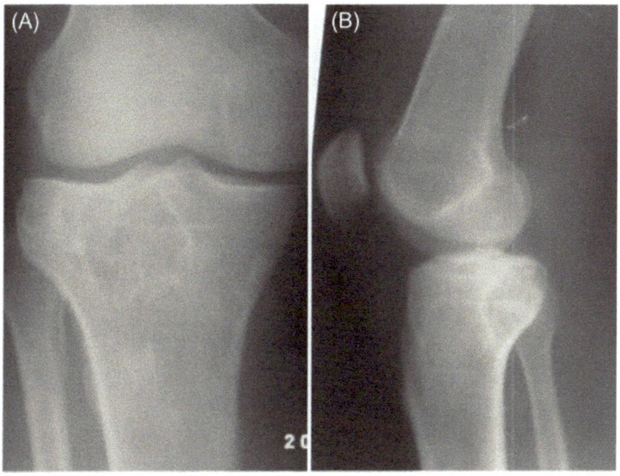

FIGURE 5.43 (A and B) show that X-ray bone cyst is located in the posterior lateral of the tibial plateau.

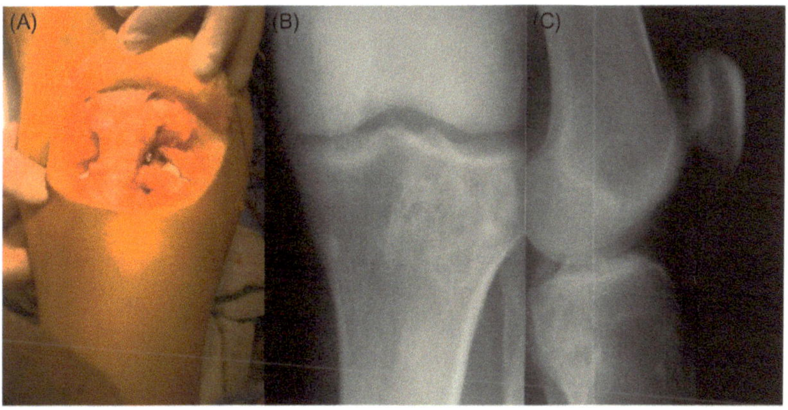

FIGURE 5.44 Intraoperative cysts and postoperative X-ray review.(A) Intraoperative. (B) Transverse position of 3 months postoperatively. (C) Lateral position of 3 months postoperatively.

the right humerus. Admission diagnosis: the middle part of the right humerus bone cyst. After admission, right humerus middle segment bone cyst curettage and bone graft internal fixation were enforced. After complete curettage in the tumor range, the MC artificial bone granule 8 cm^3 was given. The operation was smooth. All kinds of symptomatic treatment were given after the operation. The patient was discharged from hospital 2 weeks later.

The X-ray films were followed up for 4 months immediately after the operation, as shown in Fig. 5.45.

Postoperative immediate X-ray: the curettage site of the cyst filled with artificial bone MC particles; 9 months after the operation, the bone defect

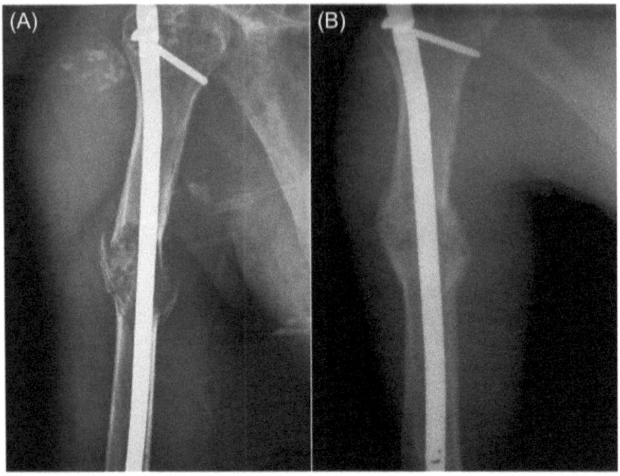

FIGURE 5.45 X-ray examination after operation and follow-up (A) Immediately after operation. (B) 4 months after operation.

sites on both sides of the humerus showed obvious bone healing. (From: General Hospital of Guangzhou Military Command of PLA.)

5.7.4 Case 4: Fibrous Dysplasia of Bone

The male, 19 years old, was admitted with fibrous dysplasia of the right humerus with. The X-ray showed that the middle and lower part of right humerus was $3 \times 4 \times 3$ cm, and the structure of cancellous bone was not clear. The hospital diagnosis was that the right humeral bone fibrous structure was bad. The patient underwent right humerus bone structure of fibrous dysplasia tumor curettage, bone grafting, and internal fixation; the tumor was completely cleared in the organization, the legacy of the bone defect area with MC artificial bone particles 6 cm^3. The defects were fully filled with intramedullary internal fixation. The operation was smooth. All kinds of symptomatic treatment were given after the operation. The patient was discharged from the hospital 3 weeks later. The follow-up was half a year after discharge.

The X-ray films of 3 months before and after the operation are shown in Fig. 5.46.

Preoperative X-ray examination showed that the middle and lower middle right humerus were $3 \times 4 \times 3$ cm. Three months after the operation, there was obvious callus hyperplasia and thickening of the cortex on both sides of the middle segment of the humerus. (From: General Hospital of Guangzhou Military Command of PLA.)

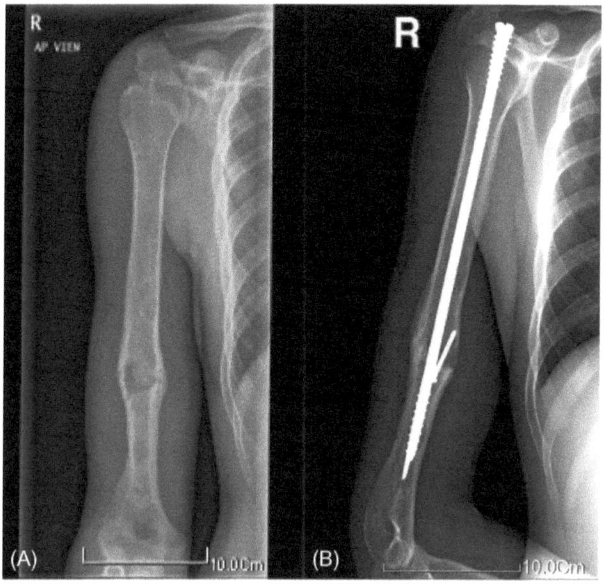

FIGURE 5.46 Preoperative and follow-up X-ray examination. (A) Preoperative. (B) 3 months after operation.

5.7.5 Case 5: Distal Femur Cyst

The patient, 27 years old, was admitted with left epicondyle cyst of the left femur. The X-ray showed the left anterolateral distal femur showed 4×3 cm low density in cortex, hardening. Admission diagnosis: left distal femur bone cyst. After admission, the tumor was curettaged and bone grafting was performed on the left distal femur cyst. Implantation of artificial bone putty mixed MC artificial bone particles 4 cm^3. Surgery was successful. The follow-up was 6 months after the operation.

The X-ray films were followed up for 4 months after the operation, as shown in Fig. 5.47.

The bone defect of the proximal part of the distal leave of the left femur was observed before operation. At 6 months after operation, X-ray showed that there were vague particles in the bone defect and unclear edges. There were new bone trabeculae in the cavity, and no obvious cortical hardening was found. (From: General Hospital of Guangzhou Military Command of PLA.)

5.8 VERTEBRAL COMPRESSION FRACTURES BY USING MINERALIZED COLLAGEN MODIFIED BONE CEMENT

Vertebral compressive fracture refers to the compression of the anterior half of the vertebra (parastyle) caused by anterior flexural force, and the posterior

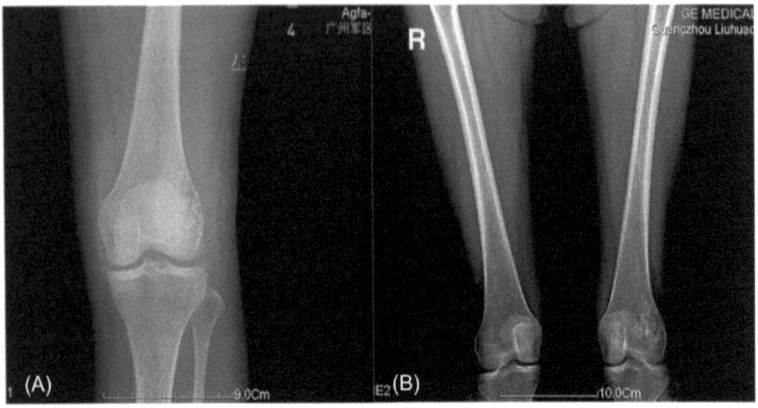

FIGURE 5.47 Preoperative and follow-up X-ray examination. (A) Preoperative. (B) 6 months after operation.

vertebral arch (posterior column) of the spine is normal, few of them have tensile damage. Disc wedge is a common injury type in spinal fractures and more common in the elderly patients with osteoporosis. Percutaneous vertebroplasty (PVP) and percutaneous kyphoplasty (PKP) have been becoming commonly used surgeries for the treatment of osteoporotic vertebral compression fractures (OVCF). Nowadays, polymethylmethacrylate (PMMA) bone cements with good injectability and high contrast effect have been widely applied in PVP and PKP. However, many disadvantages have influenced clinical performance of these PMMA bone cements. The compressive modulus is relative higher than that of the natural vertebral bone, the suddenly increased intensity of the treated vertebral body may induce secondary fracture on adjacent ones, especially for those osteoporotic bodies. On the other hand, PMMA is a bioinert material that cannot form osteointegration with the host bone at the implant site. The implanted PMMA bone cement may loosen or even dislodge inside the vertebral body. Such complications need further surgeries, which increase illness and economic burden for the patients. In this clinical observation, to improve the properties of the commercially available PMMA bone cement, we used the mineral collagen for the modification of the PMMA bone cement. Such modification could effectively reduce the hardness and improve its biocompatibility, so as to reduce the occurrence of either secondary fracture at the adjacent vertebrae or dislodgement of the implanted bone cement for the treatment of patients with OVCF [15].

5.8.1 Case 1

The female patient, 90 years old, because of the low back pain after a fall, was unable to sit for a long time. The admission was diagnosed as "L5 vertebral compression fracture." All auxiliary examinations were conducted after admission and kyphoplasty was performed for vertebral compression fractures of L5 by implant PMMA bone cement modified by BonGold. The patient's pain was relieved after the operation. After 3 days in bed, the patient was discharged from the hospital 2 weeks later.

The results of X-ray examination during the follow-up period are shown in Fig. 5.48.

The cortical compression of the posterior margin of the L5 vertebral body was seen before operation. The height of the compressed L5 vertebral body was recovered and the curvature of the lumbar spine was significantly improved after the operation. The patient was followed up for 1 year. No recompression of the adjacent segments of the vertebral body was found during the follow-up period. (From: Peking Union Medical College Hospital.)

5.8.2 Case 2

The woman, 83 years old, was admitted to the hospital for back pain and limited activity for hours. The admission was diagnosed as "L3 vertebral compression fracture." Improve the auxiliary examination after admission, L5 for vertebral compression fracture kyphoplasty operation of implantation PMMA bone cement modified BonGold bone graft material. The patient's pain was relieved after the operation. After 5 days in bed, the patient was discharged from the hospital 2 weeks later.

The results of X-ray examination during the follow-up period are shown in Fig. 5.49.

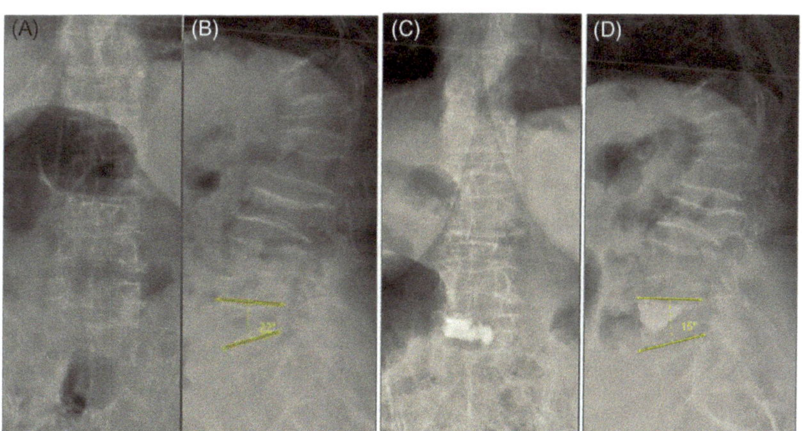

FIGURE 5.48 X-ray examination before and after surgery. (A, B) Preoperative X ray. (C, D) Immediately after the operation.

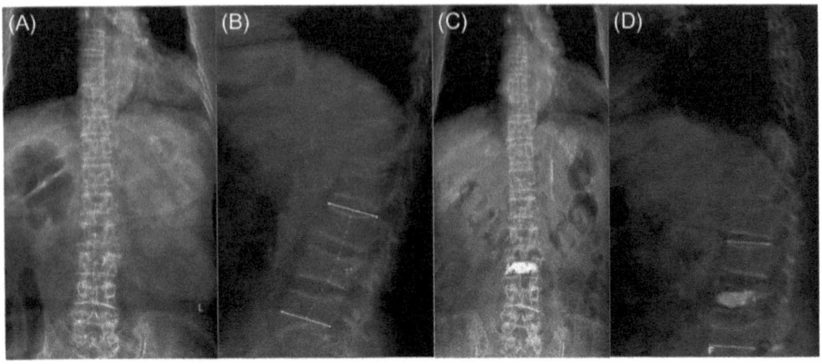

FIGURE 5.49 Before and after the X-ray examination. (A, B) Preoperative X ray. (C, D) Immediately after the operation.

L3 vertebral endplate fracture and precorticum compression were seen before operation. The height of the compressed L3 vertebral body was recovered and the curvature of the lumbar spine was significantly improved after the operation. The patients were followed up for 1 year. No recompression of the adjacent segments of the vertebral body was found during the follow-up period. (From: Peking Union Medical College Hospital.)

5.8.3 Case 3

The woman, 61 years old, was admitted to the hospital for "the pain of the back of the waist and the limited activity of 3 hours." The admission was diagnosed as "L2 vertebral compression fracture." Improve the auxiliary examination after admission, L2 for vertebral compression fracture kyphoplasty operation of implantation PMMA bone cement modified BonGold bone graft material. The patient's pain was relieved after the operation. After 4 days in bed, the patient was discharged from the hospital 10 days later.

The results of preoperative X-ray examination are shown in Fig. 5.50.

The results of postoperative X-ray examination are shown in Fig. 5.51.

II degree compression of the L2 cortices in the anterior cortices of the vertebral body was observed before operation. The height of the anterior margin of the L2 vertebral body was recovered and the curvature of the lumbar spine was significantly improved after the operation. The height of anterior vertebral body (Ant) of L2 was changed from 14.8 to 17.1 mm, the middle height (Mid) changed from 16.6 to 19.8 mm, and the posterior edge height (Post) changed from 27.9 to 28.1 mm, and the vertebral height was restored effectively. The patient was followed up for 1 year. No recompression of the adjacent segments of the vertebral body was found during the follow-up period. (From: Peking Union Medical College Hospital.)

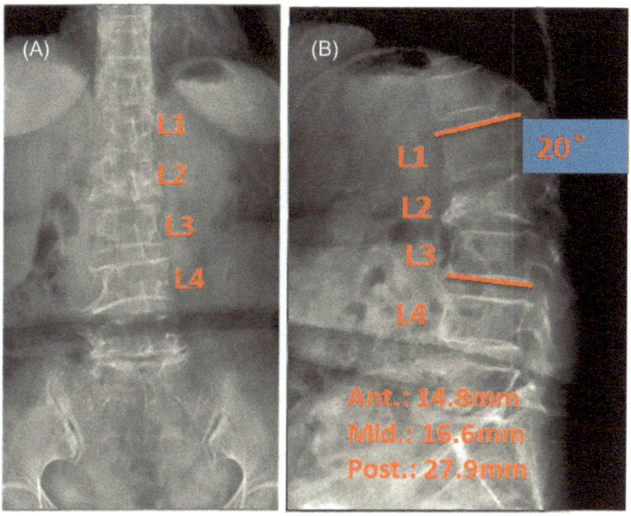

FIGURE 5.50 (A) Anterior lumbar spine orthotopic film. (B) Anterior lumbar lateral film.

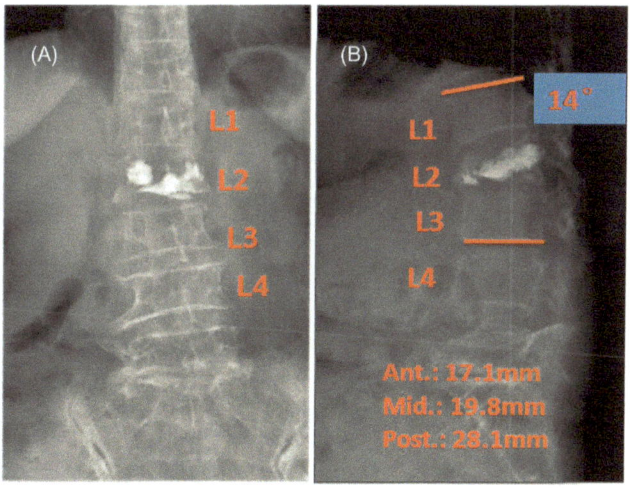

FIGURE 5.51 (A) Postoperative lumbar spine orthotopic film. (B) Postoperative lumbar lateral film.

5.8.4 Case 4

The woman, 80 years old, was admitted to the hospital for pain at the back of the waist and limited activity for 3 hours. The admission was diagnosed as "L4 vertebral compression fracture." Improve the auxiliary examination after admission, L5 for vertebral compression fracture kyphoplasty operation of implantation PMMA bone cement modified BonGold bone graft material.

The patient's pain was relieved after the operation. After 3 days in bed, the patient was discharged from the hospital 2 weeks later.

The results of X-ray examination during the follow-up period are shown in Fig. 5.52.

The left cortical compression and endplate fracture of L4 were seen before operation. The height of the compressed L4 vertebral body was recovered and the curvature of the lumbar spine was significantly improved after the operation. The follow-up was 1 year after the operation. No recompression of the adjacent segments of the vertebral body was found during the follow-up period. (From: Peking Union Medical College Hospital.)

The application of MC modified PMMA bone cement in PKP in the Second Affiliated Hospital of Inner Mongolia Medical University was observed and followed up. The study shows that the effect of bone cement composite artificial bone repair material can achieve the effect of using bone cement alone. Meanwhile, bone meal can induce new bone formation and reduce the incidence of adverse reactions of bone cement, so it has good prospects for popularization [15].

In the department of orthopedics of the Second People's Hospital of Lianyungang, the clinical application and clinical follow-up of MC modified PMMA bone cement in PVP were observed. In this clinical observation, to improve the properties of the commercially available PMMA bone cement, we used the mineral collagen for the modification of the PMMA bone cement. Mineral collagen with good osteogenic activity and degradation properties can effectively improve the mechanical properties and

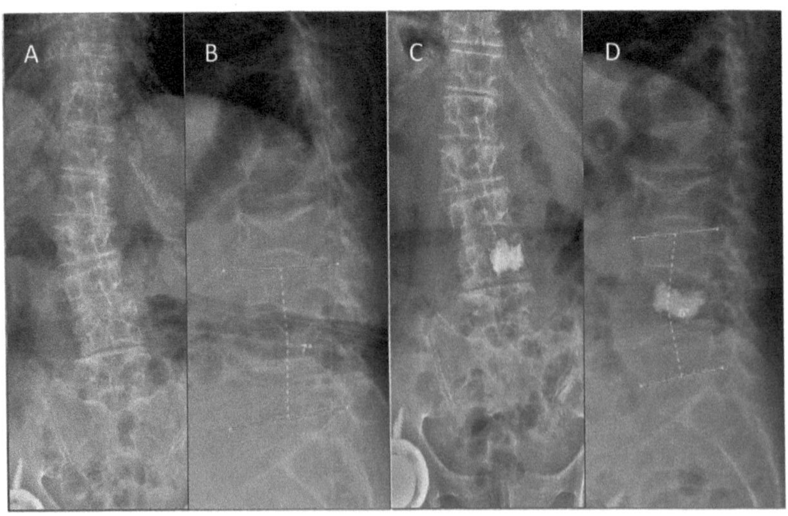

FIGURE 5.52 (A, B) Preoperative X-ray radiography. (C, D) Immediate positive side after operation.

biocompatibility of the PMMA bone cement, could effectively reduce the hardness and improve its biocompatibility, so as to reduce the occurrence of either secondary fracture at the adjacent vertebrae or dislodgement of the implanted bone cement for the treatment of patients, thus obtain better clinical results [16].

5.8.5 Mineralized Collagen Modified Polymethylmethacrylate Bone Cement was Compared With Traditional Polymethylmethacrylate Bone Cement for 1 Year

In the Affiliated Hospital of School of Medicine of Ningbo University, we evaluated the therapeutic effect of MC modified PMMA bone cement and PMMA bone cement in the treatment of vertebral osteoporotic bone, with a total of 105 patients. The results of surgery procedure showed the same clinical operation and injection performance between the MC-PMMA and PMMA groups. The study also focused on height reduction of the vertebral body. The vertebral height of MC-PMMA group also descended after 1 year, however, the degree of decline is significantly smaller than PMMA group. Our result showed the Cobb's angle decreased obviously after the surgery in both two groups and the change of angle was basically the same. In summary, we believe that after MC modified bone cement has good biocompatibility, form a stable structure in the vertebral body and improve the prognosis of patients.

CT examination showed a fuzzy boundary was observed between the bone cement composited with bone-MC and the bone tissues around it (arrow) in group MC-PMMA one year postoperatively (Fig. 5.53). However, the bone cement was still clearly visible after one year in group PMMA (Fig. 5.54).

5.9 THE APPLICATION OF MINERAL COLLAGEN BONE GRAFTING MATERIALS IN SITE PRESERVATION

Tooth extraction site preservation means taking some measures at the same time or at a later time, minimizing the absorption of alveolar ridge, and providing enough good bone for later implant restoration. MC can be made into a variety of implant materials, such as dental bone powder and filling plug, so as to meet the needs of dental extraction site preservation [17,18].

5.9.1 Case 1

MC dental bone powder for alveolar ridge bone increment.

Patients with left upper second and third teeth had long tooth loss before operation, and from the CT and intraoral images, the alveolar bone edge of

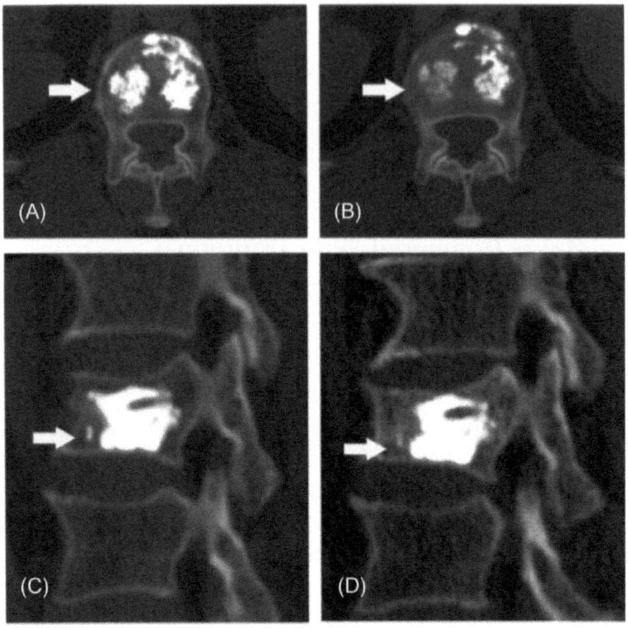

FIGURE 5.53 (A, B, C, D) show that 1 year after operation there is a fuzzy boundary between the material and the surrounding tissues.

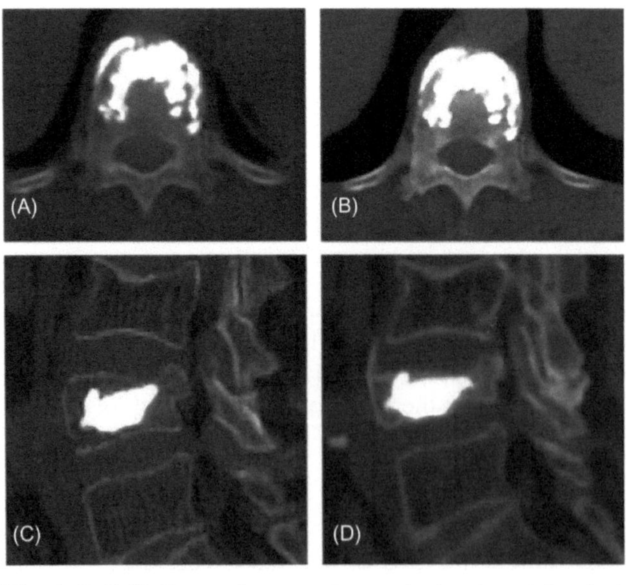

FIGURE 5.54 (A, B C, D) Computed tomography examination showed that the bone cement was still clearly visible after 1 year.

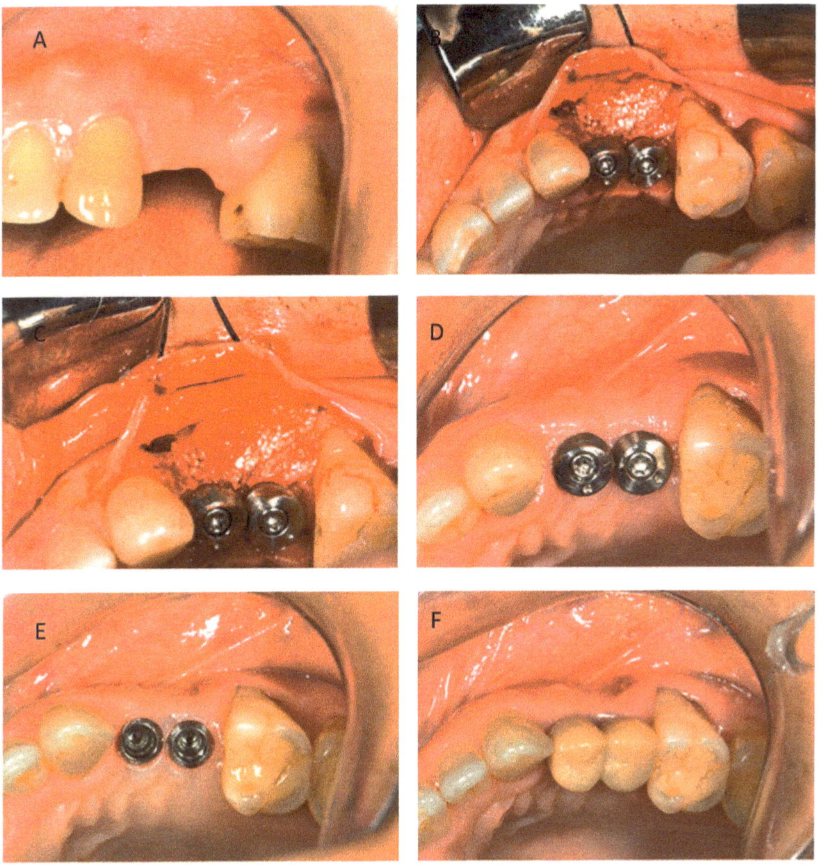

FIGURE 5.55 (A) Preoperative; (B) intraoperative implantation of dental bone powder; (C) guided tissue regeneration (GTR) film; (D) 3 months after the operation. (E) 5 months postoperatively; (F) the crown installed 5 months after the operation.

the missing teeth was visible. Therefore, during implantation, submucous implant of bone graft material of CHIBEI which was produced by Beijing Allgens medical Science and Technology Co., LTD dental bone powder 0.5 cm^3 was implanted, and implants were implanted at the same time. GTR membrane was used to suture the mucosa. After 3 months of surgery alveolar increments are obvious; seen from the CT on the surrounding of implant bone tissue appeared dense. Measurements of available buccal palatal bone thickness were 1.9 and 1.1 mm, sufficient to maintain implant stability, and bone regeneration of CHIBEI was good. Reexamination of the prosthesis during and after the operation is shown in Fig. 5.55. (From: Liu Yu, Doctor, Associate Senior Doctor, Associate professor) (Figs. 5.56 and 5.57).

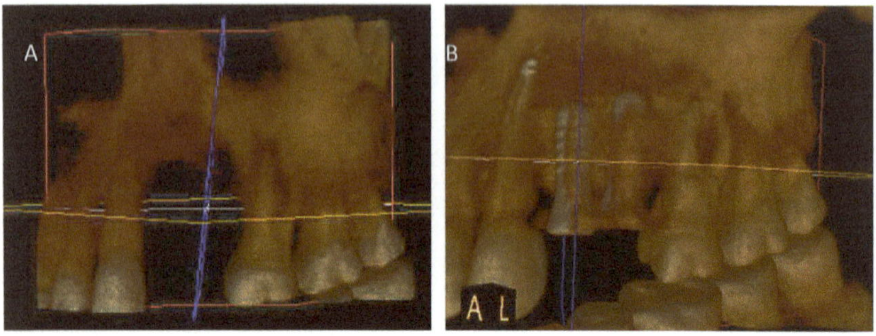

FIGURE 5.56 (A) Preoperative; (B) the results of computed tomography three-dimensional reconstruction 5 months after the operation.

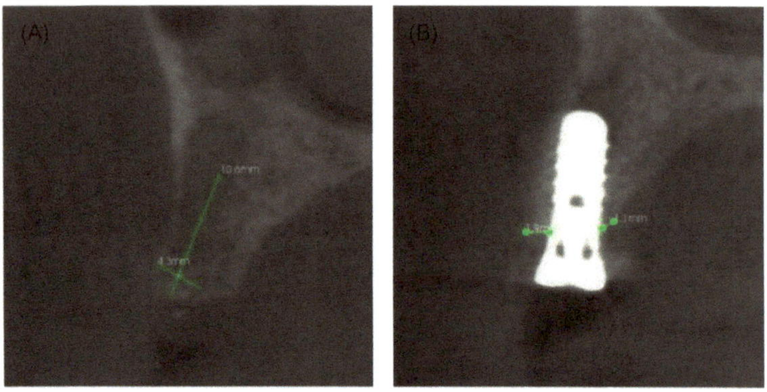

FIGURE 5.57 (A) Preoperative; (B) measurement of osteogenic thickness on the CT map 5 months after operation.

5.9.2 Case 2

MC dental bone powder for sites preservation.

With mandibular periapical of right diseases, root canal treatment caused periodontitis surrounding alveolar bone loss, so the fourth tooth cannot exercise its normal function. The chosen teeth were extracted to protect the wound healing process and guide bone regeneration for the residual bone. We implanted CHIBEI dental bone powder 0.3 cm^3. At 3 months after the operation, the alveolar ridge augmentation in the implant site was satisfied, and the implant was implanted and the crown was installed 5 months after the operation. The osteogenesis was observed at 5 months after the operation, and the effect of osteogenesis was good (Figs. 5.58–5.61).

Fig. 5.62 shows the X-ray examination for immediately after the operation, postoperative 3 months, and 7 months after operation. We can see obvious tooth extraction immediately after operation. Three months after operation, bone healing is good.

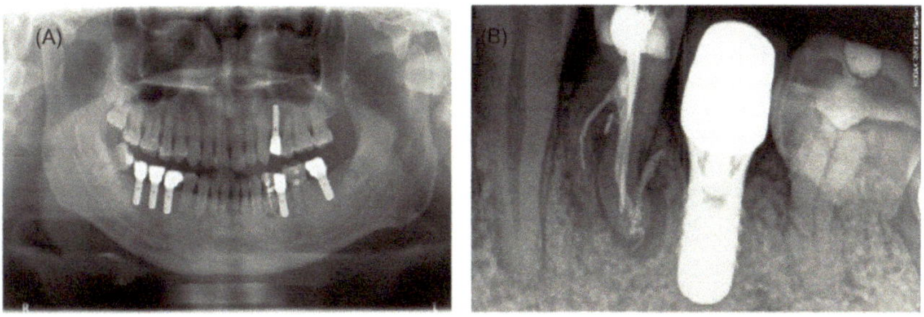

FIGURE 5.58 X-ray manifestations of periapical periodontitis after root canal therapy (A) X-ray film; (B) local X-ray.

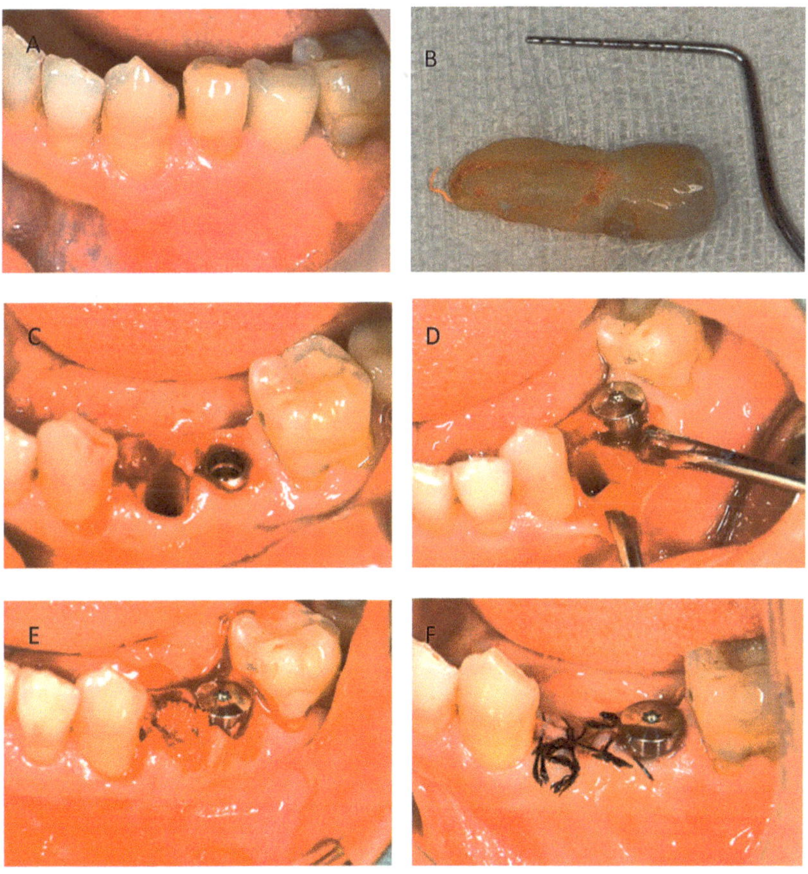

FIGURE 5.59 (A, B) Tooth extraction; (C, D, E, F) implant of CHIBEI material.

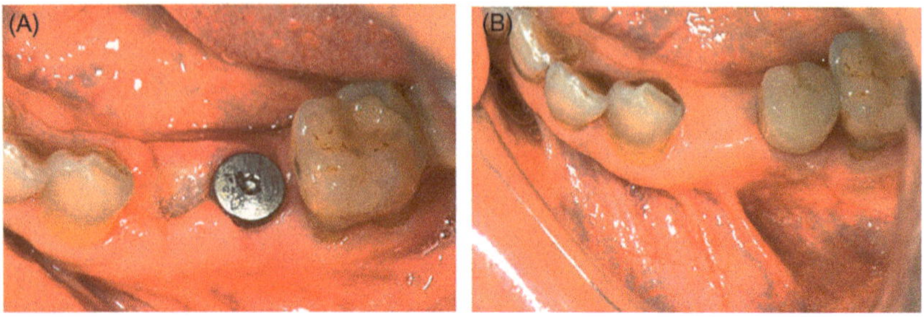

FIGURE 5.60 (A) 3 months after operation; (B) 5 months after operation.

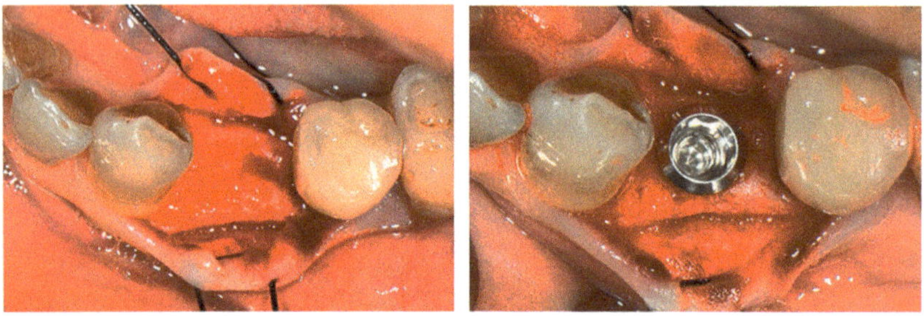

FIGURE 5.61 Osteogenesis and implantation at 5 months after operation.

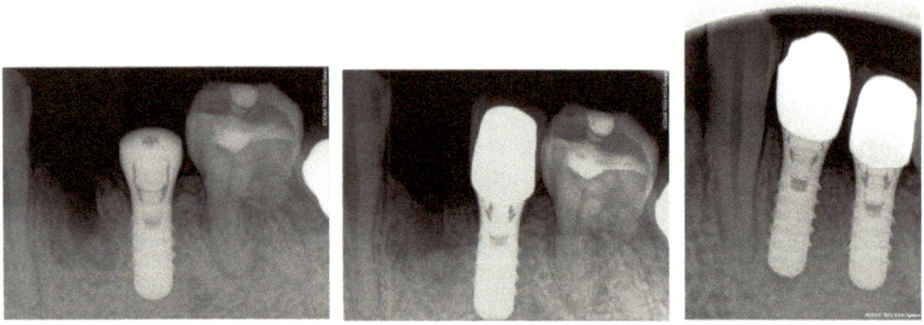

FIGURE 5.62 X-ray films immediately after operation, 3 months, and 7 months (after implantation).

Five months after operation, new bone tissue was removed and observed for pathological section. Fig. 5.63 shows that there is a lot of new bone tissue formation, and bone materials always contact with trabecular bone and gradually become autografts. (From: Liu Yu, Doctor, Associate Senior Doctor, Associate professor.)

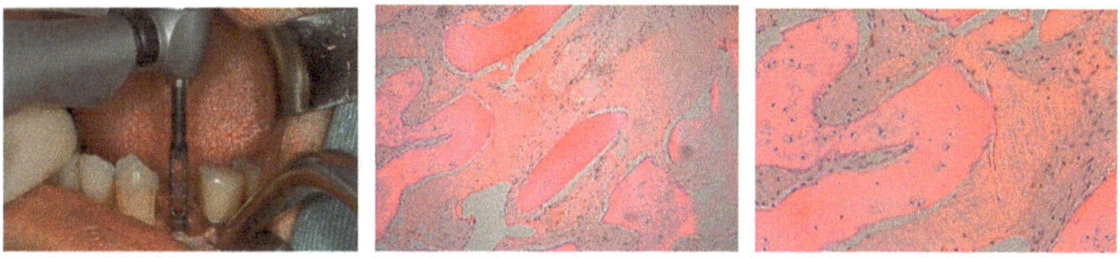

FIGURE 5.63 Histopathological observation of the new bone tissue taken out at 5 months after operation.

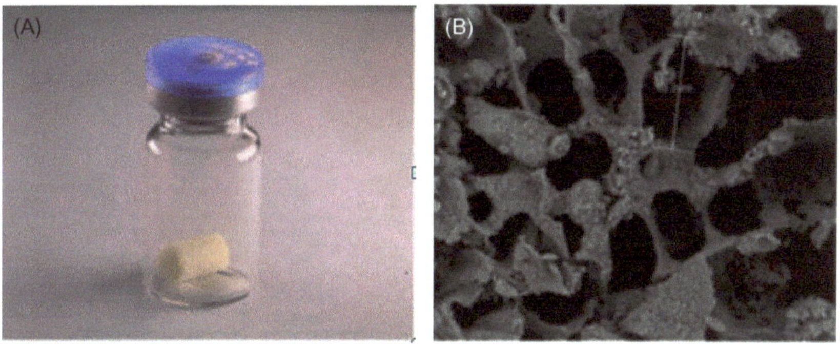

FIGURE 5.64 (A) Appearance of filling plug; (B) scanning electron microscope photograph.

5.9.3 Mineralized Collagen in the Extraction Sites Preservation

Mineral collagen based filling plug for tooth extraction is a product that is mainly used for the preservation of the tooth extraction site, which is made of MC. It can increase bone mass of the tooth socket, compensate for level and vertical bone resorption, adhere to soft tissue on the surface of bone effectively. It is beneficial to preserve tooth extraction soft tissue volume. The product for integrated design can shorten the operation time, and can adapt to all kinds of arbitrary shapes of jaw defect in dry state [17] (Fig. 5.64).

5.9.4 Case 1

MC filling plug for site preservation.

Thirty-four patients who have lost teeth due to trauma or decay were randomly selected from Department of Stomatology of Dongzhimen Hospital from December 2013 to December 2014 [17]. Therefore, the microstructure played an important role in clinical performance for the bone grafts. Compared with physically blended nHA/Col, biomimetic MC had significant promotion effect on the height of bone formation.

1. For left upper fourth tooth trauma caused by the crown and the partial root defect, the treatment of dental extraction was performed. To prevent

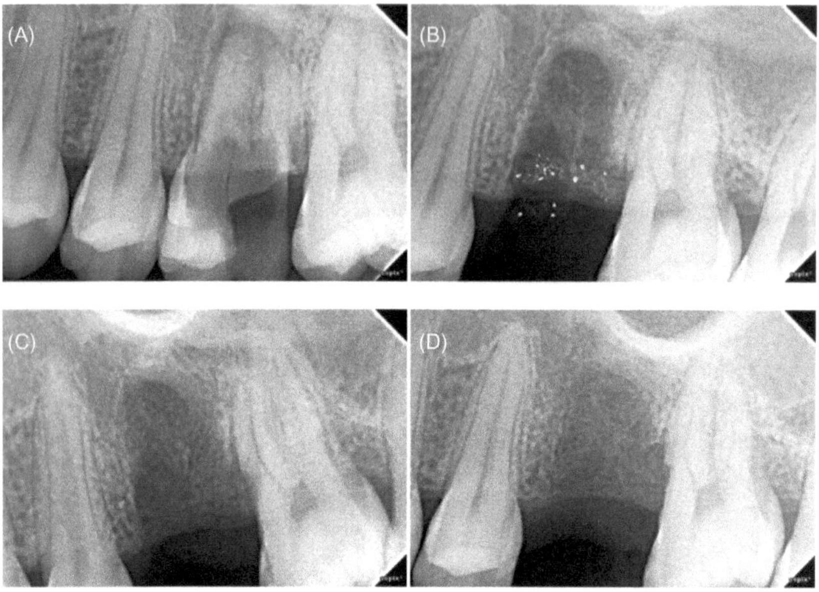

FIGURE 5.65 (A) Preextraction; (B) immediately after surgery; (C) 3 months postoperatively; (D) 5 months after the operation.

the absorption of the alveolar bone after the operation, the CHIBEI was placed after the operation. For X-ray results at different time points before and after the operation, see Fig. 5.65.

Three months after surgery, X-ray examination showed that alveolar cancellous bone formation, without adjacent teeth loosening and displacement; after 5 months, significant alveolar cancellous bone hyperplasia can be seen, the sockets are closed, and adjacent teeth are in normal position. (From: Department of Stomatology of Dongzhimen Hospital.)

5.10 THE APPLICATION OF MINERALIZED COLLAGEN BONE POWDER AND GTR MEMBRANE IN BONE GRAFT AFTER CURETTAGE OF APICAL CYST

Apical cyst is a common group of gingival diseases, often developed by apical granuloma or chronic alveolar abscess. Apical cyst causes gingival bone destruction. On the X-ray film, there are round or oval, dense, decreasing areas around the root tip. The boundary is clear and neat, surrounded by clear white opaque hardened layer. The larger cysts can oppress the adjacent teeth to absorb or shift the root of the teeth, and the infected root cysts are irregular at the edge of the light zone.

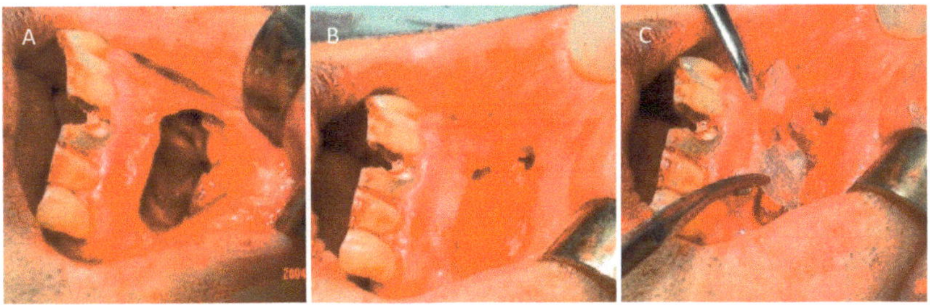

FIGURE 5.66 (A) Giant maxillary cysts; (B) implantation of dental bone powder; (C) implantation in GTR membrane.

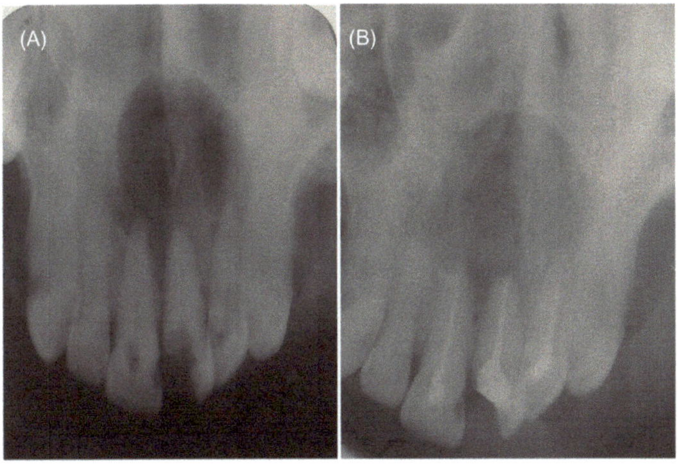

FIGURE 5.67 (A) The sclerosing edge of the maxillary cyst is clear; (B) 3 months after the operation, the trabecular bone in the cyst area was seen.

5.10.1 Case 1

Male, 69 years old, maxillary central apical cyst, CHIBEI dental bone powder 7.5 cm^3 was implanted and covered with MC membrane (GTR membrane) after curettage. The effect of bone defect repair was good 1 month after the operation.

The case of the operation was showed in Fig. 5.66.

The preoperative and postoperative review of X-ray findings are as shown in Fig. 5.67. (From: China Medical University School & Hospital of Stomatology.)

5.11 THE APPLICATION OF MINERALIZED COLLAGEN IN BONE GRAFT AFTER CURETTAGE OF CHRONIC PERIAPICAL PERIODONTITIS

Chronic periapical periodontitis is a chronic inflammatory reaction around the periapical tissue, which is characterized by inflammatory granulation tissue formation and alveolar bone destruction.

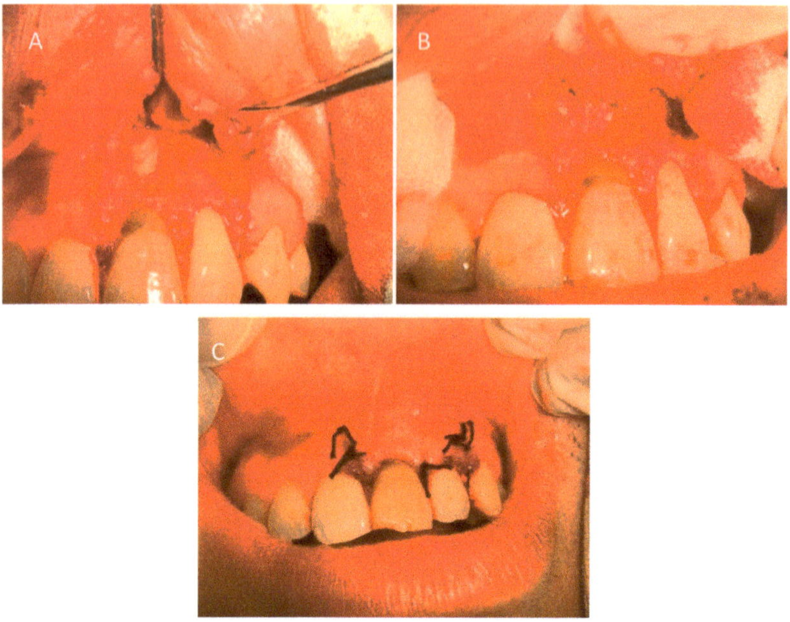

FIGURE 5.68 (A) Exposing cysts during operation; (B) implantation of artificial bone particles; (C) suture.

5.11.1 Case 1

Male, 45 years old, 21st teeth were diagnosed as chronic periapical periodontitis with root apex operation; the cavity of the bone was about 8 × 8 mm, and was filled with the CHIBEI artificial bone granules. In the 6 month reexamination, the density of the bone lumen increased significantly, and the shadow disappeared (Figs. 5.68 and 5.69).

Six months after scavenging and bone grafting, the location of the periapical cyst was blurred on X-ray, and it was filled with trabecular bone. (From: West China School/Hospital of Stomatology Sichuan University.)

5.12 REGENERATIVE REPAIR OF CRANIUM BONE DEFECT WITH MINERALIZED COLLAGEN

Skull defect caused by trauma, congenital malformation, tumor and craniotomy is a common disease seen in the Department of Neurosurgery. A variety of synthetic materials have been widely applied in bone defect repair, such as titanium alloys, calcium phosphate bioceramics, polyethylene, PEEK, PMMA, and bioresorbable polyesters. But the use of these repair materials in vivo is limited because they are not biodegradable, and can lead to thermal damage of brain tissue, injury, and skull deformity and so on, which is

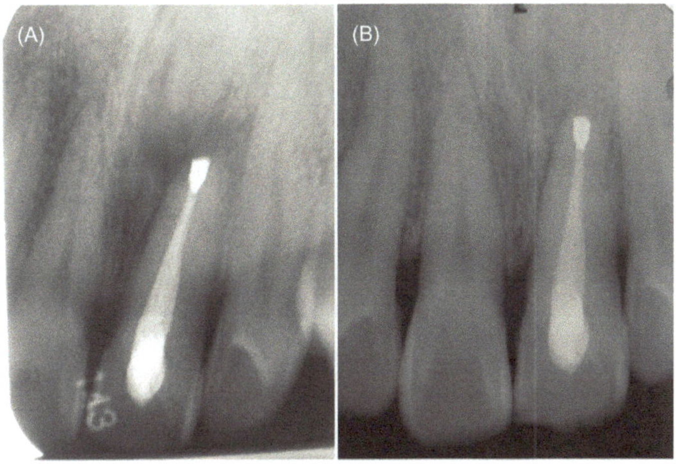

FIGURE 5.69 (A) Before bone grafting; (B) 6 months after operation.

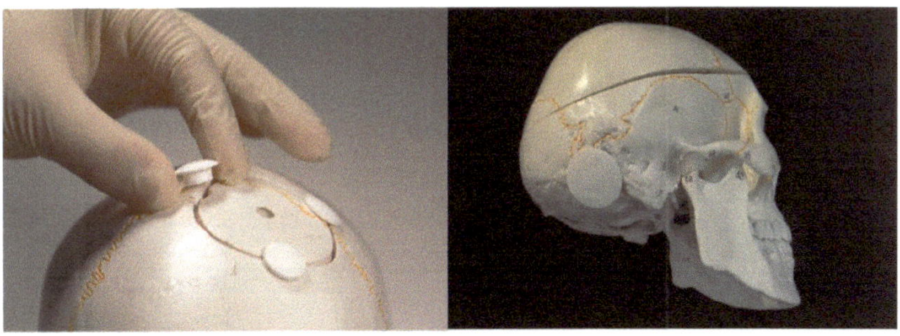

FIGURE 5.70 Mineralized collagen cranial repair plug and its schematic diagram.

adverse to the rehabilitation of patients with skull repair. A plug composed of a MC material, commonly used in clinical cranioplasty, cranial drill diameter, can effectively repair skull defect after craniocerebral operation and promote healing [19,20] (Fig. 5.70).

5.12.1 Case 1

Case 1 was a 12-year-old male. Four, 2.0 cm × 1.0 cm bone defects were produced after surgery for cyst removal at the left temporal region. The right two defects were implanted with the MC burr-hole plugs (SKUHEAL), and the left two defects were set as blank controls without any treatment. The clinical effects were evaluated by plain radiographs at the 1st, 3rd, and 10th months after surgery.

Postoperative plain radiographs from case 1 are shown in Fig. 5.71.

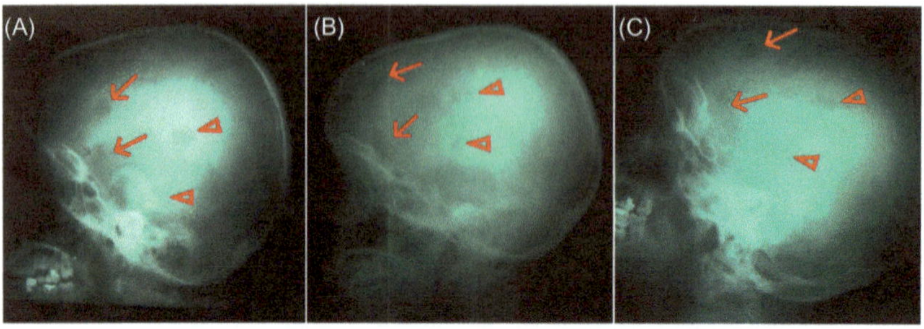

FIGURE 5.71 (A) 1-month follow-up; (B) 3-month follow-up; (C) 10-month follow-up. The sites treated with mineralized collagen burr-hole plugs (noted by triangles); the blank control sites (noted by arrows).

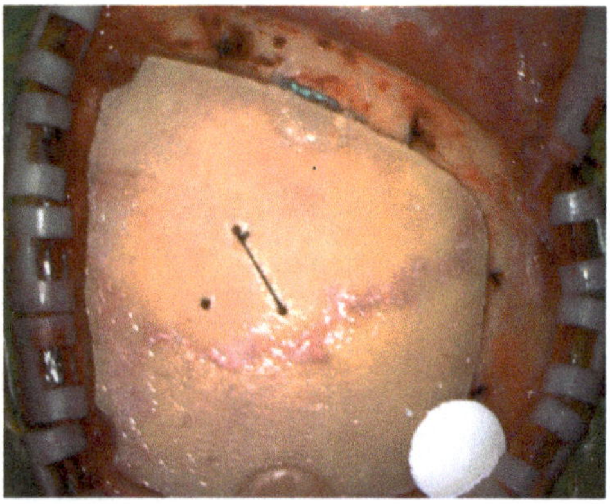

FIGURE 5.72 The mineralized collagen burr-hole plug was implanted into one bone defect after cranial bone flap reposition.

Fig. 5.71 shows plain radiographs from the patient's follow-up. At the sites treated with MC SKUHEAL burr-hole plugs (noted by triangles), bone mineral density gradually increased and approximated the host temporal bone. The interfaces between the implants and the host bone became fuzzy, indicating a remarkable osteogenesis effect. However, the bone mineral density of the blank control sites (noted by arrows) remained obviously lower than that of the surrounding normal bone tissue. (From: Tsinghua University YuQuan Hospital.)

5.12.2 Case 2

Case 2 was a 27-year-old male. Three 2.0 cm × 2.0 cm bone defects were produced after surgery for cranial bone flap reposition. The left defect was implanted with the MC burr-hole plug, while the right two defects were set as blank controls without any treatment. Fig. 5.72 shows an image of the

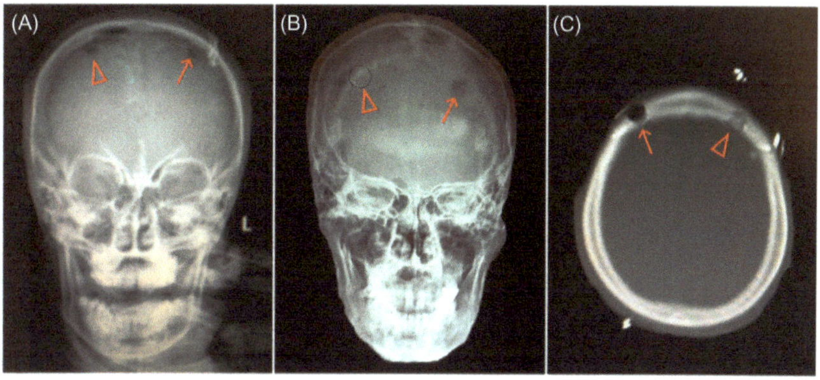

FIGURE 5.73 (A) Plain radiograph at 1-month follow-up; (B) plain radiograph at the 6-month follow-up; (C) computed tomography scan at the 6-month follow-up. The site treated with the mineralized collagen burr-hole plug (noted by triangles); the blank control sites (noted by arrows).

intraoperative repair as the burr-hole plug was implanted into the left bone defect. The clinical effects were evaluated by both plain radiography and CT at the first and sixth months after surgery.

Postoperative plain radiographs and CT scan of case 2 were showed by Fig. 5.73.

Fig. 5.73 shows plain radiographs and a CT scan from case 3's follow-up. At the site treated with the MC burr-hole plug (noted by triangles), bone mineral density gradually increased and approximated that of the host cranial bone. The interfaces between the implant and the host bone became fuzzy, indicating a remarkable osteogenesis effect. Similar to those in case 1, the blank control sites (noted by arrows) continued to have obviously lower bone mineral density compared with that of the surrounding normal bone tissue. A slight swelling was detected by palpation at both blank control sites, due to ingrowth of soft tissues. (From: Tsinghua University YuQuan Hospital.)

5.12.3 Case 3

Case 3 was an 18-year-old male. A piece of cranial bone was removed to evacuate an intracranial hematoma, forming a 2.0 cm × 3.0 cm bone defect in the skull. A MC burr-hole plug (SKUHEAL) was implanted into the bone defect, as shown in Fig. 5.68. The clinical effects were evaluated by CT at the 1st, 3th, and 12th months after the surgery.

Intraoperative scene as the burr-hole plug was implanted in Fig. 5.74.

Postoperative CT scans of case 3 were showed by Fig. 5.75.

Fig. 5.75 shows CT scans from case 2's follow-up. Bone mineral density gradually increased after surgery (noted by triangles). At the 12th month, the

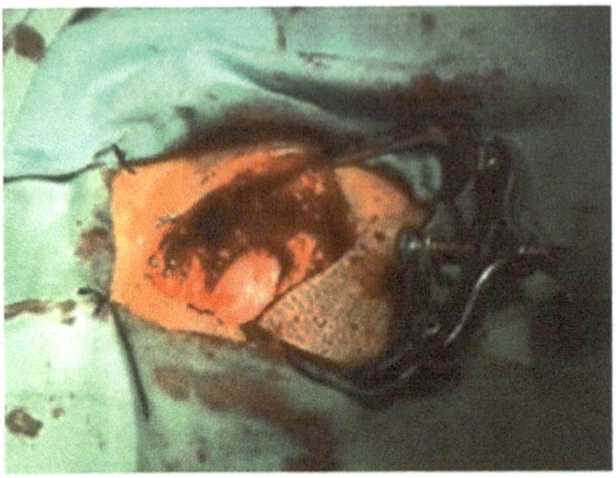

FIGURE 5.74 Intraoperative scene as the burr-hole plug was implanted.

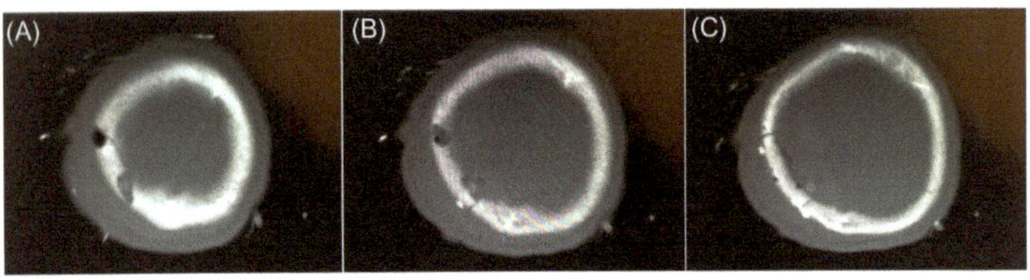

FIGURE 5.75 (A) 1-month follow-up; (B) 6-month follow-up; (C) 12-month follow-up.

outline of the implant disappeared, and bone mineral density was closed to the host skull. Therefore, the bone defect in the skull healed very well. (From: Tsinghua University YuQuan Hospital.)

5.12.4 Case 4

The female patient, 30 years old, because of "forehead bone cyst" to cyst excision surgery, bone defect after the formation of a forehead about 3×3.0 cm size fenestration, given the implantation of MC "SkuHeal repair plug" successful operation, with 3 weeks after operation. The patient was followed up for 1 year. In this case, MC SkuHeal repair plug was implanted in the case, as in Fig. 5.76.

The patients were followed up for 4 months, and the results of image examination are shown in Fig. 5.77.

Postoperative CT showed that 1.5 months after cranioplasty, the defect was partially filled with regenerated bone and the internal and external skull plates were differentiated. Four months after operation, the skull defect was completely filled, and the skull was completely differentiated. (From: Nanning Hospital of Traditional Chinese Medicine.)

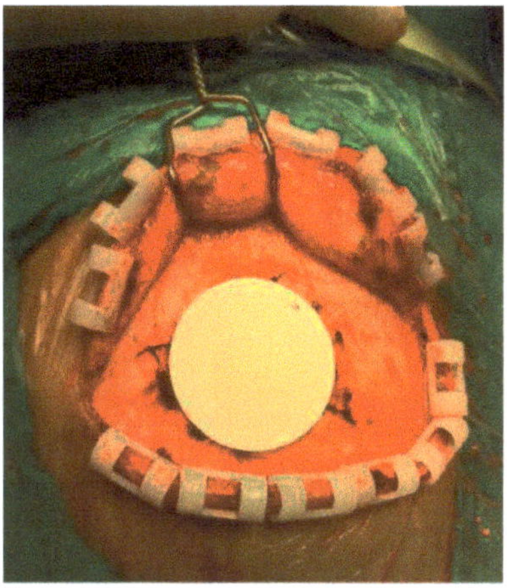

FIGURE 5.76 Implant of MC "SkuHeal repair plug".

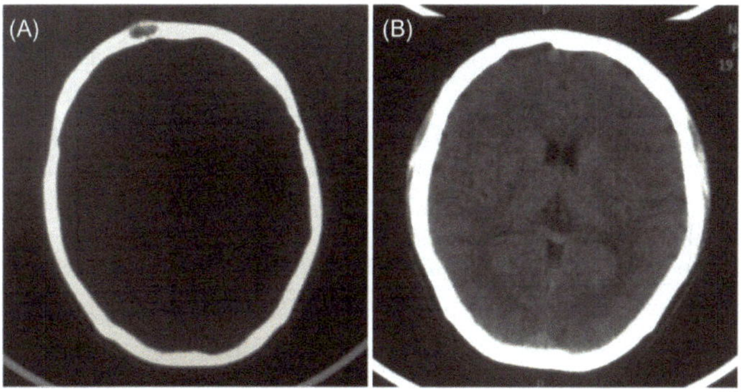

FIGURE 5.77 (A) 1.5 months postoperatively; (B) 4 months after the operation.

5.12.5 Case 5

The patient was 59 years old with right trigeminal nerve microvascular decompression for right trigeminal neuralgia; the operation was smooth and the decompression was complete. In the operation, the diameter of the right posterior mastoid was formed after the 25 mm was opened to the skull defect, and the implanted cranioplasty plug filled with MC was implanted into the defect. The filling effect was good. The patient was followed up for 1 year.

The results of postoperative and follow-up imaging findings are shown in Fig. 5.78.

Six months after operation, CT examination and 3D reconstruction showed that the cranial ear defect after implantation of SKUHEAL bone repair plug was completely filled by bone tissue and healed. (From: Tsinghua University YuQuan Hospital.)

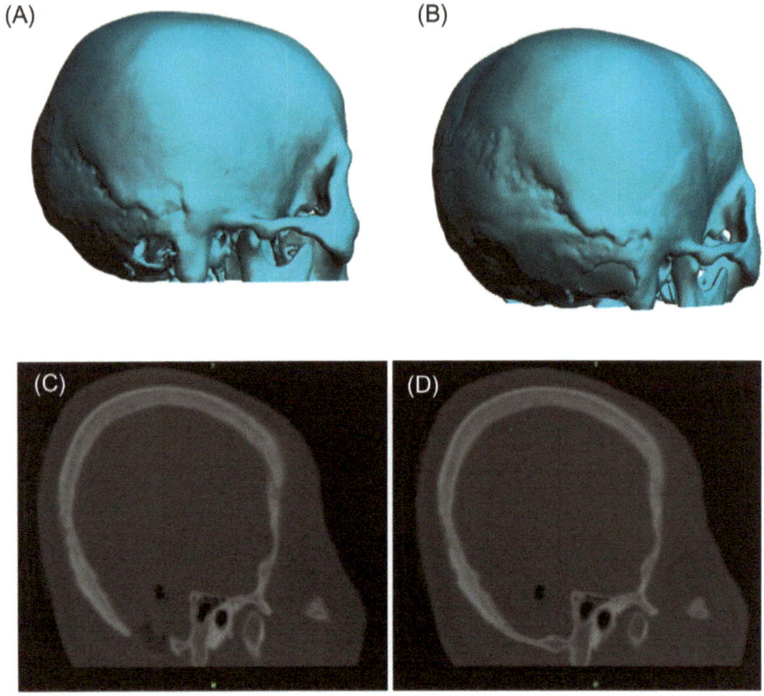

FIGURE 5.78 Images of skull defect following Microvascular decompression (MVD) operation. (A) Immediate three-dimensional reconstruction after the operation; (B) 6 months after the operation. (C) Immediate postoperatively computed tomography (CT); (D) CT 6 months after the operation.

In summary, the MC artificial bone products of Beijing Allgens Medical Technology Co. Ltd. with similar composition and microstructure to natural bone matrix, which has high biocompatibility and osteogenic ability, has a guiding and widespread role in the Department of Orthopedics, Department of Stomatology, and Department of Neurosurgery and throughout the clinic for the treatment of bone defect and bone disease resulting from a variety of causes. The material has achieved good results, including in fracture and bone defects caused by various reasons, delayed healing and nonunion of fracture, benign bone tumor, necrosis of the femoral head, joint fusion, and the treatment of cranial bone defect repair and alveolar bone augmentation in the Department of Stomatology, and its safety and effectiveness are verified.

Biomimetic mineralization of PMMA modified bone collagen products has obtained satisfactory results in reducing the elastic modulus of bone cement and solidified surface increased biological activity, and it has been recognized by many experts from many hospitals and bone cement manufacturers all over the country. It has made considerable progress in the improvement of bone cement in clinical application so that a large number of patients benefit.

In the future, the technology of biomimetic mineralization of collagen artificial bone products (based on BonGold, CHIBEI, SKUHEAL) will lead to more brilliant achievements!

REFERENCES

[1] V. Goriainov, R. Cook, J.M. Latham, et al., Bone and metal: an orthopaedic perspective on osseointegration of metals, Acta Biomater. 10 (10) (2014) 4043–4057.

[2] K. Lian, H. Lu, X. Guo, et al., The mineralized collagen for the reconstruction of intraarticular calcaneal fractures with trabecular defects, Biomatter 3 (4) (2013).

[3] X. Yu, L. Xu, F.Z. Cui, et al., Clinical evaluation of mineralized collagen as a bone graft substitute for anterior cervical intersomatic fusion, J. Biomater. Tissue Eng. 2 (2) (2012) 170–176.

[4] X. Yu, L. Xu, F.Z. Cui, Anterior cervical operation using nano-crystal/collagen bone materials, Orthop. Bromech. Mater. Clin. Study 1 (1) (2003) 14–16.

[5] X. Yu, L. Xu, L.Y. Bi, et al., Posterolateral fusion using nana-crystal/collagen bone materials in lumbar spine, Orthop. Biomech. Mater. Clin. Study 1 (7) (2004) 6–9.

[6] Z. Chen, J. Wang, Z.-Y. Qiu, et al., The application of mineralized collagen bone grafts in osteoporotic thoracolumbar fractures, J. Biomater. Tissue Eng. 7 (11) (2017) 1122–1129.

[7] C. Gao, J. Gao, W. Tian, et al., Clinical observation on repair of limbs bone defect by using mineralized collagen graft, Chin. J. Primary Med. Pharmacy 24 (12) (2017).

[8] C. Peng, H.P. Wang, J.H. Yan, et al., Locking system strengthened by biomimetic mineralized collagen putty for the treatment of osteoporotic proximal humeral fractures, Regen. Biomater. 4 (5) (2017) 289–294.

[9] J.M. Kou, T.Y. Fu, X.J. Jia, et al., Clinical observations on repair of noninfected bone nonunion by using mineralized collagen graft, J. Biomater. Tissue Eng. 4 (12) (2014). 1107-12(6).

[10] N.S. Ghate, H. Cui, Mineralized collagen artificial bone repair material products used for fusing the podarthral joints with internal fixation—a case report, Regen. Biomater. 4 (5) (2017) 295.

[11] C. Huang, L. Qin, W. Yan, et al., Clinical evaluation following the use of mineralized collagen graft for bone defects in revision total hip arthroplasty, Regen. Biomater. 2 (4) (2015) 245–249.

[12] Q.S. Zhang, G.H. Yan, X.H. Jin, et al., Short-term therapeutic effect of the core decompression combined with bone grafting of iliac bone and the gold ar-tificial bone on the early nontraumatic necrosis of the femoral head, Orthop. Biomech. Mater. Clin. Study 14 (1) (2017) 36–38.

[13] F.B. Mo, S.H. Yang, S.N. Ye, et al., The efficacy observation of using allogeneic bone brace combined with allograft for the treatment of the adults' early necrosis of femoral head, Chin. J. Anat. Clin. 22 (1) (2017) 37–41.

[14] B. Xie, H. Wang, J. Hao, et al., Histopathological and imageological studies on clinical outcomes of mineralized collagen reconstruction rod for femoral head necrosis with one case report, Regen. Biomater. 4 (4) (2017) 243–249.

[15] M. Bai, H.P. Yin, Y.M. Wu, et al., Application of bone cement composited with artificial bone in percutaneous balloon kyphoplasty, Orthop. J. China 24 (22) (2016) 2022–2026.

[16] X. Wang, J.M. Kou, Y. Yue, et al., Clinical observations of osteoporotic vertebral compression fractures by using mineralized collagen modified polymethylmethacrylate bone cement, Regen. Biomater. 4 (2) (2017) 105–109.

[17] L. Feng, L. Zhang, Y. Cui, et al., Clinical evaluations of mineralized collagen in the extraction sites preservation, Regen. Biomater. 3 (1) (2016) 41–48.

[18] Y. Xia, L. Xie, Y. Zhou, et al., A new method to standardize CBCT for quantitative evaluation of alveolar ridge preservation in the mandible: a case report and review of the literature, Regen. Biomater. 2 (4) (2015) 251–260.

[19] Z. Qiu, Y. Zhang, Z. Zhang, et al., Biodegradable mineralized collagen plug for the reconstruction of craniotomy burr-holes: a report of three cases, Trans. Neurosci. Clin. 1 (1) (2015) 3–9.

[20] M. Chen, H.Z. Wang, Z.J. Huang, et al., Nanocomposites are a period of repairing skull defect children clinical studies, Suzhou Univ. J. Med. Sci. 30 (6) (2010) 1320–1321.

Index

Note: Page numbers followed by "*f*" and "*t*" refer to figures and tables, respectively.

B

C

D

I

J

T

U

V

W

X

Z